2/2/96

CHANGING
THE ODDS

CHANGING
THE ODDS

Cancer Prevention
Through Personal Choice
and Public Policy

R. GRANT STEEN

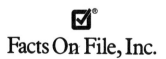

Facts On File, Inc.

AN INFOBASE HOLDINGS COMPANY

Changing the Odds: Cancer Prevention Through Personal Choice and Public Policy

Copyright © 1995 by R. Grant Steen

Facts On File, Inc.
460 Park Avenue South
New York NY 10016

Library of Congress Cataloging-in-Publication Data

Steen, R. Grant.
    Changing the odds : cancer prevention through personal choice and public policy / R. Grant Steen.
        p. cm.
    Includes bibliographical references and index.
    ISBN 0-8160-3167-3
    1. Cancer—Prevention. 2. Cancer—Risk factors. 3. Cancer—
    Prevention—Government policy—United States. I. Title.
    RC268.S74 1995
    616.99'4052—dc20   94-25291

Facts On File books are available at special discounts when purchased in bulk quantities for businesses, associations, institutions or sales promotions. Please call our Special Sales Department in New York at 212/683-2244 or 800/322-8755.

Text design by Donna Sinisgalli
Jacket design by Dorothy Wachtenheim
Printed in the United States of America

MP TT 10 9 8 7 6 5 4 3 2 1

This book is printed on acid-free paper.

Dedicated to the patients and families
of
St. Jude Children's Research Hospital,
in the hope that all cancers will someday be preventable.

CONTENTS

TABLES

ACKNOWLEDGMENTS

My wife, Wil O'Loughlin, has been a patient and gracious partner during the writing process, and she and my children, Alena and Mariel, have provided love, light, warmth, and perspective. My parents, Noreen and Ralph Steen, have been very encouraging and supportive throughout the process of capturing evanescent ideas with real words. Dr. Leonard Muscatine, Dr. George Laties, and Dr. Margaret McFall-Ngai, all of the University of California at Los Angeles, played large roles in teaching me to think like a scientist while writing like a person. Dr. Jerry Glickson helped me to start my career in cancer research and has been a consistent friend along the way. I also want to thank Matthew Galvez and Dr. Linda Porter, who encouraged me to follow this path; Dr. Barry Fletcher and Dr. June Taylor, who've made it possible for me to continue; and Jeanne Fredericks, who helped in the practical aspects of book publication.

*For to win one hundred victories
in one hundred battles is not the acme of skill.
To subdue the enemy without fighting is the acme of skill.*

—Sun Tzu
The Art of War

1

....

THE NATURE OF THE
PROBLEM

Cancer is probably the most dreaded of all diseases; nearly everyone has close friends or relatives who have fallen victim to it. Yet even the well-informed layperson may underestimate the scope of the cancer problem (Table 1-1). In the United States, one in every three people will develop cancer in their lifetime, and one in every five people will die of it. Men born in the 1940s have twice the likelihood of death from cancer as men born 50 years earlier.[1] It has been calculated that more than 10 million Americans are now in some phase of developing a cancer that will ultimately kill them.[2] Cancer is now the leading cause of death for women, and the second leading cause of death overall, after heart disease. Cancer has been projected to become the leading overall killer in the United States by the year 2000.[3]

Since it seems that everyone must eventually die, simply determining the number of people killed by a particular disease gives an incomplete picture of the tragedy. To give a more telling picture of the burden of suffering caused by cancer, one must examine the average number of years of life lost for the major causes of death.[4] This is actually a measure of how many years of life were lost due to premature death. From 1973 to 1989, accidents caused the greatest damage, as about 34.4 years of life were lost prematurely by each victim of a fatal accident. But the average patient who died of cancer could have expected to live an additional 15.3 years had he or she been able to prevent cancer. In fact, cancer was the leading cause of premature death from disease. The average number of years of life lost to heart disease was less, at 11.5 years.[5] This reflects the fact that heart disease seldom strikes the very young, while cancer is less sparing of youth.

It has been concluded that about 75% of all deaths in the United States are premature, caused by "degenerative diseases," which result from abuse and disuse. In fact, all of the top 10 killers in the United States are, at least in part, preventable (this list, in order, is: heart disease, cancer, stroke,

1

TABLE 1-1 MAJOR TYPES OF CANCER				
TYPE OF CANCER	U.S. CASES (1992)	RANK	RELATIVE FREQUENCY	KNOWN CARCINOGENS
Breast	181,000	1	5	Hormones, radiation
Lung	168,000	2	5	Chemicals, radiation
Colorectal	156,000	3	5	Diet, heredity
Prostate	132,000	4	4	Hormones
Bladder	51,600	5	4	Chemicals
Uterus	45,500	6	3	Viruses, hormones
Lymphoma	41,000	7	3	Viruses, radiation
Melanoma	32,000	8	3	Lifestyle, heredity
Oral cavity	30,300	9	3	Chemicals
Pancreas	28,300	10	3	Chemicals
Kidney and urinary	26,500	11	3	Chemicals
Stomach	24,400	12	2	Diet, bacteria
Ovary	21,000	13	2	Hormones
Brain and CNS	16,900	14	2	Injury, heredity
Liver	15,400	15	2	Chemicals, viruses
Multiple myeloma	12,500	16	2	Unknown
Larynx	12,500	17	2	Chemicals
Thyroid	12,500	18	2	Chemicals
Lymphocytic leukemia	11,800	19	2	Radiation
Granulocytic leukemia	11,300	20	2	Radiation
Esophagus	11,100	21	2	Chemicals
Hodgkin's disease	7,400	22	1	Viruses
Testis	6,300	23	1	Unknown
Connective tissue	5,900	24	1	Heredity

The major types of cancer are ordered by rank, so that the most common cancers appear at the top of the list.[19] Only cancers that were estimated to affect more than 5,000 people are tabulated, and those cancers that affect an approximately equal number of people (multiple myeloma, larynx, and thyroid), were ranked in order of severity, as judged by the estimated number of deaths in 1992. Relative frequency is based on the total number of expected cases, categorized as follows: extremely common cancers affecting >150,000 people per year were ranked as 5; very common cancers affecting between 50,000 and 150,000 people per year were ranked as 4; common cancers affecting between 25,000 and 50,000 people per year were ranked as 3; less common cancers affecting between 10,000 and 25,000 people per year were ranked as 2; and relatively rare cancers affecting fewer than 10,000 people per year were ranked as 1. Relative frequency values will be used in the calculation of risk weight. Known carcinogens are listed, but this is not an inclusive list, and only the most important carcinogens are listed.

accidents, chronic lung disease, pneumonia, diabetes, suicide, liver disease, and atherosclerosis). Perhaps 60% of all premature deaths could be significantly postponed, which would amount to 500,000 people a year spared from dying prematurely.[6] These numbers should convince even the hardiest skeptic that disease prevention in general, and cancer prevention in particular, is a compelling goal, both personally and nationally.

LEARNING ABOUT CANCER PREVENTION

Although cancer prevention is a goal that almost everyone would agree is worth achieving, most people are very confused about what to do to achieve the goal. This confusion is not the fault of the lay public—when dealing with issues as complicated as cancer prevention, confusion is inevitable and arises for many reasons. Cancer prevention is a relatively new field of study, which has so far provided us with many more questions than answers, and genuine confusion exists within the field. Just as most movies, most books, and most car models are workmanlike but undistinguished, most scientific studies are also workmanlike but undistinguished. Almost never is a study so well executed that it is widely accepted as the last word on a subject. Sincere scientists, acting in good faith, can mistakenly report data that later prove to be incorrect, while other scientists may attempt ambitious studies that ultimately fail to obtain a clearcut answer to any question. Overcautious scientists may be reluctant to report their findings, while other scientists may report preliminary findings from small studies as if these findings were established fact. Members of the media may be gullible enough to accept preliminary findings at face value, failing to see the problems that ultimately undermine a poorly executed study. Many newspapers and television news shows are guilty of presenting an oversimplified summary of a complicated issue, in order to fit the story into limited newspaper space or airtime. The lay person is bombarded with utterly fallacious pseudo-science while standing in the grocery checkout line, and many stories presented in respectable newspapers are incomplete or incorrect. Most people don't have the time, energy, or inclination to separate grains of scientific truth from the chaff of disinformation.

The subject of cancer prevention is both complex and emotionally charged, and many people end up feeling overwhelmingly confused about the subject. This book will try to bring clarity to a subject that has been too often obscured with a haze of unconnected facts, partial truths, and outright lies.

ECONOMIC INCENTIVES TO EMPHASIZE
CANCER PREVENTION

In addition to the personal reasons for emphasizing cancer prevention, many economic incentives also exist. Until very recently, our health care system has largely ignored disease prevention. This is true even of the insurance companies that, from a financial standpoint, have the most to gain. The Medicare budget of the United States was greater than $131 billion in 1992, and the estimated budget for 1997 is $226 billion. Health care costs now make up more than 12% of the federal budget, and this may increase to 30% of the federal budget by 2020 unless the health care initiatives currently being discussed are successfully implemented. Fraud and abuse account for more than 10% of all medical costs in the United States, which translates into an annual loss of about $80 billion. Despite this staggering cost to the taxpayer, adequate health care is still often unavailable to the poor. This probably is the reason why poverty itself is a risk factor for breast cancer.[7]

IS CANCER REALLY PREVENTABLE?

Recently a fossil dinosaur leg bone was found that preserved evidence of an unusual tumor that may have caused the death of the dinosaur. This fossil tumor was about 140 million years old, so the problem of cancer is neither recent nor limited to humans. In fact, cancer has been described in virtually every major group of plants and animals. Ancient Egyptian hieroglyphics show that early physicians had experience with cancer, and at least one Egyptian mummy appears to have died of cancer. The ubiquity and antiquity of cancer as a health problem suggest that somehow living organisms are vulnerable to processes that result in cancer.

Accordingly, cancer will probably never be completely preventable. Yet it has been calculated that about two-thirds of all human cancers could be prevented.[8] This is only an estimate, subject to all manner of errors, and it must be noted that no one really knows to what extent cancer is actually preventable. Let us consider, however, one example of a major cancer killer: as recently as 1930, lung cancer was a medical oddity, affecting about three men in 100,000.[9] By 1982, lung cancer incidence had increased nearly 30-fold, and lung cancer is now the second most common cause of cancer death, and one of the leading causes of death overall. The change from medical oddity to major killer has been caused by widespread exposure to cigarette smoke. Since it is within our power to eliminate human exposure to cigarette smoke, lung cancer is largely a preventable disease.

It is fair to say that certain cancers, including lung cancer, could be virtually eliminated, while many cancers could be significantly reduced in incidence. A great many sweeping changes will be required, on both a personal and a societal level, to achieve these goals. Such changes will not be easy, nor will they be inexpensive, but they can be achieved. What is needed is a personal determination to minimize risk exposure, and a societal consensus that cancer prevention is a worthy and achievable goal. Since exposure to most cancer risk factors is largely preventable, people could benefit substantially from a better understanding of how to avoid or minimize exposure to the known risk factors for cancer.

The recent decline in mortality from heart disease can serve as a model for what can be achieved for cancer. Mortality from heart disease has declined by 45% since 1950.[3] This remarkable decline has come about, in part, because of improved treatment for many of the manifestations of heart disease. But there has also been a striking reduction in prevalence of the three major risk factors: tobacco use (in any form), untreated hypertension, and high blood cholesterol. The decline in mortality from heart disease shows clearly the impact of both lifestyle choices and improved medical treatment and suggests that cancer incidence can also be strongly affected by prevention efforts.[11]

WHAT IS CANCER?

In order to better understand cancer prevention, it is important to better understand cancer. A cancer can be defined as any growing mass of cells that is both invasive and metastatic.[12] An invasive cancer is one that is able to grow into surrounding normal tissues, thereby interfering with the function of these normal cells. A metastatic cancer is one that is able to seed cancerous cells into normal tissues that are remote from the original tumor, so that secondary tumors are initiated. Unless a tumor is both invasive and metastatic at some point in its history, it is benign and should not be considered a malignant cancer.

There is clear evidence that virtually every cancer arises from a single cell that somehow becomes transformed, and that this founder cell then divides innumerable times to establish a clone of cells. The clone of cells forms a tumor that, to meet the definition of cancer, must be both invasive and metastatic. It therefore becomes important to ask, what properties of a single cell enable it to form an invasive and metastatic tumor?

Recent work shows that cells capable of forming a tumor generally have one or more mutated oncogenes or tumor suppressor genes. These are a diverse collection of genes that normally are critical for regulating cell growth and differentiation. If such a gene somehow mutates, it can become involved in the process of creating a tumor. In fact, a single mutated oncogene or tumor suppressor gene within a cell is often sufficient to cause that cell to become malignant. Most oncogenes contain the information necessary to make proteins that act as growth factors or growth factor receptors and that indirectly affect the normal cell growth rate. However, some oncogenes and most tumor suppressor genes encode proteins that directly control cell division or stimulate the growth of a "founder cell." If the function of each such gene could be determined, we would know what properties of a cell actually cause cancer. Since mutated genes can cause cancer and since they are usually involved in regulation of normal cell growth, then the conclusion is simple: cancer is a disease caused by abnormal regulation of cell growth.

To say that cancer is a disease of abnormal cell growth regulation does not imply that all cancers grow rapidly. Certain leukemia cells have an average doubling time of seven days, whereas the average doubling time of comparable normal cells is only 18 hours. Thus, these normal cells grow more than nine times as fast as leukemic cells. Yet uncontrolled cell growth results because leukemic cells are unresponsive to those factors that modulate the growth and maturation of normal cells. Leukemia occurs when certain cells are unable to assume their normal function, yet they are able to continue dividing indefinitely, unlike normal cells, which cease to divide at maturation. Each leukemic cell typically produces a large number of abnormal cells, explaining why the disease is characterized by an overabundance of one or a few primitive cell types in the blood.

THE ROLE OF CARCINOGENS IN CANCER CAUSATION

Extensive research has shown that the causes of cancer fall into two broad categories: causes that are intrinsic to the patient and causes that are extrinsic to the patient. Intrinsic causes of cancer can include heredity and hormones, while extrinsic causes of cancer can include chemicals, dietary factors, radiation, or viruses. These causative agents are usually referred to as carcinogens, since they are responsible for the "genesis" of cancer. There are frequently interactions among different carcinogens, as, for example, people with a prior exposure to a virus may be more prone to develop cancer after a subsequent chemical exposure. Alternatively, people with a particular genetic inheritance may be more sensitive to DNA damage produced by radiation or chemicals. But it is an important point that cancer is usually caused by exposure to carcinogens, so it may be possible to reduce the incidence of cancer by reducing exposure to carcinogens.

Although many different carcinogens have been identified, most of them share certain similarities. Transformation of a normal cell to a malignant state is usually caused by exposure of that cell to some agent that increases the normal rate of cell growth. For example, chemicals can induce an increase in the rate of cell division, which is the basic mechanism of chemical carcinogenesis. Rapidly dividing cells are more at risk of mutation than are nondividing cells, since the cellular DNA is not as well protected during cell division. Therefore, rapid cell growth increases the odds that a normal cell will transform to the malignant state. Certain carcinogens can also cause cancer by directly inducing mutations in the cellular DNA or by interfering with the ability of cells to repair damaged DNA. But even after mutation of the DNA in a cell has occurred, cancer does not automatically result. In fact, such a mutation of DNA cannot produce a tumor unless the cancerous cell continues to reproduce, because the mutation would be limited to a single cell unless that cell produced offspring.

Cancer induction is believed to be a multiple-step process, and it is thought that an absolute minimum of two steps is required. A "two-hit" model of cancer induction has been proposed, in which each "hit" is a mutation of the cellular DNA. These two hits often correspond to two separate exposures to carcinogens: the first exposure acts as a tumor initiator, while the second exposure promotes tumor development. However, the "two-hit" model of cancer induction also explains certain types of cancer that run in families. In hereditary cancers, the "first hit" may be a genetic mutation that is passed down from one generation to another, while the "second hit" is a more conventional exposure to a carcinogen. Alternatively, the first hit could be an inherited mutation, while the second hit is a spontaneous mutation. In any case, the necessity for two separate events in cancer induction implies that development of a tumor is a lengthy process.

Since cancer induction seems to be a multiple-step process, it may be feasible to block one step of the process and thereby block the whole process. Thus, to prevent cancer, it may not be necessary to completely eliminate all carcinogens. Instead, eliminating interaction among carcinogens may be sufficient. In practice, this might not really be very different from eliminating all carcinogen exposures; it is not usually possible to determine whether someone has already been exposed to a given carcinogen, and for those individuals with an inherited tendency to develop cancer, one carcinogen exposure may be enough. However, blocking the mechanism that allows carcinogens to interact with one another may also be possible. This strategy of cancer prevention will be discussed more fully in the chapter on chemical prevention of cancer.

UNDERSTANDING CANCER RISK FACTORS

In 1989 there was a widely publicized health scare involving apples tainted with traces of an insecticide called Alar. These apples were indicted as a cause of cancer by several influential television shows and a series of ill-informed witnesses testifying before Congress. At the height of the panic, a Chicago television station interviewed a mother who had heard about the dangers of Alar-tainted apples and had driven to her son's school to retrieve an apple from his lunch. The interviewer emphasized the woman's concerns about cancer and portrayed these concerns as legitimate. Yet, throughout the interview, the woman was smoking a cigarette while she described her fears about cancer. The risk of developing cancer as a result of habitual cigarette smoking is more than 10,000-fold greater than the risk of developing cancer from the amount of Alar on an apple or in a glass of apple juice. The fact that the interviewer was unaware of this irony indicates that there is a profound lack of understanding about cancer risk factors.

A risk factor can be defined as any action, exposure, or genetic pre-disposition that increases the odds of developing cancer. The study of risk factors for disease is the core of a branch of science called epidemiology, which analyzes the prevalence and spread of disease in a community. Therefore much of our discussion will be drawn from the medical literature specifically related to epidemiology, and this text will necessarily incorporate some concepts and terminology from epidemiology. However, the terminology is generally fairly straightforward, and the concepts are often intuitively obvious.

A measure of the strength or importance of a risk factor can be given by the concept of "relative risk."[13] Relative risk is defined as the proportional increase in cancer incidence caused by a single risk factor. In other words, how does any one particular risk factor affect the odds that an individual will get cancer? Relative risk is calculated by comparing cancer incidence in a group of individuals who have a particular risk factor versus cancer incidence in a group of individuals without the risk factor in question. A ratio is calculated to compare the number of sick individuals with the risk factor to the number of sick individuals without the risk factor. For example, a relative risk factor equal to 1.0 would imply that the risk factor under study did not actually lead to any increase in cancer incidence. But a study of women who survived the atomic bomb blasts in Japan showed that such women were about three times as likely to develop breast cancer as women who were not exposed to radiation. Therefore, the relative risk of breast cancer from high-dose radiation exposure is calculated to be 3.0.

Typically, the relative risk from a risk factor exposure is rather small, often being only somewhat larger than 1.0. For example, the relative risk of breast cancer in obese women over the age of 50, compared to nonobese women over the age of 50, is only 1.2. This means that, although obesity is considered to be a major risk factor for breast cancer, an obese woman is only 20% more likely to get breast cancer than a woman who is not obese. To consider these numbers in another way, about 12% of women (1 in 8) will get breast cancer at some point during their lives. But in a group of obese women, more than 14% will get breast cancer. While this may seem like a relatively small increase in risk, these numbers must be extrapolated to the population level—with more than 130 million women in the United States, a 20% increase in risk could mean an enormous increase in the number of new breast cancer cases.

The concept of relative risk becomes particularly important when considering risks that interact with one another. For example, the risk of cancer of the mouth is increased in people who smoke cigarettes, and risk increases with the number of cigarettes smoked per day.[14] In addition, among persons who do not smoke, the risk of cancer of the mouth increases with the level of alcohol intake. However, in people who both smoke and drink, the relative risk is elevated in a way that suggests that the separate risks for smoking and drinking are multiplicative, rather than merely additive. Among people who smoked two or more packs of cigarettes and drank more than four alcoholic beverages per day, the relative risk of oral cancer was elevated more than 35-fold. In fact, it was calculated that smoking and drinking combine to account for approximately three-fourths of all oral cancers.[15] Scientists have been studying risk factors for many years now, but the concept of interactive or multiplicative risk is fairly new. It is probable that the next decade or so will show that interactive risks are extremely important in cancer causation. In fact, since the "two-hit" model requires at least two genetic mutations for the expression of cancerous traits, it is possible that interacting risks may be required to explain all cancers.

RISK WEIGHT: A NEW WAY OF LOOKING AT CANCER RISK

The concept of relative risk is complicated enough that, if risk is not considered in a sufficiently broad context, it can be very misleading. For example, the risk of developing cancer in a part of the kidney called the renal pelvis is increased by drinking more than six cups of coffee a day.[16] The relative risk for heavy coffee drinkers is 1.8, compared to nondrinkers, meaning that heavy coffee drinkers have an 80% higher chance of developing this cancer. This increase in risk was reported in the media, and it made quite a stir because a large number of people fall into the category of heavy coffee drinkers. Yet cancer of the renal pelvis is a rare cancer, with fewer than 2,000 cases diagnosed each year. If there are 2,000 new cases per year among 250 million people, then the odds that any one person will develop the disease in a given year are only one in 125,000. If these odds are increased by 80%, due to heavy coffee consumption, then the odds that any one person will get the disease are still only about one in 69,444. So, while there has been a large increase in relative risk, there has not been much change in what might be called the "absolute risk" of getting cancer of the renal pelvis. Thus, even a rather strong risk factor can have a small effect on society as a whole if it increases the risk of a very rare cancer. Therefore, relative risk really tells only a part of the story, since it can reveal the risk to an individual from exposure to a particular risk factor, but it cannot reveal the risk to society from a particular risk factor.

The concept of risk weight is introduced here for the first time; this is a new way of calculating cancer risk that takes into account the effect of a risk factor on society as well as on the individual. Risk weight is simply the relative risk caused by a particular risk factor, multiplied by the relative frequency of the associated cancer. The method by which weighted risk is calculated is shown in Table 1-2 using lung cancer as an example. This calculation of weighted risk reveals that tobacco smoke is the single most important risk factor for lung cancer and, because this risk factor increases the risk of a very common cancer, that tobacco smoke has a tremendous impact on society as a whole.

THE IMPORTANCE OF IDENTIFYING CANCER RISK FACTORS

Hundreds of millions of dollars of taxpayer money have been spent identifying and studying cancer risk factors. This vast expenditure of money, time, and effort is important because a better understanding of cancer risk factors should enable us to modify exposure to these factors and so reduce cancer risk.[17] However, it is also possible that a better understanding of cancer risk factors will enable us to have a better general understanding of the mechanisms of cancer causation. This will be needed if we are ever to improve our ability to prevent new cancers or treat established ones.

TABLE 1-2 RISK FACTORS FOR LUNG CANCER				
RISK FACTOR	RELATED CANCER	RELATIVE RISK	RELATIVE FREQUENCY	RISK WEIGHT
Tobacco smoke	Lung	65	5	325
Tobacco × asbestos	Lung	50	5	250
Very high radon levels	Lung	13	5	65
Saturated fat	Lung	6.1	5	31
Low intake of β-carotene	Lung	2.4	5	12
Second-hand tobacco smoke	Lung	2	5	10
Low intake of selenium	Lung	2	5	10
Low intake of Vitamin E	Lung	2	5	10
Asbestos fibers	Lung	5	5	25
Air pollution	Lung	1.4	5	7
Average radon (home)	Lung	1.1	5	6

Sample relative risk weight calculations performed for lung cancer as an example. The relative importance of a risk factor is quantified by considering three factors: the relative risk associated with the risk factor; the relative frequency of the related cancer; and the statistical power of the study which linked the risk factor with the cancer. Relative risk is simply the relative increase in risk associated with a particular risk factor, and is defined as the proportional increase in cancer incidence caused by a single risk factor exposure. The tabulated value for relative risk is generally selected from the largest (and statistically most powerful) study discussed in the chapter text. Frequency is a measure of how common a particular cancer is, so that the relative importance of a particular risk factor can be assessed; if a risk factor causes an increase in a rare cancer, this is not as important as those that cause an increase in a common type of cancer. Relative frequency is based on the total number of expected cases, from Table 1-1. This table has the same form as tables presented in the following chapters, in which risk factors are summarized irrespective of the type of cancer they cause.

There are several other important potential benefits from identifying previously unknown causes of cancer.[18] A fuller knowledge of cancer risk factors may enable us to identify patients at greater risk of developing cancer; such individuals would thus benefit from closer medical surveillance for disease. Identifying unknown cancer risk factors may also allow us to identify patients for whom preventive treatment is appropriate; such preventive treatments could involve mastectomy for women at very high risk of developing breast cancer or prostate removal for men at a greatly elevated risk of prostate cancer. These prophylactic treatments are inappropriate unless a person is known to be at a greatly elevated risk of cancer, so it is important to be able to accurately predict cancer risk. Finally, a better understanding of cancer risk factors would enable us to discover subjects at high risk of developing cancer for whom it would be appropriate to participate in clinical studies aimed at assessing the effectiveness of intervention. At present, it is often somewhat unclear which subjects are at an elevated risk of cancer, so it is difficult to assess whether an anticancer intervention has been successful. This may explain why the few intervention studies that have already been attempted have often produced results that are difficult to interpret.

SUMMARY

Cancer causes untold amounts of pain, suffering, and premature death, and it annually drains billions of dollars from our economy. Yet cancer is largely preventable; a disease whose annual incidence could be reduced by relatively simple lifestyle changes and whose annual mortality could be reduced by a set of simple public health measures. The prevention of cancer is therefore a compelling goal, both at a personal and at a national level. Prevention of cancer requires a better understanding of the disease process itself, so that the causes of cancer can be eliminated. But it also requires that government agencies provide more leadership, and that cancer researchers do a better job of providing guidance to both the public and the government.

NOTES TO CHAPTER 1

1. D.L. Davis, G.E. Dinse, and D.G. Hoel, "Decreasing cardiovascular disease and increasing cancer among whites in the United States from 1973 through 1987," *J. Amer. Med. Assoc.* 271 (1994): 431–438.
2. L.W. Wattenberg, "Prevention-therapy-basic science and the resolution of the cancer problem," *Cancer Res.* 53 (1993): 5890–5896.
3. B.E. Henderson, R.K. Ross, M.C. Pike, "Toward the primary prevention of cancer," *Science* 254 (1991): 1131–1138.
4. B.F. Hankey, "Average years of life lost per person," *J. Natl. Cancer Instit.* 84 (1992): 1311.
5. *Ibid.*
6. H.B. Simon, *Staying well: Your complete guide to disease prevention,* (New York: Houghton Mifflin Co., 1992), 13–14.
7. R. Hand, S. Sener, J. Imperato, J.S. Chmiel, J. Sylvester, A. Fremgen, "Hospital variables associated with quality of care for breast cancer patients," *J. Amer. Med. Assoc.* 266 (1991): 3429–3432.

8. Wattenberg, "Prevention-therapy-basic science," 5890–5896.
9. J.D. Minna, "Neoplasms of the lung," in *Harrison's principles of internal medicine*, E. Braunwald, et al., editor. (New York: 1987), McGraw-Hill Book Co., 1115–1123.
10. Henderson, "Toward the primary prevention of cancer," 1131–1138.
11. *Ibid.*
12. R.G. Steen, *A conspiracy of cells: The basic science of cancer* (New York: Plenum Press, 1993), 353.
13. J.R. Harris, M.E. Lippman, U. Veronesi, W. Willett, "Breast cancer (Part 1)," *N. Engl. J. Med.*, 327 (1992): 319–328.
14. W.J. Blot, J.K. McLaughlin, D.M. Winn, D.F. Austin, R.S. Greenberg, et al., "Smoking and drinking in relation to oral and pharyngeal cancer," *Cancer Res.* 48 (1988): 3282–3287.
15. *Ibid.*
16. R.K. Ross, A. Paganini-Hill, J. Landolph, V. Gerkins, B.E. Henderson, "Analgesics, cigarette smoking, and other risk factors for cancer of the renal pelvis and ureter," *Cancer Res.*, 49 (1989): 1045–1048.
17. Harris, "Breast cancer (Part 1)," 319–328.
18. *Ibid.*
19. American Cancer Society. *Cancer facts & figures—1992* (Atlanta: American Cancer Society, 1992), 6.

2

....

DEFINING THE CAUSES
OF CANCER

A search for the causes of cancer has engaged physicians and scientists for hundreds of years. The first notable success occurred in 1700, when Bernardino Ramazzini noticed that nuns had a higher incidence of breast cancer than other groups of women. He attributed this to the celibacy of nuns, thereby making the first connection between cancer incidence and lifestyle. The potential of tobacco to cause cancer was first noted in 1761, when John Hill attributed development of nasal cancer to the use of snuff.

These early findings depended upon an observant physician making an intuitive connection between disease incidence and a potential risk factor. Yet even today, when science has matured and the "scientific method" holds sway, observation and intuition remain important tools for the scientist. But observation and intuition are not enough. Potential cancer risk factors may initially be identified by observation and intuition or by sheer luck, but scientific methods are then used to determine the importance of the potential risk factor.

SCIENTIFIC APPROACHES TO STUDYING
CANCER CAUSATION

Epidemiologists are the scientists most often involved in studying cancer risk factors. Typically they study disease by examining large groups of people to determine why disease incidence in one particular group is either higher or lower than normal. This can be done in one of two main ways, which sound superficially similar, but are really quite different in one aspect: the point of the observer in time with respect to the observed event, the diagnosis of cancer (Table 2-1).

In a case-control study, patients (or cases) who have already been

14

TABLE 2-1
HOW DO SCIENTISTS DETERMINE WHAT CAUSES CANCER?

METHOD OF STUDY	STRENGTHS	WEAKNESSES
Case-control	Relatively inexpensive Can identify risk factors quickly Sensitive to rare risk factors Rare cancers can be studied	Study is retrospective Possible memory bias Exposures hard to measure Insensitive to common risks Cannot control all variables Exposures can vary over time Insensitive to mechanisms
Cohort	Study is prospective Eliminates memory bias Exposures measured accurately Sensitive to common risks	Extremely expensive Very time consuming Insensitive to rare risk factors Rare cancers cannot be studied Cannot control all variables Exposures can vary over time Insensitive to mechanisms
Laboratory	Study is prospective Exposures measured accurately Most cancers can be studied Can identify risk factors quickly Exposures do not vary over time Dose-response can be determined Relatively inexpensive Potentially sensitive to any risk Sensitive to mechanisms Can control all variables	Must extrapolate to humans Chronic exposures impossible Spontaneous cancers common Acute exposures usually used Poor reflection of human risks

diagnosed with cancer are compared to similar individuals (controls) who do not have cancer. The controls are chosen to be similar to the cases in terms of age, sex, environment, and any obvious variables such as smoking habits. Both groups of people are then asked the same set of questions, to determine whether consistent differences emerge between cases and controls. This is done to determine whether there is one particular difference between the groups that is correlated with or predictive of cancer. Because scientists are comparing individuals who already have cancer with similar individuals who do not have cancer, they must determine whether a cause in the past can be correlated with a cancer in the present. This is therefore a retrospective study since the scientist is essentially looking back in time.

Unfortunately, this type of study has several major weaknesses.[1] Cases are more motivated than controls to remember risk factor exposures that occurred in the past. Risk factor exposures in the past are difficult to measure in any reliable way. If exposure to a particular risk factor is commonplace, determining whether cases had significantly greater exposure than controls is nearly impossible. Exposure to one risk factor is often associated with exposure to a second risk factor. For example, people who smoke heavily are more likely to drink heavily as well, compared to a group of non-smokers. Finally, both cases and controls may not remember, or even be aware of, the most critical risk factor exposure.

In a cohort study, a very large group of people is selected, all of whom are symptom-free at the start. This cohort of people is closely studied over time, under the assumption that some will develop cancer while most will not. Those individuals who do develop cancer are then compared to the rest of the cohort who have not developed the disease. Because this type of study is initiated before any of the cohort have cancer, the scientist must determine whether causes in the present are correlated with cancers in the future. This type of study is therefore prospective, because the scientist is looking forward in time.

A cohort study can avoid the "memory bias" problem inherent to a case-control study, but cohort studies also have their weaknesses.[2] To obtain information from a reasonable number of cancer patients in the future, thousands of cohorts may have to be enrolled at the beginning of a study. There is always a risk that few of the cohorts will develop cancer, so it may be impossible to obtain valid information on the differences between cases and controls. If a study is too small it may fail to adequately test that a suspected risk factor is in fact actually related to a particular cancer. For this reason, it is the usual practice to enroll huge numbers of people in a cohort study. This makes a cohort study inherently very expensive, since thousands of people must be followed for years to see if they develop cancer.

Although the retrospective and prospective type of study each have weaknesses, both types are still commonly done. Generally when there is not a strong suspicion as to the cause of a particular cancer, and especially if a cancer is relatively rare, a retrospective study will be done. Such a study may identify potential risk factors quickly, but there is always a possibility of bias or error if the researcher did not properly match cases with controls. Furthermore, a retrospective study may permit the scientist to attribute a cause for a particular cancer, but it does not permit the scientist to manipulate that cause experimentally. Therefore, if there is already a suspicion that some risk factor is causative of a particular cancer, it is more likely that a prospective study will be done. This type of study allows data to be recorded in a more unbiased fashion and also provides more scope for manipulating the factor presumed to be causative.

Retrospective and prospective studies both have several additional weaknesses. Risk factor exposure can vary over the years, so determining the exact relationship between risk factor exposure and cancer development is often difficult. Both types of study are vulnerable to errors in design, so that both may fail to identify high-risk subgroups in a population. Furthermore, both types of study may identify spurious correlations, so that cancer risk is attributed to a factor that is actually unrelated. The cancer literature is full of instances in which cancer risk was attributed to some risk factor, but larger or better-designed studies that followed were unable to confirm the initial finding.

Although there have been instances in which cancer risk was attributed to the wrong risk factor, there are also instances in which a risk factor was identified that was counterintuitive, but still apparently correct. For example, women who fracture their forearms are less likely to develop cancer, and are specifically less likely to get breast or genital cancer.[3] This is certainly not what one would predict, but there appears to be a sound biological reason for this observation. Arm fractures are often indicative of bone weakening, and bone weakening is associated with estrogen deficiency. Since estrogen is a risk factor for breast and genital cancer, it makes sense that low estrogen levels should be associated with bone fractures and a reduced incidence of these cancers. However, other associations have been found in epidemiological studies that cannot yet be rationalized. For example, exposure to fluorescent lights was identified as a risk factor for melanoma in men, while ovarian cancer risk is reduced in women with allergies to pollen.[4] These findings are currently unexplainable and may, in fact, be spurious. This is why it is imperative that scientists properly replicate important findings, so that greater confidence can be placed in the results.

The recent revolution in molecular biology has enabled scientists to study cancer risk by a novel technique called linkage analysis. This very powerful technique uses the tools of molecular biology to examine families of people who are at high risk of developing cancer. These familial groups, or kindreds, are examined to determine what feature of their shared genes predisposes them to develop cancer.[5] Linkage analysis often makes it possible to identify a particular gene in a person even when that gene does not manifest an obvious effect. However, this type of study is really retrospective, because it is only ever attempted with kindreds who have an elevated incidence of cancer. The major weakness of this type of study is that the risk factors for these kindreds may differ from the risk factors for a normal group of people.

Because each type of epidemiologic study we have discussed has shortcomings, independent scientific confirmation of potential cancer risk factors is critical. This is one reason why laboratory research, particularly with animal models of cancer, is generally so important. If we are ever to understand in depth the mechanisms of cancer causation, that understanding will emerge from the laboratory.

Laboratory experimentation offers a clear advantage over any of the other types of study we have discussed because a properly designed experiment can control all of the variables. Typically, a laboratory experiment is done with an animal, such as a rat or mouse, that has been specifically bred so that all of them are genetically similar, if not identical. Thus, a major source of variation, the individual complement of genes, is eliminated because all animals in the experiment share the same genetic information. Furthermore, all animals are chosen to be exactly the same age and to have had exactly the same life history prior to the experiment. When animals are kept in cages, various features of the environment (e.g., diet, availability of water, extent of crowding, exercise schedule, light regime, bacterial or viral exposure, handling history, and carcinogen exposure) can be precisely controlled. All of these variables can potentially contribute to differences in cancer incidence between a group of cases and a group of controls.

The results of a laboratory experiment are usually much simpler to interpret than the results of an epidemiological study. Thus, laboratory experiments often permit scientists to precisely determine the relationship between a cancer and a carcinogen exposure. It is sometimes possible to determine what is known as a "dose-response relationship" for a particular carcinogen. Since the extent of exposure to a carcinogen should determine the extent or rapidity of cancer development, an understanding of the dose-response relationship is important. All agents that cause cancer are thought to show a dose-response relationship. In fact, if a dose-response relationship cannot be found between a supposed carcinogen and the cancer that it is thought to cause, then it is often concluded that the "carcinogen" does not really cause cancer.

GENERAL MECHANISMS OF CANCER CAUSATION

Many different causes of cancer have been identified, and each of these major causes will be examined in greater detail in the chapters to follow.

However, worth noting is that most of the different cancer-causing agents share certain similarities. Cancer is usually associated with some mechanism that increases the rate of normal cell growth. A growing and dividing cell is apparently more at risk of mutation than is a non-dividing or quiescent cell, and chronic stimulation of cell division is clearly involved in many types of human cancer. For example, chemical induction of an increased rate of cell division has been implicated as the basic mechanism of chemical carcinogenesis. This is demonstrated by studies of the induction of skin cancer following application of a carcinogenic chemical to the skin surface. Typically, if the dose level of the chemical is increased, so that the rate of cell division is increased in a dose-dependent fashion, then the time period before appearance of a tumor is shortened. Thus the rate of tumor progression is increased if the rate of cell division is increased. This is a clear example of a dose-response relationship, since a higher dose of carcinogen causes an earlier onset of cancer. Generally, any agent that increases the likelihood that a cell can divide rapidly or in an uncontrolled manner increases the likelihood that a tumor will be formed.

ASSESSING CANCER RISK

From a public health standpoint, cancer cannot be prevented without an understanding of the level of danger posed by each carcinogen. But how does one actually measure the carcinogenic potential of a chemical? Having an objective yardstick of hazard associated with a carcinogen is important because we are constantly exposed to a range of potential carcinogens. Since we cannot eliminate all carcinogens simultaneously, we need to know which are the most important to control. But how do we quantify the degree of hazard so as to prioritize hazard mitigation?

Generally, the cancer risk associated with a potential hazard is quantified using laboratory data rather than epidemiological data. This laboratory data may involve measurement of the incidence of cancer in animals exposed to a carcinogen, or of the ability of a carcinogen to induce mutations in cultured cells. Any experiment designed to characterize the dose-response relationship of a carcinogen, as a way of characterizing carcinogen hazard, is called a bioassay.[6] A bioassay should be able to predict cancer hazard accurately, and, ideally, it should do so rapidly and cheaply. However, no bioassays are yet available that are accurate, fast, and cheap. In fact, many would argue that no bioassays are available that are even accurate.

Data on the induction of cancer in rats or mice may predict the risk of cancer in humans fairly accurately, but it is prohibitively time-consuming and expensive to test all potential carcinogens in rodents. It can take weeks or months for a particular carcinogen to induce a cancer in a rodent, so enormous numbers of animals must be housed and fed for a long time, often at great expense. Testing for the induction of mutations in cultured cells is faster and cheaper than testing in animals, but it is unclear that this test accurately predicts cancer risk in humans. Typically, cell bioassays are used to identify an agent as a potential carcinogen, then that agent is investigated in more depth with an animal bioassay. But extensive use of cell bioassays can potentially cause major problems; in several studies, cell bioassays have failed to identify a substantial fraction of known or suspected carcinogens.[7] For this reason, it is now commonplace to employ several different cell bioassays to identify potential carcinogens for further study. Animal bioassays remain the standard by which the carcinogenicity of an agent is finally determined.

But several problems associated with animal bioassays tend to weaken the utility of these tests. Each animal in a bioassay is essentially serving as a surrogate for a person, and the animal must accurately mirror the response of the person to carcinogen exposure. But, if a common environmental pollutant is tested in a bioassay involving 1,000 animals, each animal is serving as a surrogate for 200,000 people.[8] It seems unlikely that these few animals could adequately reflect the range of responses possible in a large human population. Furthermore, a significant number of rodents reared in captivity fall victim to spontaneous cancers. This could be because of the genetic make-up of the animals or because of unsuspected carcinogen exposures in food or water. Nevertheless, if a substantial number of control animals develop cancer spontaneously, then the fact that cancer can be induced in experimental animals is less compelling. A very large number of animals may be needed to be sure that experimental animals that were exposed to a carcinogen really do suffer a higher incidence of cancer than control animals.

Animal bioassays may systematically underestimate the cancer risk to humans simply because of differences in size between animals and humans. Imagine a carcinogen that has an effect on only one cell in 100 trillion cells.[9] This carcinogen might be able to induce cancer in only one rat in 250, since rats are rather small and are composed of substantially less than a trillion cells. Yet humans have roughly 75 trillion cells, so the hypothetical carcinogen might be able to transform one cell in the human body. Scientists believe that one cell that is transformed to malignancy may be sufficient to cause cancer. Therefore, this hypothetical carcinogen would cause cancer in only one out of 250 rats, but it might be capable of causing cancer in half the people exposed to it. Thus far we have no evidence that such a thing happens, but the possibility cannot be completely dismissed.

As well as the obvious differences in size between rats and humans, there also differences in metabolism. Perhaps humans have a more sophisticated immune system than rats or are better able to metabolize certain carcinogens. In any case, a direct comparison between two different species is always difficult; we must always bear in mind the potential for differences in response to a carcinogen, since there are manifest differences in the physiology of humans and rodents.

An even greater problem with animal bioassays is the type of animal experiments that are done. Animal bioassays usually involve exposing rodents to very high concentrations of a suspected carcinogen, because if low concentrations of carcinogen are used, it may take an extremely long time for the animals to develop cancer. High-level carcinogen exposures are therefore used to shorten the time to development of cancer. Yet humans are usually exposed to very low concentrations of a carcinogen for long periods of time. It is highly problematic to estimate cancer risk from low-level or chronic carcinogen exposure, using data from high-level or acute exposures to a carcinogen, because there is a great deal of controversy about the "threshold" of carcinogenic effects.[10]

A dose-response relationship assumes that, for each dose increment there is an incremental increase in the risk of developing cancer. If this is true, then the risk from low-level exposure can be accurately estimated from high-level exposures. But it is possible that low-level exposure to a "carcinogenic" chemical may not be harmful. This could happen if, for example, the liver was able to detoxify low levels of a particular carcinogen, while at high levels of exposure the detoxification system was overwhelmed. Alternatively, if there was a substance in cells that could inactivate carcinogens, then the cell would be safe from carcinogen exposure until the protective chemical was depleted, when the cell would quickly become vulnerable to damage.

These problems are compounded by the fact that there are chemicals that are not carcinogenic by themselves, but that are capable of promoting tumor development in animals previously exposed to a certain carcinogen. If an animal was previously exposed to the relevant carcinogen, then exposure to the "promoter" will induce cancer, while if the animal was not previously exposed to the carcinogen, the promoter will not induce cancer. If a group of animals differs in its prior exposure to carcinogen, then it would be essentially impossible to derive a dose-response relationship for the promoter. A given level of promoter might interact with a variable level of carcinogen, so that some animals would develop cancer rapidly while others might not develop it at all. This is why it is so critical to control the life history and carcinogen exposure of animals even prior to the beginning of an experiment.

A final problem with animal bioassays is that they do not reflect a real-world situation very well. Humans can be exposed to many different carcinogens simultaneously, whereas experimental animals are usually exposed to only one carcinogen at a time. If there is any interaction between carcinogens, then the single-exposure data will not accurately predict the incidence of cancer following multiple carcinogen exposures. In fact, interacting carcinogens are known to exist and to increase cancer risk dramatically over what would be predicted on the basis of single-agent exposures.

Nevertheless, with all of these caveats, animal bioassays remain vital to the prediction of human cancer risk. It is unethical ever to do experiments on humans, it is impractical to do low-dose experiments on animals, and it is inaccurate to do cell bioassays. Yet there is a pressing need for the prediction of human cancer risk. Therefore, the best approach is to employ a range of different techniques: cell bioassays should be used to screen many different potential carcinogens, then animal bioassays should be used to follow up on any suspected carcinogens. Finally, epidemiological research on cancer incidence in human populations remains vital as a way of identifying unsuspected carcinogens. This many-faceted approach is currently being used by the National Cancer Insitute, which screens tens of thousands of chemicals a year. Such work will remain essential unless a way can be developed to predict carcinogenic potential on the basis of theory alone.

ASSESSING PUBLIC HEALTH IMPACTS

Once a dose-response relationship has been determined for a particular carcinogen in an animal bioassay, that data can be used to estimate the risk for humans exposed to the same carcinogen. To simplify this calculation, it is generally assumed that the effects of a carcinogen are irreversible, so that the actions of minor carcinogens can combine with each other to increase overall cancer risk.[11] Furthermore, it is assumed that there is no threshold below which a carcinogen has no effect. This is a good assumption to make for two reasons: first, we have no evidence that such a threshold exists; and second, assuming that there is no threshold ensures that the estimate of risk will be very conservative, and will err towards overestimation of risk. Finally, it is assumed that all carcinogens are capable of inducing cancer by themselves, without requiring interactions with other carcinogens. This also is a conservative assumption, since chemicals that are merely promoters (i.e., unable by themselves to induce cancer) can be regulated as if they are able to induce cancer by themselves.

The use of bioassay data to extrapolate human risk from carcinogen exposure is very difficult and controversial. When doing this extrapolation, several questions must be carefully considered:[12]

1. Were the key studies well designed, so that the results are believable?
2. Has the experimental data been extensively replicated, so that the results can be accepted with a high degree of confidence?
3. Is there consensus among scientists that the data have been correctly analyzed and interpreted?
4. Has a clear dose-response relationship been derived, so that the relative level of risk from each exposure can be calculated?
5. Do the dose levels used in animal experiments roughly correspond to the doses likely in human exposures?

Generally, the answer to the last question above is no; the dose levels used in animal studies seldom correspond to the doses likely in human exposures. Consequently, when an agent is found to be carcinogenic at high levels of exposure, it is usually necessary to assume: one, that exposure at any level entails risk and, two, that low-level risks can be calculated from high-level exposures. Several different mathematical models have been developed, each using experimental dose-response data to extrapolate the risk of cancer from human carcinogen exposure.

The goal of governmental regulation of carcinogen exposure is generally to assure that individuals exposed to a given carcinogen for 70 years will have less than one chance in a million of developing cancer as a result of that exposure. This may not be realistic since the excess cancer risk of an improper diet is about 70,000-fold higher than the goal.[13] Even if this goal is realistic, it is unclear if we could ever obtain it. This is because it may not be possible to ever determine that a potential carcinogen is truly "safe." If 100 animals are tested in a bioassay and none of them develop cancer, then the agent to which they were exposed might be considered "safe."[14] Yet, from a statistical standpoint, the absence of cancer in a group of 100 animals actually means only that we can be 99% sure that the true incidence of cancer in this test is less than 5%. If a substance causes no cancer at all, when fed to mice at a dosage of 1% of the diet, then we can extrapolate that the risk of cancer at a dose level of 10 parts per million might be less than 5×10^{-5}. However, if this level of risk is accepted, many people might still be at risk. Consider that the population of the United States is 2.5×10^8; if 5×10^{-5} of these people are at risk, this translates to 1.25×10^4 people at risk. Therefore the finding that no mice develop cancer in this experiment might actually mean that no more than

12,500 people in the United States will develop cancer. This is true even though the human exposure occurs at a lower level, where risk is less. This example makes it clear why so much contention exists in the area of government regulation of carcinogen exposure.

Occasionally an agent is identified that is carcinogenic at high doses, but that is also strongly beneficial at doses closer to what humans are likely to encounter. This situation can be extremely difficult to resolve, since there is seldom enough information available to do a formal risk-benefit analysis. A good example of such a quandry is seen with nitrite, a chemical that is used as a food preservative. Several studies, done more than 20 years ago, show that sodium nitrite is carcinogenic to rats when added in large amounts in the diet. Yet this preservative is commonly used in packaged meats to stop the growth of the bacteria that cause botulin poisoning. Botulin poisoning results from a toxin secreted by bacteria as they grow, and this toxin is one of the most poisonous substances known. Although a formal risk-benefit analysis of nitrite was never done, the risks of this chemical should be considered in context with the benefit from its use. Since botulin poisoning is almost invariably fatal, the benefit of nitrite use is clear, while the human risks from low level exposure to nitrite are less well established. Clearly, this is a difficult regulatory problem.

There is now a growing recognition that cancer risk is not always additive, as was assumed in the past. Several recent studies of cancer risk show that carcinogens can strongly interact with one another, so that the risk associated with each individual factor is multiplied when the risk factors co-occur. A good example of this is the risk of oral cancer in people who smoke tobacco and drink alcoholic beverages. Tobacco and alcohol use each appear to cause a 2- to 3-fold increase in the risk of oral cancer. But tobacco and alcohol use combined cause a 15-fold elevation of oral cancer risk, in contrast to individuals who neither smoke nor drink. Among people who smoke two or more packs of cigarettes per day and consume more than four alcoholic beverages per day the relative risk of oral cancer is increased 35-fold over a control population.[15] Alcohol abuse increases the risk of cancer at every site in the oral cavity that normally comes in contact with fluid, while adjacent sites that do not come in contact with fluid do not have an elevated risk of cancer. This interaction is especially interesting because alcohol is not a carcinogen in animal tests. It is quite likely that many other multiplicative cancer risks have not yet been identified.

SUMMARY

Epidemiological methods of identifying potential carcinogens are the most important tool in an effort to identify new carcinogens. Yet epidemiologic methods alone are insufficient; it is critical that independent scientific confirmation of potential cancer risk factors be made. This is one reason why laboratory research with animals is generally so important. Animal models of cancer can help us to understand the mechanisms of cancer causation, so that we may eventually be able to block the process of cancer formation.

While our methods of defining the causes of cancer are flawed, they are still essential if we are to reduce or eliminate cancer. Unless we can correctly identify carcinogens in the environment, we are powerless to mitigate the hazard from these exposures. Given that each of the various methods available to us has inherent strengths and weaknesses, a responsible approach is to utilize all of the techniques in a concerted program to identify new carcinogens. The National Cancer Institute has already undertaken a very sophisticated program of screening chemicals for carcinogenicity. However, this should not lull us into complacency, since new chemicals are being produced and released into the environment faster than they can be tested.

NOTES TO CHAPTER 2

1. C.D. Sherman, K.C. Calman, S. Eckhardt, I. Elsebai, D. Firat, et al., "Aetiology," in *Manual of Clincial Oncology.* (New York: Springer-Verlag, 1987), 13–29.
2. *Ibid.*
3. S. Jenks, N. Volkers, "Razors and refrigerators and reindeer—oh my!" *J. Natl. Cancer Instit.* 84 (1992): 1863.
4. *Ibid.*
5. J.R. Harris, M.E. Lippman, U. Veronesi, W. Willett, "Breast cancer (Part 1)," *N. Engl. J. Med.* 327 (1992): 319–328.
6. H.C. Pitot, "Evaluation of toxic and carcinogenic environmental agents: scientific and societal considerations," in *Fundamentals of Oncology.* (New York: Marcel Dekker, 1986): 273–294.
7. *Ibid.*
8. S. Weinhouse, "Problems in the assessment of human risk of carcinogenesis from chemicals," in *Origins of Human Cancer: Human Risk Assessment*, H.H. Hiatt, J.D. Watson, J.A. Winsten, editors (Cold Spring Harbor, N.Y.: Cold Spring Harbor Laboratory, 1977): 1307–1309.
9. T. Sugimura, "Multistage carcinogenesis: A 1992 perspective," *Science* 258 (1992): 603–607.
10. B.N. Ames, L.S. Gold, "Mitogenesis increases mutagenesis," *Science* 249 (1990): 970–971.

11. Pitot, "Evaluation of toxic and carcinogenic environmental agents," 273–294.
12. *Ibid.*
13. P.H. Abelson, "Pesticides and food," *Science* 259 (1993): 1235.
14. Weinhouse, "Problems in the assessment of human risk of carcinogenesis from chemicals," 1307–1309.
15. W.J. Blot, J.K. McLaughlin, D.M. Winn, D.F. Austin, R.S. Greenberg, et al., "Smoking and drinking in relation to oral and pharyngeal cancer," *Cancer Res.* 48 (1988): 3282–3287.

3

··

STRATEGIES OF CANCER PREVENTION

Cancer prevention is a deceptively simple phrase, describing a goal that many would argue cannot be obtained. To a certain extent, the critics are right—it will probably never become possible to eliminate cancer as a cause of death. But it has been estimated that between 50% and 80% of all human cancers can be prevented.[1]

CANCER PREVENTION DEFINED

Progress in the war against cancer is measured in various ways, with cancer incidence, cancer survival, and cancer mortality being the most commonly reported statistics. Probably the most important and meaningful measure of the success of a cancer prevention effort is a reduction in the mortality.[2] The only feasible ways to reduce cancer mortality are to reduce the incidence of cancer and to increase patient survival after cancer is diagnosed.

A reduction in the incidence of cancer will be achieved principally through a general reduction in the exposure of people to various cancer risk factors.[3] Reduction of risk factor exposure has been called "primary prevention," since it is the first step in prevention. Reduction of risk factor exposure will occur principally by educating people about the risk factors that should be avoided and by inducing people to make necessary lifestyle changes.

An increase in patient survival after cancer diagnosis will be attained through increasing the success of early cancer detection. If cancer is diagnosed before it becomes extensively invasive or widely metastatic, then the cure rate is dramatically higher. For example, the five-year survival rate for eight major cancers (bladder, breast, colorectal, larynx, lung, oral, prostate, and uterus) averages 70% if the tumor is diagnosed when it is localized. However, if there is even regional involvement (i.e., not wide

27

metastasis), five-year survival for these same cancers drops to only 38%.[4] If there is widespread metastasis at diagnosis, the expected five-year survival rate for these cancers is substantially worse. The most reasonable way to increase the rate of early cancer diagnosis is through widespread implementation of various cancer screening programs and through increasing general awareness of the early symptoms of cancer. An increase in the early detection rate for cancer has been called "secondary prevention," but this terminology will be avoided here because it is confusing.

PRACTICAL GOALS OF CANCER PREVENTION

The human condition dictates that we cannot eliminate cancer mortality, since mortality is a given. But many cancer prevention goals could be achieved in an incremental fashion, so that a series of small gains would lead to a major victory.

One major incremental goal of cancer prevention should be postponement of the first incidence of cancer. Cancer is generally a disease of older persons so, as the average age of the population of the United States increases, cancer will probably become increasingly common. This is because the rate at which persons of a specific age get cancer has changed little over the past few decades. However, if the average age at incidence of any type of cancer could be postponed by even a single year, this would have a large effect on both personal and public health. Thus, each year added to the average age at which a particular cancer occurs should be seen as a major victory. Currently, the only effective means to achieve this goal is through risk factor reduction, although in the future postponement of the first incidence of cancer may involve other interventions. A secondary goal of "cancer postponement" might be the eventual elimination of all childhood and young adult cancers.

Another major goal of cancer prevention should be postponement of mortality in patients who have already developed cancer. This can be achieved principally through cancer screening, which enables the detection of cancer when tumors have not yet metastasized. When tumors are only locally involved, the chances of achieving a cure are greatly improved. Even when a cure cannot be obtained, early diagnosis generally enables the patient to have a better quality of life for a longer time before the cancer becomes terminal. A secondary goal of "mortality postponement" might be the transformation of cancer into a chronic disease. This involves learning how better to treat cancer patients, so that the disease becomes survivable, even if not curable, over the long term. This will only be achieved through medical advances that enable patients to survive despite their disease.

These practical goals of cancer prevention will be reached by combining three separate strategies: reduction in exposure to cancer-causing agents (passive prophylaxis); intervention in the process that results in cancer (active prophylaxis); and early and aggressive response to any newly diagnosed cancers.

PASSIVE PROPHYLAXIS

Passive prophylaxis is a process of identifying what we should avoid if we want to prevent cancer. Passive prophylaxis includes the identification of risk factors for cancer and the reduction in exposure to these risk factors. Since many cancer risk factors are still unknown, research into the epidemiology of cancer (to identify new and previously unknown risk factors) will play an important part in passive prophylaxis. Epidemiological research alone, however, will not be sufficient.

Passive prophylaxis will also involve an ongoing and coordinated attack on cancer in the laboratory. There is a continuing need for conventional studies of cancer causation augmented with new research initiatives. For example, several recent studies have suggested that many cancers are caused by two or more risk factors that strongly interact with one another. This type of multiplicative risk may be common in cancer causation, but relatively little, as yet, is known about multiplicative risk.

Finally, passive prophylaxis will also involve effective public education programs to disseminate information from the laboratory to the street. Cancer prevention will only become possible if new findings are made known to the public; there is a need for reliable source of information, so that people are not duped by the false or exaggerated claims commonly seen in supermarket tabloids. "Science by press conference" will not become useful until reporters become more sophisticated about science, because an unknowledgeable reporter is simply unable to report science objectively or in context. This leads to misleading or frankly inaccurate news reports—a confirmation of an old idea may be reported as a new finding, or an incremental new result may be reported as the resolution to a long-standing debate.

ACTIVE PROPHYLAXIS

Active prophylaxis is a term that denotes any effort to actively intervene in the process that results in cancer. This could include surgery undertaken to eliminate the possibility of cancer developing in a particular organ, or it could include chemical intervention in the carcinogenic process itself.

Chemoprevention of cancer is a relatively new idea, but it has achieved a small measure of success in certain cases such as breast cancer.[5]

Another important area that falls under the heading of active prophylaxis is cancer screening. This includes any effort to detect lesions at a pre-cancerous stage. This approach has achieved a striking degree of success in some cases such as cervical cancer. Detection of a lesion before it becomes cancerous is the best way to prevent progression to malignancy. Similarly, an early response to an established cancer is the best way to increase survival among patients who already have cancer. It is imperative to make a diagnosis when the cancer is still small and amenable to treatment. This can only be achieved by the full implementation of existing cancer screening tests, combined with development of new screening efforts. It is anticipated that cancer screening will become increasingly common as new and more effective screening techniques become available.

Another possible method of active prophylaxis, which is far more speculative at present, is the possibility that cancer can be prevented by vaccines. Several cancers appear to be the result of infection by disease-causing organisms. Thus the incidence of these cancers might be reduced by vaccinations against the disease-causing organism. Possibilities include vaccines against the viruses that cause liver and cervical cancer and against the bacteria that may cause stomach cancer.

MAKING CANCER A CHRONIC DISEASE

There have been several recent advances in cancer symptom management, in the control of cancer pain, and in psychosocial counseling of the cancer patient. These advances suggest that symptom management and long-term cancer control may become a viable alternative to cure in some cases. Many of the major human diseases, including hypertension, coronary artery disease, diabetes, arthritis, Parkinson's disease, ulcerative colitis, manic depression, and schizophrenia, cannot be cured. However, disease progression can be blocked and symptoms can be managed. Similarly, it may be unreasonable to expect cancer to be curable in every case. If disease progress can be arrested, while symptoms are controlled, then even an inoperable cancer might become a chronic disease. The goal of cancer control in such a case would be to reduce cancer to a condition that might limit a person's activity but would not significantly shorten expected lifespan.

A shift toward regarding cancer as a chronic, rather than a terminal, disease could result in changing perceptions of the goal of cancer treatment. Little research emphasis has been placed on controlling the systemic manifestations of cancer, yet it is just these manifestations that most often result in the death of a cancer patient. A good deal of evidence suggests that tumors, even relatively small ones that are still local rather than regional, can have broad systemic effects on the patient.[6] This may result from inappropriate hormone secretion by the tumor, or it may occur by some as-yet-unsuspected mechanism. If we are to succeed in making cancer a survivable chronic disease, then the mechanisms of systemic failure seen in advanced cancer patients must be better understood. This implies that more research should be done on the development of sophisticated patient management techniques.

WHY HAS SURVIVAL IMPROVED FOR SOME CANCERS?

These various strategies for cancer prevention are expensive and difficult to implement. Since cancer prevention requires the expenditure of federal monies and the broad-based support of taxpayers, there must be a good prospect of success before funds are committed. Therefore, we need some way to judge whether our proposed cancer prevention strategies have a reasonable probability of success. Perhaps the best way to determine whether cancer prevention efforts can succeed in the future is to look at the past: has the survival rate for any cancer improved as a result of a cancer prevention effort?

A careful study, covering the period from 1973 to 1986, has shown that cancer mortality decreased strikingly for five of the most dreaded cancers: breast cancer; stomach cancer; cervical cancer; testicular cancer; and colorectal cancer.[7] These five cancers together accounted for roughly 34% of the new cancer cases diagnosed in 1990, so a reduction in their mortality is important. Real increases in overall cancer survival can occur by only two mechanisms: either the cancer is detected at an earlier stage, when it is more responsive to treatment (and when survival is longer even without treatment); or else more effective treatments are available for the cancer, even if it is diagnosed at an advanced stage. These different mechanisms of improved cancer survival will have very different effects on stage-specific incidence, stage-specific survival, and overall incidence and survival. For example, if cancer is simply diagnosed earlier, but is not treated any more effectively than in the past, then stage-specific survival would be unchanged, but stage-specific incidence would shift dramatically. Alternatively, if cancer is treated more effectively than before, then stage-specific survival and overall survival would improve, while incidence might be unchanged. The patterns of change in incidence and survival were examined for each of these five cancers to determine which factors accounted for the striking improvements in cancer survival.

Between 1974 and 1986, breast cancer mortality declined by 8% for women under the age of 65.[8] This decline arose because of a shift in the stage-specific distribution of breast cancer: in 1974, only 46% of cancers were localized at the time of diagnosis, whereas in 1986, 53% were localized at diagnosis. Yet the two-year survival rate changed little for each of the stages, and overall breast cancer incidence increased slightly. This pattern of change is most consistent with early detection of breast cancer leading to a better overall survival rate. During this same period, mammography became increasingly widespread as a screening technique for early diagnosis of breast cancer. The overall decrease in breast cancer mortality suggests that mammographic screening has had a beneficial effect on breast cancer survival.

There was also a 26% decrease in mortality from stomach cancer between 1974 to 1986.[9] This decrease arose because of a decrease in overall incidence, without a decrease in the incidence of advanced cancers. This pattern of change is most consistent with a reduction in risk factor exposure, so that there are simply fewer cases of stomach cancer. Unfortunately, it is not yet clear what all the risk factors are for stomach cancer, so we do not know which risk factor reduction actually acccounted for the decline in stomach cancer mortality.

Between 1974 and 1986, there was a 43% decrease in mortality from cervical cancer.[10] This occurred because of a striking decline in the overall incidence of cervical cancer, and a decline in the incidence of the earliest stage of cervical cancer. This cancer actually paints a confusing picture, because of an apparent increased incidence of advanced cancer: in 1974, only 7% of cervical cancers were diagnosed after they were metastatic, whereas in 1986, 12% of cancers were metastatic at diagnosis. However, these figures are very misleading because, over the same period, the number of cervical lesions that were detected before they became cancerous increased dramatically. The Pap test was used more and more widely over the years of this study, and this test is remarkably effective at detecting precancerous cervical lesions. The increased incidence of advanced cancers presumably arose because some women did not have access to regular medical care and did not have a Pap test performed; these same women are probably more likely to wait until their cancer is advanced before seeing a physician.

Over the 13-year period from 1974 to 1986, the mortality rate from testicular cancer declined by 72%.[11] Yet the incidence rate for this cancer actually increased, with no evidence of a significant shift toward early diagnosis. Therefore, increased survival is not the result of a decline in risk factor exposure or of detection of lesions before they become cancerous. Instead, the improvement in overall survival arose because of a major increase in two-year survival for advanced cancers: in 1974, only 24% of men with metastatic cancer survived for two years, while in 1986, 74% of men with metastatic disease survived at least two years. This pattern is most consistent with major advances in the treatment of testicular cancer. In fact, chemotherapy for advanced testicular cancer, based on use of an agent called cisplatin, was introduced in 1974.

Between 1974 and 1986, the overall mortality rate for colorectal cancer declined by 14%.[12] Yet there was a slight increase in overall incidence of this cancer, combined with a slight shift toward diagnosis of this cancer before metastasis. The two-year survival rate for colorectal cancer increased, from 56% overall in 1974 to 64% overall in 1986, with the greatest increases in survival seen in early stage cancer. The fact that overall incidence increased shows that risk factor exposures for this cancer have not declined, despite the fact that the risk factors for colorectal cancer are fairly well understood. This somewhat confusing pattern is most consistent with early detection of colorectal cancer, together with more effective treatments for all stages of the cancer. During the time covered by this study, there was more widespread use of the sigmoidoscope and the fecal occult blood test for colorectal cancer screening. In addition, advances were made in treatment for colorectal cancer as it became more common to combine aggressive surgery with adjuvant chemotherapy.

The fact that mortality from these major cancers has declined significantly in only 13 years argues strongly that cancer prevention strategies can be effective. On a personal level, untold amounts of pain and suffering were prevented by these striking reductions of cancer mortality. Thus, it is imperative that individuals be willing to make the (often simple) lifestyle changes that can help prevent cancer. On a societal level, the fact that mortality for these cancers was reduced resulted in a savings of billions of dollars. There are huge annual losses to the gross national product caused by lost worker productivity and medical care for the terminally ill. In fact, the economic burden of cancer to the United States is more than $80 billion a year.

OVERVIEW OF CANCER PREVENTION

What can actually be done to prevent cancer? As we shall see, the odds associated with any given risk factor are usually elevated only slightly (2–4-fold) in most epidemiologic studies. For this reason, it may seem that such risks are low level and perhaps even unimportant. But this impression is untrue. Some people are apparently better able to resist the effects of a cancer risk factor; if such "cancer-resistant" people are included in an epidemiologic study, then that study will underestimate the risk associated with a particular risk factor. Since epidemiologic studies generally cannot identify "cancer-resistant" people, these studies provide a very coarse level of resolution. Yet, since one never knows one's own state of vulnerability to a particular risk factor, it is very unwise to ignore a known risk.

Some risk factors are so well-known and so damaging that everyone should avoid them. This list includes dietary fat, excessive alcohol consumption, and obesity, but foremost among the known cancer risk factors is tobacco. Carcinogens in tobacco and tobacco smoke have been implicated in the causation of about one in every three cancers in the United States, including cancers of the oral cavity, larynx, esophagus, stomach, pancreas, lung, kidney, bladder, prostate, and cervix. The human body can activate certain tobacco smoke components to produce carcinogens with the capacity to affect internal organs distant from the site of smoke exposure. Recent research has shown that, in pregnant women who smoke, there are even carcinogenic effects on the placenta. Banning the sale of tobacco would be vastly more effective as an anti-cancer measure than all of the environmental remediations proposed as a part of the Environmental Protection Act.

Despite the fact that certain risk factors are well-known to increase the risk of cancer, many risk factors are still unknown. This makes it impossible to avoid all cancer risk factors, especially since there may be interactions among risk factors that could increase cancer risk in a multiplicative fashion. Since it is impossible to avoid unknown risk factors, it is even more important to avoid the known risk factors, so as to minimize any potential multiplicative interactions among risk factors.

Multiplicative risks are likely to be a major feature of cancer risk and often may involve genetic susceptibility to cancer. A good example of a genetic susceptibility to cancer is provided by a strain of laboratory rat that has a gene mutation that predisposes the rats to develop kidney cancer. When male rats bearing this mutation are exposed to a kidney carcinogen known as DMN (dimethylnitrosamine), these rats develop an average of 23 kidney tumors per animal, whereas only one in three normal male rats exposed to DMN develops a tumor. Thus, a mutation affecting a single gene caused a 70-fold increase in susceptibility to kidney carcinogenesis.[13] In the future, it may become possible to analyze cancer risk genetically, so as to identify individuals at higher risk of cancer. Until that day, it is important to avoid the known risk factors.

SUMMARY: GENERAL CANCER PREVENTION RECOMMENDATIONS

Much of what we know about cancer prevention is common sense. Everyone should eat a balanced diet and practice moderation in all things. It is fair to say that cancer is a disease of abuse or disuse, and moderation may be key to avoiding both extremes.

Everyone should avoid tobacco in any form, whether chewed, smoked, or inhaled as second-hand smoke. If this book serves no other purpose than to get a few smokers to quit, then it has been a worthwhile effort.

Everyone should also be careful about diet and nutrition.[14] It is generally wise to cut down on total fat intake and eat more high-fiber foods such as fruits and vegetables. High-fiber foods tend to be low in fat, so eating fruits and vegetables may actually accomplish two purposes. The American Cancer Society has recommended that everyone eat at least five helpings a day of fruits and vegetables; it is probably not possible to eat too much of these foods, since they are low in fat, high in fiber, high in various vitamins and nutrients, and generally not fattening. It is also important specifically to eat foods rich in vitamin A, vitamin C, and a vitamin A precursor known as beta-carotene. Foods rich in these vitamins include dark green leafy vegetables (spinach), red, yellow, and orange fruits and vegetables, citrus fruits, and juices made from them.

Vegetables from the cabbage family (cruciferous vegetables) seem to offer special protection from cancer, and they are also good sources of fiber. For this reason, vegetables such as bok choy, broccoli, Brussels sprouts, cabbage, cauliflower, collard greens, kale, kohlrabi, mustard greens, rutabagas, turnips, and turnip greens should be included in the diet. Eating a wide range of different fruits and vegetables is beneficial, since scientists simply do not know which are the best sources of protection from cancer. It may also be desirable to supplement the diet with multivitamins, although there is somewhat less evidence that multivitamins are actually beneficial. Use of fiber supplements in the diet is probably unwise, since it is unclear whether fiber supplements actually have the same effect as dietary fiber.

In general, it is wise to avoid highly processed foods and to eat more foods made with whole grains and flours. This means that whole-grain breads should be substituted for breads and other baked goods that are made with bleached or refined flours, processed grains, and refined sugars. Baked goods are also worth avoiding because they tend to have a very high content of dietary fat and refined sugar. However, it is not necessary to eliminate these elements of the diet; the object is to avoid cancer, not to avoid all the foods that make life worth living.

Other foods that should be minimized in the diet include salt-cured, smoked, or nitrite-cured foods, including processed meats, bacon, sausage, ham, smoked fish and smoked meat. These foods are generally high in dietary fat and cholesterol, and low in various essential nutrients; to the extent that they add flavor and palatability to the diet, they are good, but they should not become a major part of the diet. If it is possible to substitute lean fresh meat or fish for processed meats without a significant loss of flavor, the exchange is worthwhile. There is no indication that meats should be eliminated from the diet, but substitution of white meat for red meat may be generally beneficial.

It is preferable to use cooking methods that do not add fats to the foods. Fried foods should be avoided, especially in cases where other cooking methods do not lead to a loss of flavor. Many recipes call for foods to be baked, steamed, poached, or roasted, and these cooking methods add less fat to food during the cooking process. In fact, steaming, poaching, and roasting can even remove small amounts of fat during cooking. Using a microwave oven to reheat leftovers, rather than frying them, can substantially reduce intake of dietary fat. If meats are to be grilled, broiled, or barbecued, then fat should be carefully trimmed from the meat beforehand. Use of extremely high cooking temperatures that result in the charring of fat and meat can result in the production of potent carcinogens, so lower cooking temperatures are favored. There is often no adverse affect on flavor if meats are grilled slowly at a lower heat, since relatively low temperatures are sufficient to sear the meat and prevent loss of meat juices.

Alcoholic beverages should be consumed in moderation. There is certainly no need to eliminate wine and beer, or even hard alcohol, from the diet, but these elements should not become a regular source of calories. Too often, people feel that they haven't had dinner if they don't have a drink. Regular indulgence in any type of alcohol is not recommended, since such consumption can lead to cancer, heart disease, and alcoholism.

Certain lifestyle choices also reduce the overall risk of cancer. Regular exercise is necessary, both to maintain body weight at a desirable level and to increase the rate at which food moves through the digestive tract. Regular exercise also has the benefit of reducing the risk of heart disease. Regular exercise is much more effective, and generally more beneficial, than constant dieting as a way to avoid obesity and to obtain an ideal weight. Ideal weight for an individual must be determined by considering age, sex, bone structure, and muscle mass, and should only be done in consultation with a physician.

Whenever possible, people should learn more about their personal risk factors. If there is a family history of cancer, especially if cancer has affected a particular organ in a large number of family members, special care should be taken to avoid known risk factors for that cancer. It would also be wise to be screened for that cancer whenever possible. In the absence of specific screening tests for a particular cancer, regular visits to a family physician can substantially reduce cancer risk. However, there is no substitute for common sense, moderation, and personal knowledge of cancer risk factors.

NOTES TO CHAPTER 3

1. I.B. Weinstein, "Cancer prevention: recent progress and future opportunities," *Cancer Res.* 51 (1991): 5080s–5085s.
2. K.C. Chu, B.S. Kramer, C.R. Smart, "Analysis of the role of cancer prevention and control measures in reducing cancer mortality," *J. Natl. Cancer Instit.*, 84 (1991): 1636–1643.
3. C.D. Sherman, K.C. Calman, S. Eckhardt, I. Elsebai, D. Firat, et al., "Prevention," in *Manual of clinical oncology* (New York: Springer-Verlag, 1987), 30–37.
4. C.D. Sherman, K.C. Calman, S. Eckhardt, I. Elsebai, D. Firat, et al., in *Manual of clinical oncology.* 4th ed. (New York: Springer-Verlag, 1987), 372.
5. J.R. Harris, M.E. Lippman, U. Veronesi, W. Willett, "Breast cancer (Part 3)," *N. Engl. J. Med.* 327 (1992): 473–480.
6. R.G. Steen, *A conspiracy of cells: the basic science of cancer* (New York: Plenum Press, 1993), 427.
7. Chu, "Analysis of the role of cancer prevention and control measures," 1636–1643.
8. *Ibid.*
9. *Ibid.*
10. *Ibid.*
11. *Ibid.*
12. *Ibid.*
13. C. Walker, T.L. Goldsworthy, D.C. Wolf, J. Everitt, "Predisposition to renal cell carcinoma due to alteration of a cancer susceptibilty gene," *Science* 255 (1992): 1693–1695.
14. Sherman, "Prevention," 30–37.

4

···

CANCER AND THE FAMILY
HISTORY

Most people are familiar with the idea that smoking causes lung cancer. However, smoking cannot be the whole story; although 90% of lung cancer patients are smokers, only about 10% of smokers actually get lung cancer. This suggests that other factors can interact with smoking to increase or decrease lung cancer risk in an unpredictable manner. Evidence is now beginning to emerge suggesting that family history plays an important role in determining which smokers are most vulnerable to the carcinogenic effects of tobacco smoke.

IS THERE EVIDENCE FOR CANCER PRONENESS?

If genes and the family history are important in determining cancer proneness, then certain people will be more vulnerable to cancer than others. A recent study examined a large group of people who had been diagnosed with lung cancer to determine whether they showed any evidence of unusual proneness to lung cancer. [1] Scientists reasoned that lung cancer proneness might manifest itself in the occurrence of a second lung tumor of the same type as the first; since lung tumors are somewhat unusual, two of the same type should be a rare event. But this is a very difficult type of study to do, since most lung cancer patients are smokers. Because the whole lung surface is exposed to tobacco smoke, it should not be too surprising that lung cancer patients are vulnerable to the occurrence of a second tumor elsewhere in the lungs. Furthermore, it is difficult to know whether this second lung tumor is really another "primary" (new) cancer, or just a metastasis from the first cancer. To deal with these complex issues, this study examined only those tumors that had been carefully evaluated by microscope, so that the type of cancer each patient had developed was known. This is important because there are four major types of lung cancer: squamous cell carcinoma, adenocarcinoma, small cell lung cancer, and large cell carcinoma.

Scientists used a huge database to collate information on patient history, clinical diagnosis, and treatment outcome for cancer patients across the nation.[2] This database covers an area within which 10% of the population of the United States lives and included 111,616 patients diagnosed with primary lung cancer during the 14-year period between 1973 and 1987. Scientists found that if a person develops adenocarcinoma of the lung, that person is nearly three times as likely to get a second lung adenocarcinoma as to get any other type of lung cancer. Similarly, if a patient develops squamous cell carcinoma of the lung, he or she is nearly three times as likely to get a second squamous lung carcinoma as any other type of lung cancer. In fact, if a patient developed squamous cell carcinoma at a site outside the lungs, that person is still more prone to get squamous cell lung carcinoma than any other type of lung cancer. This held true even when a long time has elapsed between the first and second diagnosis of cancer, implying that the second cancer could not have been a metastasis from the first cancer. To put it another way, if a person develops two separate primary tumors, odds are that the two tumors will be of the same type.[3] What this suggests is that certain people are vulnerable to certain types of lung cancer. It is reasonable to conclude that this is the result of a hereditary vulnerability, and that some people are simply more prone than usual to develop certain types of cancer.

More generally, it seems that people who develop any kind of cancer may be somewhat more susceptible than usual to a second malignancy. A large number of cancer patients have been treated at the National Cancer Center in Tokyo, and recent statistics from that institution indicate that 8% of its patients are receiving treatment for a second malignancy.[4] Most of these second malignancies are neither metastases nor recurrences of earlier disease, but rather are second primary cancers. Development of second primaries is not always due to the carcinogenic effects of cancer therapy, since many such cancers arise in patients who received neither radiation nor chemotherapy as treatment for their first tumor. This same cancer center reported that, in 1962, only 2% of its patients were being treated for a second primary tumor. The increased incidence of second primary tumors could be attributable to any of several factors: perhaps tumor treatment is simply more effective, so that more patients survive to develop a second tumor; or perhaps the incidence of multiple primary neoplasia is actually increasing, as a result of some unknown cause.

There is now strong evidence that most types of cancer aggregate in families.[5] This is consistent with the idea that family members can inherit a tendency to develop certain types of cancer. In general, close relatives of a cancer patient should be considered at risk, at least for that specific type of cancer, and perhaps, more generally, for other cancers as well. The elevation in risk associated with most familial cancers is small; typically, the site-specific cancer risk is elevated two- to three-fold if there is a family history of cancer at that site. But certain cancer syndromes can have a very dramatic effect on cancer risk, although usually these syndromes are associated with very rare forms of cancer. However, there is also a growing suspicion that certain very common forms of cancer can be hereditary, even though familial suceptibility is very difficult to pinpoint. Since there are 240 million people in the United States, and since roughly one in every three Americans will develop cancer, many striking family aggregates of cancer will be due to chance alone. In fact, cancer is so common that a family history of cancer is the rule rather than the exception. It is often extremely difficult to determine whether a particular family aggregate is the result of inherited susceptibility or just plain bad luck.

EVIDENCE FOR HEREDITARY CANCER SYNDROMES

About 50 different hereditary cancer syndromes are now known in which there is often a dramatic familial increase in cancer incidence.[6] Hereditary cancers are more likely to arise at an early age and are more likely to affect several sites simultaneously. Most of these cancer syndromes are themselves rare but were recognized because they cause cancers that are extremely rare in the general population. One of the best-known examples of a hereditary cancer syndrome is retinoblastoma, a cancer of the eye that afflicts young children. This cancer can be transmitted by a mutated retinoblastoma gene, which is responsible for about 40% of all cases of retinoblastoma. A child born without the retinoblastoma gene mutation has only a 1 in 30,000 chance of developing this cancer, while the probability that a child with the mutation will develop retinoblastoma is about 95%. This translates to a 28,500-fold higher retinoblastoma risk in children with a mutated gene. Nevertheless, about 5% of patients who carry the retinoblastoma gene never develop retinoblastoma. Furthermore, retinoblastoma patients typically develop no more than three or four tumors among the millions of cells in the retina, all of which carry the mutation. Therefore, transformation of a cell to the malignant state appears to be a rare event.

Close relatives of children who develop retinoblastoma have an increased risk of a range of different cancers.[7] This was shown in a study that examined the incidence of non-ocular cancer among 4,101 parents and other relatives of retinoblastoma patients. In this large group of relatives, a total of 117 people were identified who were known to be carriers of the retinoblastoma gene mutation, but who had not themselves developed retinoblastoma. Among these people, the incidence of non-ocular cancer was nearly 10-fold higher than expected for a normal population. Retino-blastoma gene carriers were specifically at risk for brain tumors (74-fold elevation in risk), melanoma of the skin (73-fold elevation in risk), bladder cancer (29-fold elevation in risk), and lung cancer (16-fold elevation in risk). This strongly suggests that the retinoblastoma gene is very important in suppression of cancer in those people who are fortunate enough to have a normal version of the gene.

Another example of a very rare hereditary cancer syndrome is known as von Hippel-Lindau disease.[8] This unusual syndrome is associated with an elevated risk of kidney cancer, which is commonly multifocal and often affects both kidneys. The disease is characterized by a malformation of blood vessels in the retina and cerebellum, and symptoms of this syndrome include progressive loss of muscular coordination, headache, accumulation of fluid in the retina, and progressive blindness. Kidney cancer is often the cause of death in patients with this syndrome, and one von Hippel-Lindau family had 17 members afflicted with kidney cancer, even though kidney cancer is a relatively unusual cancer.[9] Very recently a gene was discovered that appears to be a "tumor suppresser gene" that specifically suppresses development of von Hippel-Lindau disease.[10]

Evidence has recently been obtained that certain relatively common cancers may also be associated with rare cancer syndromes. For example, Li-Fraumeni syndrome causes an increased susceptibility to soft tissue tumors, breast cancers, brain tumors, and several other cancers that afflict children and young adults. Li-Fraumeni syndrome can cause a substantial elevation of risk for some of these tumors: risk of sarcoma is elevated 25- to 37-fold, with respect to normal; breast cancer risk is elevated nearly two-fold; and brain tumor risk is elevated four- to seven-fold.[11] Ironically, the risk of various other cancers is actually reduced four-fold, probably because Li-Fraumeni syndrome patients die at a young age of syndrome-associated cancers. This syndrome was first identified because an astute physician noted a cluster of rare cancers in one family. In this particular family, three young patients developed a type of soft tissue tumor that ordinarily affects only one in 100,000 persons in the general population. Upon questioning family members, it was found that the mothers of two of these patients had breast cancer at a young age, while the father of the third patient had acute leukemia. In addition, other family members developed cancers of the breast and other sites at an early age. Subse-quently, the physicians who first noted this "coincidence" surveyed the medical records of 700 children with similar cancers. They found another three patients with an unusually high incidence of cancer in the family. No environmental factors appeared to account for these cancer clusters, so it was proposed that these patients were examples of a new cancer-prone syndrome.[12]

Nearly 50 families with Li-Fraumeni syndrome have now been identified and studied to determine to what extent the syndrome is responsible for the cancers that afflict these patients. One study followed 545 members of 24 different Li-Fraumeni families, with the only condition being that subjects were cancer-free at the beginning of the study.[13] These subjects were followed for an average of 14 years, to determine whether the incidence of cancer was higher in them than in the general population. Cancer risk was found to be much higher in this group, with a lifetime cancer risk two-fold higher than normal. The greatest excess cancer risk was seen in young people, as those below the age of 20 were 21-fold more likely to get cancer. Although cancer risk declined with age, this could simply be because everyone who inherited the mutated Li-Fraumeni gene died at a young age. Cancer risk was most profound for those cancers that were already attributed to the syndrome, since the relative risk for these cancers was 18-fold higher than normal. Among family members under age 45, at least 87% of all cancers occurred in those persons most likely to be carrying the mutated gene. While this does not prove that all cancers are caused by the mutated Li-Fraumeni gene, it does show that a large majority of cancers could be attributed to the gene. The mutated gene is apparently dominant to the normal gene and confers susceptibility to a wide range of different cancers.[14] Scientists have found that Li-Fraumeni syndrome is associated with mutation of a specific tumor suppresser gene, called p53.[15] This finding may eventually make it possible to identify persons with the mutated gene, so that they can be regularly screened for cancer. In addition, a better understanding of this mutation may have general implications for defining the causes of cancer, since many of these same tumors arise in families that do not have Li-Fraumeni syndrome.

INHERITED SUSCEPTIBILITY TO BREAST CANCER

It has been known for more than 100 years that a maternal history of breast cancer is a major breast cancer risk factor. A recent study, which followed 20,341 women for six years, showed that women were about twice as likely to develop breast cancer if their mothers had the disease.[16] If two or more close relatives were afflicted with breast cancer, a woman is four to six times more likely to develop the disease.[17] Cancer risk is heightened if several close relatives developed breast cancer at an early age, or if the cancer affected both breasts. For a woman with a sister who had bilateral breast cancer before the age of 50, the lifetime cumulative risk of breast cancer may be higher than 50%, and this risk is further increased if the sister was afflicted before the age of 40. Excess risk declines with increasing age of the relative at diagnosis. Thus, for the most common case of a woman whose mother had unilateral breast cancer diagnosed after the age of 60, the risk of breast cancer is only about 40% higher than for the rest of the population.[18]

About 5% of all breast cancers appear to be due to a specific genetic defect that was recently identified in several families devastated by breast cancer.[19] Identification of this breast cancer susceptibility gene was extraordinarily difficult, because breast cancer is common in the general population. Consequently it was difficult to determine which of the many breast cancer cases were associated with the rare gene mutation, and which of these cancers arose as a result of unrelated causes. The breast cancer susceptibility gene (BRCA1) was finally identified by examination of blood samples and thorough medical histories from over 1,500 families of breast cancer patients. Women with the gene defect tend to develop breast cancer at an early age; more than 50% of these women have breast cancer before they are 50 years old, and the lifetime risk of breast cancer is about 85%.[20] For women who carry the mutation, breast cancer risk increases dramatically: risk before the age of 40 is increased 32-fold, while lifetime breast cancer risk is increased nearly nine-fold. This is not to imply that all breast cancer patients carry the mutation; only about one in 200 women have it, and about 95% of all breast cancers appear to be unrelated to the mutation. Even in families with an abnormally high incidence of early onset breast cancer, fewer than 45% of the cancers are actually linked to this specific mutation of the breast cancer susceptibility gene. Nevertheless, if one in 200 women in the United States has the mutation, this means that 600,000 women are at a substantially greater risk of breast cancer. Furthermore, it is possible that other mutations of this gene will be found.[21] Some researchers have speculated that several mutations may be affecting the same gene, and that these mutations may each predispose to breast cancer.

Several studies have examined the relationship between family history and risk of breast cancer using databases that include very large numbers of women. One study, which used women involved in the Nurses' Health Study, was a prospective study of 117,988 women who were followed for 12 years.[22] Thus there were over 1.3 million person-years of follow-up in this study, which should make the results of this study very strong. Over the follow-up period, a total of 2,389 women were diagnosed with invasive breast cancer. The family histories of these women were compared to the family histories of women in the study who did not develop breast cancer, with all other variables carefully controlled. It was found that age-adjusted relative risk of breast cancer was highest among women whose mother was diagnosed with breast cancer before the age of 40. Women in this risk category were twice as likely to develop breast cancer as other women. The risk of breast cancer for daughters decreased as the age of the mother at diagnosis increased. The relative risk for a daughter was only 1.5-fold higher than normal if the mother was diagnosed after the age of 70. Having a sister with a history of breast cancer increased risk also; comparing women with one sister who has cancer to women with one sister free of cancer, the relative risk was 2.3-fold higher for women with an affected sister. For women who had both a mother and a sister with breast cancer, the relative risk of breast cancer was increased 2.5-fold above normal. This level of increased risk due to family history is somewhat smaller than had been suggested by several studies in the past, but there is still an appreciable increase in risk associated with a positive family history. Thus breast cancer probably has both a hereditary component and a component involving exposure to some carcinogen. The hereditary component of risk is likely to induce breast cancer at a relatively young age, while the environmental component may take decades to induce breast cancer. Based on the numbers presented above, it was calculated that only 2.5% of all breast cancer cases are attributable to a family history of breast cancer.[23]

Another study used an even larger group of women to examine the relationship between family history and breast cancer risk.[24] This study used the Utah Population Database, which is a database containing geneological information on descendents of Mormon pioneer families. Accordingly, this study was limited to women of similar genetic background and was not prospective, since it examined cancers that had been diagnosed, in some cases, many generations in the past. However, well over a million people are included in this database and some of the medical and geneological data go back seven generations, so this study has both advantages and disadvantages when compared to the other study. A total of 4,083 women were diagnosed with a primary breast cancer between 1966 and 1989, and these women were randomly paired with women from the same database who were free of breast cancer. Overall, a three-fold increase in risk was seen for women with the highest rate of breast cancer in the family. For women with only one first-degree relative (i.e., mother or sister) having breast cancer, the risk was increased 2.5-fold with respect to women without a family history of breast cancer. If the nearest relative with breast cancer was a second-degree relative (i.e., grandmother or aunt), then the relative risk of breast cancer declined to 1.8-fold higher than normal. If the nearest relative with breast cancer was a third-degree relative (i.e., cousin or great grandmother), then the relative risk further declined to only 1.4-fold higher than normal. There was a slightly greater risk if a woman's mother had breast cancer than if her sister had breast cancer (2.4-fold vs. 2.0-fold). Women who developed breast cancer in both breasts were nearly 10 times as likely to have a first-degree relative with breast cancer than women who did not develop cancer. Furthermore, women who had a first-degree relative with colon cancer were 1.3-fold more likely to develop breast cancer. Based on these risk estimates, it was calculated that between 17% and 19% of all breast cancer in this population could be attributed to family history.[25]

At this point it is not clear how to resolve the discrepancies between these two studies. Both studies were apparently well-executed, and both examined very large populations of women. Both studies found a roughly two-fold higher risk of breast cancer for women with a positive family history, but some of the details of risk were discrepant between the two studies. It is possible that Mormon women as a group have a breast cancer risk that differs from other white women, and it is quite likely that their breast cancer risk differs from other races. Therefore, more caution should perhaps be used in generalizing the results of the second study. However, the real surprise in both these studies was that the familial risk of breast cancer was substantially lower than has been reported in the past.

INHERITED SUSCEPTIBILITY TO OVARIAN CANCER

Unfortunately, women with the breast cancer susceptibility gene also appear to have an increased risk of ovarian cancer. Genetic analysis suggests that ovarian cancer will afflict at least 10% of those women who have the breast cancer susceptibility gene. In practical terms, this means that about 5% of the sisters of patients with inherited breast cancer will get ovarian cancer by the age of 60. [26] This amounts to more than a 300-fold elevation of ovarian cancer risk with respect to women who do not have the breast cancer susceptibility gene. The connection between breast and ovarian cancer is poorly understood at present, although it is worth noting that both the breast and the ovary are responsive to the same stimulus—the female hormone estrogen. There is a possibility that the mutation affects a cellular protein to which this hormone binds, so that cellular response to the hormone is aberrant.[27] Scientists now suspect that men carrying a mutation of the breast cancer susceptibility gene may be more vulnerable to cancer of the prostate. Prostate tissue is another tissue that is responsive to hormones, although the prostate responds to male hormones, while breast and ovarian tissue respond to female hormones.

INHERITED SUSCEPTIBILITY TO COLON CANCER

Another example of a hereditary cancer syndrome is familial adenomatous polyposis (FAP; also called polyposis coli). In this syndrome, affected individuals develop numerous tiny mushroom-like growths, called polyps, in the colon. The tendency to develop these polyps is inherited, and roughly half the children of a patient with FAP will also have the disease. Although FAP polyps are initially benign, they tend to progress to a malignant state over time. About 50% of all individuals with FAP will develop colon cancer by age 30, and virtually all FAP patients develop colon cancer by the time they reach 40. But FAP is a rare syndrome, accounting for only about 1% of all new cases of colon cancer.

Newly obtained evidence suggests that there is another type of inherited susceptibility to cancer, which may account for up to 13% of all new cases of colon cancer.[28] Since colon cancer killed more than 55,000 people in the United States in 1992, finding a specific gene associated with it makes this gene potentially one of the most important in human cancer. Furthermore, susceptibility to colon cancer is associated with susceptibility to several other cancers as well, including cancer of the uterine endometrium, stomach, pancreas, and urinary tract. The colon cancer susceptibility gene may be the most common cause of inherited disease, and it may be carried by about one person in every 200. Yet this cancer susceptibility gene was as difficult to study as the breast cancer susceptibility gene, for the same reason: inherited susceptibility explains relatively few of the many colon cancer cases that are diagnosed each year. Furthermore, most colon cancers are linked to an obvious risk factor, since improper diet remains a major cause of colon cancer.

Careful investigation of the colon cancer susceptibility gene has revealed a startling property of the gene that appears to have a major effect on the cell in which it is found.[29] DNA is a molecule within the cell that encodes all of the information necessary for cell function. Since a cell is a precisely adjusted miniature machine, any substantive changes in the cellular DNA are likely to be disastrous. Scientists compared tumor cell DNA, isolated from patients with familial colon cancer, and tumor DNA, isolated from patients with colon cancer unrelated to family history. They found that DNA from patients with familial cancer tended to have a large number of "errors."[30] In fact, about 28% of all colon tumors tested were found to contain a specific type of error, repeated over and over and scattered throughout the genome.[31] These errors may have arisen during replication, which is the process of making more DNA whenever a cell prepares to divide into two new cells.

Apparently the colon cancer susceptibility gene is not a tumor suppressor gene, but is rather an entirely new type of gene associated with cancer. Tumor suppressor genes act to restrain cell growth, so that mutation of a suppressor gene can release cells from inhibition and permit them to grow in an uncontrolled fashion. However the colon cancer susceptibility gene apparently maintains the accuracy of DNA replication during cell division, so that mistakes cannot creep into the DNA. Any mutation of this gene would allow widespread errors to occur during DNA replication, so that mutation of the colon cancer susceptibility gene should be associated with mutation of many other genes as well. In fact, cells with an altered colon cancer susceptibility gene may have thousands of other errors scattered throughout the cellular DNA. This is a remarkable finding, because it suggests that many different mutations may all be caused by one original mutation. It is still much too early to tell whether there are other examples of this type of cancer susceptibility gene. Nevertheless, these findings are consistent with a very simple conclusion: cancer is caused by mutation or loss of cellular DNA.

INHERITED SUSCEPTIBILITY TO OTHER CANCERS

Evidence is beginning to accumulate that other cancers besides breast and colon cancer can be familial. For example, prostate cancer seems to affect certain families more frequently than others. A recent study of the male relatives of 691 prostate cancer patients showed that men with prostate cancer in the family were more likely to get the disease.[32] If the affected relative was a first-degree (i.e., father or brother) or second-degree (i.e., uncle) relative, then the risk of prostate cancer was elevated two-fold. But if a man has both a first-degree and second-degree relative affected, then the relative cancer risk increases 8.8-fold with respect to a normal population of men. Relative risk tends to increase progressively with the number of affected first- and second-degree relatives. Familial prostate cancer tends to affect younger men than normal, and a substantial fraction of cases in men under 50 are probably familial in origin.

BROAD-SPECTRUM CANCER VULNERABILITY

Very recently, a study identified an association between a relatively common mutation and a broad spectrum of different cancers.[33] A gene that is largely composed of repetitive DNA of unknown function was analyzed in a large number of individuals. It was found that one of four different forms of this gene is found in about 94% of the white population, while the remaining 6% has a number of different rare forms of the gene.

A study was conducted, in which 736 cancer patients were compared to 652 individuals free of cancer, to determine which individuals had rare forms (alleles) of the gene in question (HRAS1). Rare alleles of the HRAS1 gene were associated with cancer, as persons with cancer were about twice as likely as normal to have a rare allele. Rare alleles were particularly associated with bladder cancer, leukemia, colorectal cancer, and breast cancer. An individual with a single rare allele was roughly 2.3-fold more likely to get bladder cancer or leukemia than normal, 2.2-fold more likely to get colorectal cancer, and 1.7-fold more likely to get breast cancer than normal. It was calculated that about one in 11 of all cancers of the breast, colorectum, and bladder could be attributed to this set of mutations. This means that more than 50,000 cases of cancer a year may be attributed to these rare alleles. It is not known how these alleles contribute to cancer risk, but some scientists think that the alleles somehow interfere with normal gene regulation.[34]

These striking findings have been replicated in a series of 23 smaller studies conducted by a wide range of different researchers. Generally, the results were inconsistent among the studies, probably because each study worked with a relatively small sample of cases and controls. However, if the results of these studies are statistically combined into a single large meta-analysis, the combined results are consistent with the most recent study. However, despite the strength of the combined meta-analysis, these results will require extensive corroboration. None of the studies yet conducted is prospective, few of the separate studies have an adequate sample of individuals, and meta-analyses that combine several separate studies in order to achieve significance are inherently unsatisfying. Nevertheless, if the results of these studies can be confirmed, the cancer risk attributable to this set of mutations is about double the cancer risk attributable to the recently described breast cancer susceptibility gene.

INSIGHTS INTO INTRINSIC MECHANISMS OF CANCER CAUSATION

The insight that cancer is caused by mutation or loss of cellular DNA is strongly confirmed by findings from the study of several unusual cancer syndromes. For example, critical insight into the hereditary factors that can cause cancer was provided by a genetic disorder called xeroderma pigmentosum (XP). XP is characterized by extreme sensitivity of the skin to sunlight, and patients with XP have an estimated 1,000-fold increase in risk of various skin cancers. The basic problem is an impaired ability of cells to fix the damage to DNA that can be induced by exposure to sunlight.

DNA repair ability may be impaired by 50% to 90% compared to normal individuals, and the extent of impairment correlates well with disease severity. Virtually all XP patients develop some form of skin cancer during their lives, and these patients are also much more vulnerable to certain chemicals that induce DNA damage. XP is perhaps the most direct evidence that genetic mutations can cause cancer.

Further insight into intrinsic mechanisms of cancer causation has come from study of another inherited cancer syndrome called ataxia-telangiectasia (AT).[35] This syndrome is associated with loss of physical coordination, rapid aging of the skin, defects in the immune system, and abnormalities of the endocrine and reproductive organs. About 10% of patients with AT go on to develop leukemia, so the risk of leukemia is elevated more than 700-fold with respect to a normal population. In addition, people with AT develop other cancers about 100-fold more frequently than normal. Genetic stability of normal and AT cells was studied by infecting them with DNA derived from viruses. It was found that DNA from AT cells was, on average, about 180-fold more likely to change or mutate than DNA from normal cells. The profound instability of DNA from AT cells may arise from an inability of these cells to repair damaged DNA, much as in XP cells. However, there are significant differences between XP and AT. In XP, cells may be partially unable to perform one particular type of DNA repair. In AT, cells are probably able to repair all types of DNA damage. However damaged AT cells do not stop growing long enough for these repairs to be made; the cells simply continue to grow, whether or not the DNA is damaged, so that damaged DNA is passed on to newly produced cells.[36]

In general there appear to be four intrinsic mechanisms that can produce cancer. These mechanisms include: an impaired ability to repair damaged DNA; an inherited instability of the chromosomes; accidental activation of genes that stimulate uncontrolled cell growth; or loss of genes that suppress tumor growth.[37] All of these mechanisms have in common that they affect individual cells and they result in the mutation or loss of cellular DNA. As the individual cell with the mutated DNA grows, that cell becomes the founder cell of a tumor.

INTERACTIONS BETWEEN GENES AND OTHER RISK FACTORS

As we have seen, many different gene mutations can result in the formation of a tumor. Furthermore, nonhereditary risk factors can interact with hereditary mutations to increase cancer risk greatly in an unpredictable manner. Family history probably plays a major role in determining who is most vulnerable to the effects of a carcinogen. Several examples of inherited sensitivity to carcinogens have been described within the last few years, and it is possible that most cancers are the result of an interaction between genes and other risk factors.

Although lung cancer is almost always the result of tobacco use, new evidence is accumulating to suggest that certain smokers may be more prone than others to lung cancer.[38] Tobacco smoke itself is toxic, but the body metabolizes chemicals in the tobacco smoke to an even more toxic form. Therefore, if a person was unable to metabolize the constituents of tobacco smoke to their more active form, that person would be relatively protected from the harmful effects of smoking. The ability to metabolize a chemical called debrisoquine appears to be correlated with the ability to metabolize the constituents of tobacco smoke. Therefore, the extent of debrisoquine metabolism may be able to identify those individuals most at risk for lung cancer. Debrisoquine metabolism was measured in 104 men newly diagnosed with lung cancer and 104 men without lung disease. Lung cancer patients tended to be better able to metabolize debrisoquine, suggesting that they may also be better able to form toxic products from tobacco smoke. Slow metabolism of debrisoquine, which should be protective against lung cancer, was seen in 8.7% of men without lung cancer, but in only 1.9% of men with lung cancer.[39] This suggests that a test of debrisoquine metabolism might be able to reveal which smokers are at greatest risk of developing lung cancer.

A genetic analysis of 337 families affected by lung cancer has confirmed that there is a genetic predisposition to lung cancer.[40] However, the best predictor of lung cancer risk is the number of pack-years of cigarette use, and lung cancer is rarely diagnosed in the absence of exposure to tobacco. But, if the strength of the smoking habit is factored into the lung cancer risk calculation, another pattern begins to emerge. When individuals who died of lung cancer before the age of 60 are compared to individuals who died after age 60, younger victims were more than twice as likely to have a father or mother also afflicted with lung cancer. This suggests that early onset of lung cancer is associated with some type of heritable vulnerability. The pattern of inheritance of lung cancer is best explained as the result of inheritance of a specific genetic vulnerability. When the frequency of the gene conferring vulnerability was calculated, it became apparent that up to 60% of the population may carry the lung cancer vulnerability gene. The cumulative probability that a person who lacks this gene will develop lung cancer before age 80 is almost zero, which implies that virtually all lung cancer occurs among gene carriers. However, this does not mean that lung cancer is principally a genetic disease. The risk for non-smoking gene carriers is very low, as the cumulative probability of lung cancer before age 80 among non-smoking gene carriers is only one in 1,923. This level of risk is increased nearly 42-fold if the gene carrier is a smoker. Therefore the genetic predisposition to lung cancer is inherited, but the trait is only expressed when the gene interacts with a carcinogen such as tobacco smoke. Smokers without a family history of cancer cannot conclude they are resistant to lung cancer unless both their parents also indulged in long-term tobacco use without evidence of disease. If this cancer susceptibility gene could be identified, it might become possible to identify those individuals at highest risk of lung cancer.[41]

Another example of inherited sensitivity to a carcinogen is seen with ataxia-telangiectasia (AT). AT can cause a 700-fold elevation in leukemia risk, and it is also associated with about a 100-fold elevation in risk of other cancers. An important new study examined cancer incidence over the course of six years in 161 different families, all of which had family members diagnosed with AT.[42] Cancer incidence in 1,599 blood relatives, each of whom was potentially carrying a copy of the AT gene, was compared with cancer incidence in 821 spouses, each of whom had experienced the same environment as the family members with the AT gene. It is important to note that carriers, or people with only one copy of the AT gene, do not have AT or any other obvious symptoms, although they make up nearly 1% of the Caucasian population in the United States. It was found that carriers of the AT gene were at significantly greater risk of cancers of the breast, pancreas, stomach, bladder, ovary, lung, gall bladder, and stomach. Overall lifetime risk for all types of cancer combined was elevated 3.8-fold for men and 3.5-fold for women. However, the lifetime risk of breast cancer specifically was elevated 5.1-fold for women.

This same study confirmed that carriers of the AT gene may be unusually sensitive to low levels of radiation.[43] Among probable carriers of the AT gene, a total of 19 women developed breast cancer during the six years of the study. When these AT carriers were compared to other AT carriers who did not develop breast cancer, it was found that breast cancer patients were nearly six-fold more likely to have been exposed to radiation. Radiation exposure most frequently was for diagnostic or therapeutic purposes, so the overall radiation exposure was generally quite low. Past studies have shown that women exposed to the low levels of radiation typical of a modern mammographic examination have no significant increase in breast cancer risk. Nevertheless, for women who carried an AT gene, the low level radiation in a mammographic examination seemed to be a source of breast cancer risk. Hence the implication that these women are unusually sensitive to low levels of radiation.[44]

Carriers of the AT gene may make up as much as 1.4% of the

population of the United States.[45] If the overall cancer risk for AT gene carriers is really 3.5-fold higher than that of other people, then as much as 4.7% of all cancers that affect people between the ages of 20 and 79 may be associated with the AT gene. Yet we have no specific test that can identify AT gene carriers with certainty. Thus, it is impossible to determine whether the AT gene puts carriers at significantly greater breast cancer risk after mammography. Accordingly, some impetus has developed toward tests that do not use radiation for the diagnosis of breast lesions, such as magnetic resonance imaging (MRI). There is also good reason to be prudent about mammographic examinations; while such exams are known to have great value for women over 50, the benefit for women under 50 is less clearcut. Therefore, it may be wise to minimize the number of mammographic examinations for women under 50 years of age.[46]

RACE AS A RISK FACTOR FOR CANCER

If there are significant interactions between genes and other risk factors for cancer, then it is possible that racial differences could put people at a significant risk for cancer. Recently, with the increased emphasis on studying diverse ethnic groups, evidence has been obtained that cancer risk differs among the races. These differences may mean that race is actually a risk factor for cancer, especially in the presence of other risk factors. This type of study is very controversial, and very difficult to do properly, because Americans are so sensitive to race as an issue. Nevertheless, these studies are important, precisely because race should not be an issue in determining health care delivery. If all races are to have equal access to quality health care, then a better understanding of cancer risk factors for all persons, regardless of race or ethnicity, is essential.

A recent study examined the risk of invasive cancer amongs whites, blacks, and mulattos in Sao Paulo, Brazil.[47] Sao Paulo has a population of more than seven million, and the study examined cancer incidence over five years (1969–1974), so a total of 73,529 cases of cancer were included in the study. For each of these cases, diagnosis, medical history, and ethnic group was known, so that cancer cases could be classified by race and diagnosis. Overall, cancer risk was higher among the non-white races: black and mulatto males were, respectively, 7% and 9% more likely to get cancer than white males, while black and mulatto females were, respectively, 18% and 22% more likely to get cancer than white females. The pattern of cancer risk was also quite different among the races, in ways that could not be predicted or explained. Cancer risk was calculated for each of the races separately and risk was corrected for age, marital status, birthplace, and socio-economic status, but racial differences still remained a significant cancer risk factor. For example, black males were half as likely to get colon cancer as white males, but mixed race males were 1.4-fold more likely to get colon cancer than whites, and 2.8-fold more prone to colon cancer than blacks. Overall, blacks and mulattos were at a higher risk than whites for cancers of the esophagus, stomach, prostate, cervix, and uterus, but at a lower risk for cancers of the lung, bladder, and breast. For some of these cancers, such as lung and colon cancer, lifestyle plays a clear and dominant role in cancer causation, so differences in cancer risk could be explained by risk factor exposures. However, for many of these cancers, the major risk factors are unknown. While it is unclear why cancer risk should differ so strikingly between the races, the patterns seen in Sao Paulo, Brazil are largely similar to patterns seen in the United States.[48] This suggests that differences in cancer risk among the races may be caused by differences in vulnerability to carcinogens.

Clearly, smoking is a major risk factor for lung cancer, but racial or ethnic differences in lung cancer risk of smokers may imply that certain races are more vulnerable to the carcinogens in cigarette smoke. A recent study examined ethnic differences in lung cancer risk associated with smoking, and found striking differences that could not be attributed simply to cigarette use.[49] A total of 740 lung cancer cases in Hawaii were compared to 1,616 controls, and information was obtained for each participant in the study about number of pack-years of cigarette smoking, occupation, age, and education. When these variables were factored in, it was found that Hawaiian, Filipino, and Caucasian male smokers were all at significantly greater risk of lung cancer than Japanese male smokers. In fact, lung cancer risk was 2.2-fold higher in Hawaiian men, and 1.5-fold higher in Filipino and Caucasian men than in Japanese men. Native Hawaiians thus appear to be particularly susceptible to the carcinogenic effects of smoking, while Japanese men appear to be unusually resistant to the effects of smoking. This is consistent with an unusually high incidence of lung cancer in the Pacific Islands and an unusually low lung cancer incidence in Japan. While the reasons for these ethnic differences are unknown, results clearly show that there can be an interaction between the genes and certain other risk factors.

Another recent study has shown a relationship between race and vulnerability to chemical carcinogens.[50] This study was conducted in the United States to examine the relationship between bladder cancer and cigarette smoking and to determine whether race had a significant effect on this relationship. A total of 2,160 cases of bladder cancer were compared with a control group of 3,979 cases of colorectal cancer. Complete medical and personal histories were obtained from each person and special attention was paid to past tobacco use. It was found that bladder cancer risk was increased 2.4-fold if people had ever smoked. In fact, bladder cancer risk was elevated even in persons who no longer smoked. A dose-response relationship was shown between bladder cancer risk and cigarette use; risk was related to the number of years spent smoking, the number of packs smoked, and the usual number of cigarettes smoked per day. The study also showed significantly greater risk of bladder cancer due to cigarette smoking among black males or females than among white males or females. These results show that there can be strong interactions between race and a major cancer risk factor such as smoking.

In the past, epidemiologic studies of ovarian cancer have focused on white women, since white women have a much higher incidence of this cancer than black women. In fact, the incidence of ovarian cancer in black women is 33% lower than in white women, for unknown reasons. Recently a study of ovarian cancer risk in black women was undertaken, to determine whether factors that affect cancer risk in white women similarly affect cancer risk in black women.[51] To identify risk factors, a group of 110 black women with ovarian cancer were compared to a group of 365 healthy black women. In addition, to determine whether differences in reproductive history could explain the different cancer incidence between the races, the reproductive histories of 246 black women were compared with those of 4,378 white women. Interviews were used to obtain information from all women on age at pregnancy, number of pregnancies, oral contraceptive use, and use of breast-feeding. It was found that having four or more children reduced the risk of ovarian cancer by 47%, that breast feeding for six months or longer reduced cancer risk by 15%, and that use of oral contraceptives for six years or longer reduced cancer risk by 38%. Black women were more likely than white women to have had four or more children and to have nursed each child for six months or longer, but white women were more likely to use oral contraceptives. Yet even when these various influences were factored in, scientists were unable to explain why the risk of ovarian cancer is lower among black women. These findings suggest that black women are somehow inherently less likely to get ovarian cancer than white women.[52]

Finally, another recent study has shown a relationship between race and vulnerability to certain bacteria that appear to act as carcinogens. A study compared 186 case patients with stomach cancer to 186 control subjects who did not have gastric cancer to determine what proportion of cases and controls had been exposed to the bacterial carcinogen.[53] It was found that 84% of the patients had previously been infected with the bacteria, while only 61% of the controls had been similarly infected. Bacterial infection elevated the risk of stomach cancer 3.6-fold overall, but bacterial infection specifically elevated risk nine-fold in blacks and 18-fold in all women. It is unknown why blacks and women should be particularly vulnerable to the effects of this bacterium. Nevertheless, it should be possible to screen large groups of people to determine which have been infected and are therefore at an increased risk of gastric cancer. Since infection with this bacterium appears to be so widespread, it is unknown whether a screening test would provide any useful information. If two-thirds of a large population of people is at an elevated risk for a relatively uncommon cancer, it is unclear what course of action should be taken.

WHAT IS THE SIGNIFICANCE OF UNDERSTANDING FAMILIAL CANCER SUSCEPTIBILITY?

A better understanding of familial cancer susceptibility would help us to predict which persons are most at risk of developing cancer. The prediction of individual cancer risk is a very new science, which has been christened "molecular epidemiology" because of its reliance on the techniques of molecular biology and epidemiology. Molecular epidemiology actually integrates laboratory models of cancer with molecular biology, biochemistry, and epidemiology, to infer individual cancer risk. Individual cancer risk assessment is important because many studies have identified a great deal of variation from one person to another in the features that can make someone susceptible to cancer. Given the pace of developments in the last decade, it has been predicted that, within the next 10 years, we will be able to accurately predict an individual person's cancer risk.[54] This will enable molecular epidemiologists to strengthen cancer risk assessments and to focus cancer prevention strategies where they are most needed. However, the effort to predict individual cancer risk can raise thorny moral issues. In some cases, the familial risk of cancer may be so high that a course of action is literally forced upon the individual, even when the best course of action is unclear.

SUMMARY

Despite the fact that familial risk factors were first described more than 100 years ago, they are still not well understood. But exciting new developments have taken place in understanding familial cancer susceptibility within the last few years. Scientists now suspect that familial cancer susceptibility is responsible for many more cancer cases than are produced by the familial cancer syndromes. In fact, cancer susceptibility is responsible for some of the most common cancers, while cancer syndromes tend

TABLE 4-1
WEIGHTED RISK CALCULATIONS FOR HEREDITARY RISK FACTORS

RISK FACTOR	RELATED CANCER	RELATIVE RISK	RELATIVE FREQUENCY	RISK WEIGHT
Rb gene mutation	Retinoblastoma	28,500	1	28,500a
Ataxia-telangiectasia (AT)	Leukemia	769	2	1,538b
Xeroderma pigmentosum	Skin	1,000	1	1,000a
Breast cancer suscept. gene	Ovary	300	2	600a
Ataxia-telangiectasia (AT)	All cancers	100	5	500b
Lung cancer suscept. × smoking	Lung	42	5	210b
Rb gene mutation	Brain	73.7	2	147a
Rb gene mutation	Bladder	28.8	4	115a
Familial adenomatous polyposis	Colon	20	5	100a
Rb gene mutation	Lung	16.4	5	82a
Rb gene mutation	Skin (melanoma)	73.3	1	73a
Rb gene mutation	All cancers	9.9	5	50a
BRCA1 susceptibility gene	Breast	8.6	5	43b
Father and uncle with disease	Prostate	8.8	4	35b
AT gene carrier × radiation	Breast	5.8	5	29a
Li-Fraumeni syndrome	Soft tissue	27.8	1	28c
AT gene carrier	Breast	5.1	5	26a
Li-Fraumeni syndrome	Breast	4.5	5	23c

RISK FACTOR	RELATED CANCER	RELATIVE RISK	RELATIVE FREQUENCY	RISK WEIGHT
Li-Fraumeni syndrome	Brain	11.5	2	23c
AT gene carrier	All cancers	3.6	5	18a
Neurofibromatosis (NF-1)	Brain and CNS	7	2	14c
Mother & sister with disease	Breast	2.5	5	13a
Sister with disease	Breast	2.3	5	12a
Li-Fraumeni syndrome	Leukemia	6	2	12c
HRAS1 cancer gene	Colon	2.2	5	11b
Mother with disease by age 40	Breast	2.1	5	11a
Li-Fraumeni syndrome	All cancers	2.1	5	11a
HRAS1 cancer gene	Bladder	2.3	4	9b
HRAS1 cancer gene	Breast	1.7	5	9b
Mother with disease by age 70	Breast	1.5	5	8a
Father with disease	Prostate	2	4	8b
HRAS1 cancer gene	Leukemia	2.3	2	5b

The relative importance of a risk factor is quantified by considering three factors: the relative risk associated with the risk factor; the relative frequency of the related cancer; and the statistical power of the study that linked the risk factor with the cancer. The statistical power of a study is a function of sample size, follow-up period, and the ratio of observed-to-expected cases, and it is a somewhat subjective measure of how much confidence to place in the reported findings. Degree of confidence is determined as follows: the strongest statistical relationships ($p < 0.001$: there is less than a 1 in 1,000 chance that the relationship is accidental or untrue), which engender a great deal of confidence, are designated with an a; somewhat weaker relationships ($0.001 < p < 0.01$) are designated with a b; the weakest relationships ($0.01 < p < 0.05$), which may in fact be spurious, are designated with a c. In this table, skin cancer is given a relative frequency of one, not because it is rare as a disease entity, but because fatal cases of (non-melanoma) skin cancer are very rare.

to explain only the rarest and most unusual cancers. Within the next decade it is quite likely that molecular epidemiologists will identify the genes responsible for some of the most common cancers. This should enable scientists to design new screening tests to reveal those at greatest risk of developing cancer. However, few such screening tests are now available, so guidelines are needed for avoiding or mitigating risk now.

It is particularly frightening to realize that cancer can arise, through no fault of one's own, as a result of our particular genetic make-up, and that there isn't much we can do to change this. However, major advances in diagnosis and treatment of cancer in the last few years have given cause for much optimism. Significant improvements in cancer diagnosis and treatment are coming, so that even those persons with an elevated familial incidence of cancer are likely to have an opportunity to enjoy a full and productive life. But certain steps should be taken now to lessen cancer risk in the future. First, and most important, is that people should learn more about cancer. Everyone should know their family medical history, so that they can become aware of familial cancer risk factors. Everyone should also be aware of the signs and symptoms of cancer, so that cancers can be diagnosed when they are still amenable to treatment. Second, everyone should establish or renew a relationship with their physician. All persons should see a physician regularly, not only for detection of early signs of cancers, but also so that the physician can help the patient determine the family medical history and can answer questions about personal cancer risk factors. Seeing a physician regularly also means that people are more likely to get the benefit of recent medical advances. Over the next few years a number of new cancer screening tests are likely to be validated and used more routinely and access to these new screening tests could be especially important for someone with a family history of cancer. Finally, everyone who is predisposed to cancer should stringently avoid known cancer risk factors. While there is no substitute for good genes, a stringent program of health monitoring can allay fears and detect cancers when there is still a good probability of cure.

NOTES TO CHAPTER 4

1. A.I. Neugat, D. Sherr, E. Robinson, T. Murray, J. Nieves, "Differences in histology between first and second primary lung cancer," *Cancer Epidemiol. Biomarkers Prev.* 1 (1992): 109–112.
2. *Ibid.*
3. *Ibid.*
4. T. Sugimura, "Multistage carcinogenesis: a 1992 perspective," *Science* 258 (1992): 603–607.

5. F.P. Li, "Molecular epidemiology studies of cancer in families," *Brit. J. Cancer* 68 (1993): 217–219.
6. F.P. Li, "Cancer families: human models of susceptibility to neoplasia," *Cancer Res.* 48 (1988): 5381–5386.
7. B.M. Sanders, M. Jay, G.J. Draper, E.M. Roberts, "Non-ocular cancer in relatives of retinoblastoma patients," *Br. J. Cancer* 60 (1989): 358–365.
7. J.R. Ortaldo, G.M. Glenn, H.A. Young, J.L. Frey, "Natural killer (NK) cell lytic dysfunction and putative NK cell receptor expression abnormality in members of a family with chromosome 3p-linked von Hippel-Lindau disease," *J. Natl. Cancer Instit.* 84 (1992): 1897–1903.
9. G.R. DeLong, R.D. Adams, "Developmental and congenital abnormalities of the nervous system," in *Harrison's principles of internal medicine*, E. Braunwald, et al., editor (New York: McGraw-Hill Book Co., 1987): 2027–2035.
10. F. Latif, K. Tory, J. Gnarra, M. Yao, F-M. Duh, M.L. Orcutt, et al., "Identification of the von Hippel-Lindau disease tumor suppressor gene," *Science* 260 (1993): 1317–1320.
11. Li, "Molecular epidemiology studies of cancer in families," 217–219.
12. *Ibid.*
13. J.E. Garber, A.M. Goldstein, A.F. Kantor, M.G. Dreyfus, J.F. Fraumeni Jr., F.P. Li, "Follow-up study of 24 families with Li-Fraumeni syndrome," *Cancer Res.* 51 (1991): 6094–6097.
14. *Ibid.*
15. D. Malkin, F.P. Li, L.C. Strong, J.F. Fraumeni, C.E. Nelson, D.H. Kim, et al., "Germ line p53 mutations in a familial syndrome of breast cancer, sarcomas, and other neoplasms," *Science* 250 (1990): 1233–1238.
16. P.K. Mills, W.L. Beeson, R.L. Phillips, G.E. Fraser, "Dietary habits and breast cancer incidence among Seventh-day Adventists," *Cancer* 64 (1989): 582–590.
17. J.R. Harris, M.E. Lippman, U. Veronesi, W. Willett, "Breast cancer (Part 1)," *N. Engl. J. Med.* 327 (1992): 319–328.
18. *Ibid.*
19. J.M. Hall, M.K. Lee, B. Newman, J.E. Morrow, L.A. Anderson, B. Huey, M-C. King, "Linkage of early-onset familial breast cancer to chromosome 17q21," *Science* 250 (1990): 1684–1689.
20. M-C. King, S. Rowell, S.M. Love, "Inherited breast ovarian cancer: What are the risks? What are the choices?," *J. Amer. Med. Assoc.* 269 (1993): 1975–1980.

21. *Ibid.*
22. G.A. Colditz, W.C. Willett, D.J. Hunter, M.J. Stampfer, J.E. Manson, et al., "Family history, age, and risk of breast cancer: Prospective data from the Nurses' Health Study," *J. Amer. Med. Assoc.* 270 (1993): 338–343.
23. *Ibid.*
24. M.L. Slattery, R.A. Kerber, "A comprehensive evaluation of family history and breast cancer risk: The Utah Population Database," *J. Amer. Med. Assoc.* 270 (1993): 1563–1568.
25. *Ibid.*
26. King, "Inherited breast ovarian cancer," 1975–1980
27. *Ibid.*
28. P. Peltomaki, L.A. Aaltonen, P. Sistonen, L. Pylkkanen, J-P. Mecklin, et al., "Genetic mapping of a locus predisposing to human colorectal cancer," *Science* 260(1993): 810–812.
29. L.A. Aaltonen, P. Peltomaki, F.S. Leach, P. Sistonen, L. Pylkkanen, et al., "Clues to the pathogenesis of familial colorectal cancer," *Science* 260 (1993): 812–816.
30. *Ibid.*
31. S.N. Thibodeau, G. Bren, D. Schaid, "Microsatellite instability in cancer of the proximal colon," *Science* 260 (1993): 816.
32. H.B. Carter, J.D. Pearson, E.J. Metter, L.J. Brant, D.W. Chan, et al., "Longitudinal evaluation of prostate-specific antigen levels in men with and without prostate disease," *J. Amer. Med. Assoc.* 267 (1992): 2215–2220.
33. T.G. Krontiris, B. Devlin, D.D. Karp, N.J. Robert, N. Risch, "An association between the risk of cancer and mutations in the hRas1 minisatellite locus," *N. Engl. J. Med.* 329 (1993): 517- 523.
34. *Ibid.*
35. M.S. Meyn, "High spontaneous intrachromosomal recombination rates in ataxia-telangiectasia," *Science* 260 (1993): 1327–1330.
36. *Ibid.*
37. R.A. Weinberg, "Tumor suppressor genes," *Science* 254 (1991): 1138–1146.
38. M.R. Law, M.R. Hetzel, J.R. Idle, "Debrisoquine metabolism and genetic predisposition to lung cancer," *Br. J. Cancer* 59 (1989): 686–687.
39. *Ibid.*
40. T.A. Sellers, J.D. Potter, J.E. Bailey-Wilson, S.S. Rich, H. Rothschild, R.C. Elston, "Lung cancer detection and prevention: evidence for an interaction between smoking and genetic predisposition," *Cancer Res.* 52 (1992): 2694s–2697s.
41. *Ibid.*

42. M. Swift, D. Morrell, R.B. Massey, C.L. Chase, "Incidence of cancer in 161 families affected by ataxia-telangiectasia," *N. Engl. J. Med.* 325 (1991): 1831–1836.
43. *Ibid.*
44. *Ibid.*
45. *Ibid.*
46. *Ibid.*
47. C. Bouchardy, A.P. Mirra, M. Khlat, D.M. Parkin, J.M.P. de Souza, S.L.D. Gotlieb, "Ethnicity and cancer risk in Sao Paulo, Brazil," *Cancer Epidemiol. Biomarkers Prev.* 1 (1991): 21–28.
48. *Ibid.*
49. L. Le Marchand, L.R. Wilkens, and L.N. Kolonel, "Ethnic differences in the lung cancer risk associated with smoking," *Cancer Epidemiol. Biomarkers Prev.* 1 (1992): 103–108.
50. P.B. Burns, G.M. Swanson, "Risk of urinary bladder cancer among Blacks and Whites: the role of cigarette use and occupation," *Cancer Causes Control* 2 (1991): 371–379.
51. E.M. John, A.S. Whittemore, R. Harris, J. Itnyre, the Collaborative Ovarian Cancer Group, "Characteristics relating to ovarian cancer risk: collaborative analysis of seven U.S. case-control studies. Epithelial ovarian cancer in black women," *J. Natl. Cancer Instit.* 85 (1993): 142–147.
52. *Ibid.*
53. J. Parsonnet, G.D. Friedman, D.P. Vandersteen, Y. Chang, J.H. Vogelman, N. Orentreich, R.K. Sibley, *"Helicobacter pylori* infection and the risk of gastric carcinoma," *N. Engl. J. Med.* 325 (1991): 1127–1131.
54. P.G. Shields, C.C. Harris, "Molecular epidemiology and the genetics of environmental cancer," *J. Amer. Med. Assoc.* 266 (1991): 681–687.

5

....

CHEMICAL EXPOSURES AND CANCER

Chemical exposure can potentially involve a broad range of exposures to cancer-causing agents, but by far the most important known carcinogen is tobacco smoke. Tobacco smoke injures cells in a fashion that is fairly typical of other chemical carcinogens, so tobacco can serve as a model of chemical carcinogenesis. Most exposure to chemical carcinogens is likely to happen at work, yet occupational exposure to carcinogens probably accounts for no more than 4% of cancers in the United States.[1] This means that chemicals other than tobacco are a rather minor cause of cancer. Therefore, much of the following material will relate to tobacco as a cause of human cancer.

TOBACCO USE AND LUNG CANCER

Recently, the Centers for Disease Control in Atlanta estimated that cigarette use causes 20% of all adult deaths in the United States.[2] Admittedly, not all of these deaths are due to cancer; tobacco use has been strongly linked to deaths from many other diseases, including heart disease, bronchitis, emphysema, and even diabetes. But tobacco use does cause roughly one-third of all human cancers, and 45% of all cancers in men. Tobacco causes cancers of the nose, mouth, larynx, pharynx, esophagus, stomach, pancreas, lung, kidney, bladder, cervix, and blood. It has been estimated that smoking is responsible for: 90% of all deaths from lung cancer; 80% of all deaths from cancer of the larynx; 78% of all deaths from esophageal cancer; 48% of all deaths from kidney cancer; 29% of all deaths from pancreatic cancer; and 17% of all deaths from stomach cancer.[3] Tobacco use has even been linked recently to an increased incidence of myeloid leukemia.

Lung cancer has now surpassed coronary artery disease as the leading cause of excess mortality among smokers in the United States.[4] The death toll from tobacco-induced cancer in the United States is in excess of 200,000 people a year and, worldwide, more than a million people a year die of tobacco-induced cancer. The average smoker dies more than six years sooner than the average non-smoker.[5] In short, tobacco use accounts for more deaths than all other known cancer causes combined, even though it is one of the most preventable causes of cancer.

By comparison with non-smokers, the average smoker incurs a lifetime cost of more than $20,000 in excess medical bills and lost wages. This figure doesn't even include the actual cost of the 10,000 packs of cigarettes used by the average smoker. For smokers, the cost of excess medical bills and lost wages amounts to more than $2 per pack of cigarettes smoked.[6] A recent Congressional study reported that the public health costs due to adverse effects of smoking account for more than $100 billion a year in medical bills and lost worker productivity. In fact, tobacco abuse costs each *non*-smoker over $200 a year because of increased insurance costs and the lost productivity of smokers. It is particularly ironic that the United States government subsidizes tobacco growers to produce tobacco, then often must subsidize the medical costs of those who develop cancer because of tobacco use.

Tobacco smoke contains more than 4,700 chemicals, of which more than 40 are known carcinogens,[7] capable of inducing cancer in experimental animals (Table 5-1). A very strong dose-response relationship exists between the lung cancer death rate and the total exposure to tobacco smoke. The risk of developing lung cancer is 60- to 70-fold higher for a man smoking two packs a day for 20 years than for a non-smoking man. Even smoking a low-tar, low-nicotine cigarette does not appreciably reduce risk with respect to a non-smoker, because cigarette smoke is so damaging. The British Health Education Council has stated that smoking low-tar, low-nicotine cigarettes is "like jumping from the 36th floor instead of the 39th".

TABLE 5-1
PARTIAL LIST OF MAJOR CARCINOGENS IN TOBACCO SMOKE[65]

Nicotine	Nitrosamines
Aniline	Acrolein
Toluidine	Aminobiphenyl
Ethylaniline	Naphthylamine
Methyl-naphthylamine	Acetaldehyde
Nickel	Formaldehyde
Cadmium	Urethane
Arsenic	Hydrazine
Phenol	Polonium-210

The recent increase in incidence of lung cancer in women is almost certainly related to the relatively recent increase in smoking by women. Women who smoke have a 35-fold higher risk of developing lung cancer than non-smoking women.[8] Data on smoking prevalence and lung cancer incidence, collected for men and women in Great Britain since 1900, show a clear relationship between smoking and cancer. Tobacco use by men began to increase before the turn of the century, but lung cancer incidence did not undergo a similar increase until about 1930. The incidence of smoking by women increased in about 1940, but lung cancer incidence did not undergo a corresponding increase until about 1960. Often there is a very long lag time between exposure to a carcinogen and development of the associated cancer.

Cessation of smoking sharply reduces the risk of developing lung cancer.[9] A recent study examined the lung cancer risk of former smokers, compared with current smokers and with non-smokers who had never smoked ("never-smokers"). In general, lung cancer risk was greatly reduced for smokers who quit before they were in their mid-60s, even though risk increased slightly with age at smoking cessation. For those who quit smoking between 30 and 49 years of age, the lung cancer death rate was very nearly the same as for never-smokers. At age 75, the relative risk for never-smokers compared with current smokers was 5%, meaning that never-smokers lung cancer risk was 95% lower than for smokers. Similarly, people who quit smoking in their 30s had a lung cancer risk that was more than 90% lower than that of smokers by age 75. For those who quit smoking in their early 50s, lung cancer risk at age 75 was about 80% lower than for smokers. For smokers who quit in their early 60s, lung cancer risk at age 75 was about 55% lower, or less than half that of current smokers. Therefore, while it is clear that quitting at a young age is more beneficial than quitting at an older age, major benefits of quitting accrue even to those who quit in their 60s.[10]

Recently, a great deal of controversy has surrounded the subject of "second-hand smoke." The Centers for Disease Control have estimated that 3,000 non-smokers a year die in the United States because of the effects of second-hand smoke. The incidence of lung cancer is certainly higher in non-smoking long-term co-habitants of smokers than in a comparable non-smoking population that is not exposed to cigarette smoke on a daily basis. However, the actual level of risk associated with second-hand smoke is somewhat controversial. For example, one recent study concluded that the relative risk for non-smokers subjected to second-hand smoke is only 1.3-fold higher than for other non-smokers.[11] Another very recent report concludes that non-smokers exposed to second-hand smoke (for at least 22 years) have a lung cancer risk that is

2.4-fold higher than other non-smokers.[12] While both risk estimates are relatively low, by comparison to the risk of smoking oneself, there is still quite a discrepancy between the two risks. As yet, this discrepancy cannot be resolved because we simply do not know enough about the risks of long-term exposure to second-hand smoke. Also unclear is whether short-term or incidental contact with tobacco smoke increases lung cancer risk. However, in general, the incidence of lung cancer in non-smokers exposed to cigarette smoke is dramatically lower than the incidence of lung cancer in smokers.

TOBACCO USE AND OTHER CANCERS

In addition to lung cancer, smoking has been strongly linked to many other cancers. One study, conducted in Poland, compared 249 men, newly diagnosed with cancer of the larynx, with 965 healthy men.[13] Scientists found that cigarette use was the single greatest risk factor for laryngeal cancer, and the risk of this cancer was 60-fold higher for a man who smoked 30 cigarettes a day. This study concluded that smoking alone is responsible for more than 95% of all the laryngeal cancer cases in Poland.

Another study examined smoking as a potential risk factor for cancers of the mouth and pharynx.[14] A total of 1,114 patients with oral or pharyngeal cancer were compared to 1,268 controls, to characterize the tobacco and alcohol use of each group. It was clearly shown that cancer risk increased with the amount smoked, even among subjects who did not drink, and that cancer risk also increased with alcohol use, even among subjects who did not smoke. The relative risk of oral and pharyngeal cancer in heavy smokers (who did not drink) was more than two-fold higher than among people who neither smoked nor drank. Risk was also more than two-fold higher among heavy drinkers who did not smoke than among people who abstained. But cancer risk increased in a multiplicative fashion for people who both smoked and drank. The relative risk of oral or pharyngeal cancer was 38-fold higher for a man who consumed two or more packs of cigarettes and more than four alcoholic beverages per day. In fact, tobacco and alcohol abuse combined to account for about 75% of all oropharyngeal cancers. The risk of oropharyngeal cancer declined dramatically among those who quit smoking; among former smokers who had not smoked for at least 10 years, oropharyngeal cancer risk was the same as if they had never smoked.[15]

Very recently, cigarette smoking was identified as a risk factor for colorectal cancer in both men and women. Although epidemiological studies had identified smoking as a potential cause of colorectal cancer in men, no such relationship was known for women. In men, the relationship was statistically rather weak, because there is apparently a very long time between smoking onset and the diagnosis of colorectal cancer.[16] A group of 47,935 men who were participating in the Health Professionals Follow-up Study were followed prospectively for six years. At enrollment, these men completed a detailed questionnaire about smoking history and other potentially important variables, and these men were contacted every two years to update the information. During the follow-up interval, a total of 238 new cases of colorectal cancer were diagnosed, and a further 626 cases of colorectal adenoma were diagnosed among 12,854 men who underwent a colonoscopic examination. Complete knowledge of the smoking history of these men prior to diagnosis enabled scientists to calculate the relative risk of both colorectal cancer and adenoma on the basis of pack-years of smoking. Smoking during the preceding 20 years was associated with a three-fold elevation in risk of small adenomas, but no increase in risk of large adenomas or cancers. However, smoking did cause a two-fold elevation in risk of colorectal cancer after an induction period of more than 35 years. Thus, the interval between smoke exposure and cancer development is substantially longer than 20 years.[17]

For women, the relationship between smoking history and colorectal cancer risk is very similar.[18] A group of 118,334 women enrolled in the on-going Nurses' Health Study were followed prospectively for 14 years to assess the relationship between smoking and colorectal disease. Again, it was found that smoking in the past 20 years increased the risk of small adenomas about 1.5-fold, but no relationship was found between smoking and colorectal cancer during the 20-year interval. However, among women who started smoking more than 10 cigarettes per day 35-to-39 years in the past, the relative risk of colorectal cancer was 1.5-fold higher. Risk increased steadily with time since smoking, as women who began smoking 40-to-44 years in the past had a 1.6-fold higher risk of colorectal cancer, and women who began smoking 45 years or more in the past had a two-fold higher risk of cancer. Thus, the minimum induction period for colorectal cancer appears to be at least 35 years.[19] In a sense, this long induction period is unfortunate, because it makes it very difficult to convince a smoker of the immediate need to stop smoking.

Cigarette smoking is also a major risk factor for cancers affecting the kidneys and urinary tract. One study compared 160 people who were diagnosed with renal cell carcinoma and an equal number of people of similar age, race, and sex.[20] It was found that cigarette smoking increased the relative risk of renal cell carcinoma two-fold in men, but that cigarette use apparently did not affect kidney cancer risk in women. The reason for such a sex difference in vulnerability to kidney cancer is unknown.

Another study compared 187 people diagnosed with cancer of the urinary tract (at the renal pelvis or in the ureter) with healthy persons matched for age, sex, and race.[21] This study concluded that cigarettes are the most important risk factor for cancer of the urinary tract; subjects who smoked more than 25 years were 4.5-fold more likely to get urinary tract cancers than non-smokers. Finally, a group of 2,160 bladder cancer patients was compared to 3,979 patients with cancer of the colon or rectum.[22] It was found that people who had smoked regularly at any time in the past were more than two-fold as likely to develop bladder cancer, and there was a strong dose-response relationship between cancer risk and the total number of cigarettes smoked. Cigarettes are now thought to account for about 50% of all cases of bladder cancer.[23] Bladder cancer risk varies depending upon the type of tobacco smoked, with black tobacco being more damaging than blond tobacco. Overall, for pack-a-day smokers, bladder cancer risk is increased between three- and six-fold, depending upon the type of tobacco smoked and the duration and severity of the smoking habit.[24]

Men who smoke are also more likely to get prostate cancer.[25] A recent study followed a cohort of 17,633 men, 35 years and older, who responded to a mailed questionnaire in 1966; they were followed until 1986. The questionnaire was designed to assess the risk of cancer associated with diet, tobacco use, and other potential risk factors. During the 20-year follow-up period 149 men died from prostate cancer. When these men were compared to men in the cohort who did not smoke, smokers were found to be 1.8-fold more likely to die of prostate cancer, while users of smokeless tobacco were more than twice as likely as normal to die of prostate cancer. This study also found that dietary factors seemed to be unrelated to the risk of fatal prostate cancer. No association was found between cancer risk and frequency of consumption of meats, fish, dairy products, fruits, or vegetables, nor did coffee and alcohol consumption affect risk. The risk of fatal prostate cancer was also unrelated to marital status, education, or place of residence. There was some slight indication that dietary consumption of vitamin A and beta-carotene could decrease the risk of fatal prostate cancer, but these results were rather weak. Thus, of the many different potential risk factors analyzed, tobacco use was the only factor that significantly increased the risk of fatal prostate cancer. Because these findings came from a prospective study that followed a very large group of men for an unusually long time, the findings are especially convincing.

Women who smoke are also more likely to get cervical cancer than are non-smoking women. The risk of cervical cancer is elevated 3.4-fold among women who currently smoke, and risk remains elevated 1.4-fold even in ex-smokers.[26] In fact, cervical cancer risk is elevated nearly three-fold in women exposed to second-hand smoke (for at least three hours per day), compared to women without such exposure. Perhaps surprisingly, the risk of cervical cancer from second-hand smoke is higher among women who do not smoke themselves, than it is among smoking women.[27] This may be because women smokers are better able to detoxify tobacco carcinogens than are "tobacco-naive" women, or it may be that "first-hand" smoke is such a powerful risk that other risk factors become unimportant. While it may be difficult to accept that smoking can cause cervical cancer, good evidence exists that the body can absorb and metabolize tobacco smoke components to produce carcinogens that can affect internal organs distant from the site of actual smoke exposure. Scientists have used a very sensitive technique to measure levels of nicotine in mucus washed from the cervix and vagina of smoking and non-smoking women.[28] It was found that nicotine levels in mucus from female smokers was, on average, 22-fold higher than in non-smokers, even though many of the non-smokers were exposed to second-hand smoke.

Recent evidence shows that cigarette smoking is even a risk factor for leukemia.[29] A group of 610 case patients, all newly diagnosed with acute leukemia, were compared with 618 matched healthy controls. It was found that, for persons over 60, those who had ever smoked were at a two-fold higher risk of developing acute leukemia. For the particular sub-type of leukemia known as acute lymphocytic leukemia (ALL), smoking cigarettes increased the relative risk 3.4-fold among those over 60. The risk of ALL and acute myeloblastic leukemia (AML) increased with the number of pack-years smoked, in a dose-dependent fashion. However, these trends were not true for persons under 60 years of age, even if they had smoked cigarettes for most of their life. The reasons for such a discrepancy between older and younger persons is unknown, although it is true that the incidence of both ALL and AML generally increases with age. It may be that there are simply too few cases of acute leukemia in younger persons to detect the influence of cigarette smoking on leukemia risk. Nevertheless, the conclusion seems sound that smoking can increase the risk of developing acute leukemia.

Many smokers rationalize their smoking habit by thinking that they are not harming anyone but themselves. The news that second-hand smoke can be damaging to others came as a real shock to many smokers. Recently a paper was published that reported even more shocking news—smoking may increase the cancer risk to the unborn.[30] The paper reporting this studied a very small number of women, so the results must be treated with a great deal of caution. Nevertheless, the conclusions are potentially very important, so they are included here with the caveat that the last word has not been spoken. Scientists in Sweden studied 128 children under 16 years of age who were diagnosed with acute lymphoblastic leukemia, and compared them with 301 cancer-free children with diabetes. Maternal exposure to cigarette smoke during pregnancy was measured using a questionnaire, which is potentially a problem; mothers were asked to recall their smoking habits from as long ago as 16 years. Nevertheless, it was found that maternal smoking of 10 or more cigarettes a day increased the cancer risk in offspring by more than two-fold. If smoking was combined with prenatal exposure to X-rays, also a risk factor for childhood leukemia, then the risk to the child was increased nearly four-fold with respect to children having neither of these exposures.[31] While these results may seem somewhat farfetched, the discovery of nicotine in cervical mucus suggests how maternal smoking might affect the cancer risk of the fetus or newborn.

OTHER EXAMPLES OF CHEMICALLY INDUCED CANCER

Most chemical carcinogens other than tobacco smoke are encountered in significant amounts only by people whose occupation involves exposure. Since occupational exposure to carcinogens probably accounts for less than 4% of all cancers, all other known chemical carcinogens combined are relatively unimportant when compared to tobacco smoke. Nevertheless, many chemicals have been found to cause cancer and, for some individuals, occupational exposure to these chemicals can be a significant risk factor (Table 5-2).

In recent years, chemically induced cancer has been the center of a great deal of controversy, because of a purported increase in incidence of liver cancer among soldiers exposed to the herbicide Agent Orange in Vietnam. Agent Orange was typically contaminated with two chemicals, known as dioxin and 2,4D, both of which can cause liver cancer in laboratory rats.[32] Carcinogens can have very different effects on different organisms, however. For example, an explosion in a chemical factory in Seveso, Italy, in 1976, caused the release of a large cloud of dioxin within the city limits. Rats and rabbits were killed almost immediately by exposure to the chemical, but the worst consequence for humans seems to have been a skin irritation known as chloracne. Nearly 18 years later, cancer incidence is not significantly elevated in Seveso, even among people who as children developed severe chloracne. Nevertheless, while dioxin may not pose a major cancer risk, 2,4D may be a more serious risk factor than was first thought. This is potentially problematic, since 2,4D is an ingredient of

TABLE 5-2
OCCUPATIONAL CANCERS CAUSED BY CHEMICAL EXPOSURES[66]

OCCUPATION	CHEMICALS	AFFECTED ORGAN	RISK
Plastic workers	Vinyl chloride	Liver Brain	200x 4x
Dye makers or users; rubber workers; paint manufacturers	Auramine, benzidine, α- or β-naphthylamine, magenta, 4-aminodiphenyl, 4-nitrodiphenyl	Bladder	2–90x
Chromium manufacturers; acetylene or aniline workers; bleachers; glass, pottery, and linoleum workers; battery makers	Chromium	Nasal cavity, sinuses, lung, larynx	3–40x
Mustard gas workers	Mustard gas	Larynx, lung, trachea	2–36x
Miners; millers; textile, insulation, and shipyard workers	Asbestos	Lung, lining of body cavities	2–12x
Miners; smelters; tanners; insecticide makers or sprayers; chemical workers; vintners; oil refiners	Arsenic	Skin, lung, liver	3–8x
Herbicide applicators; farmers; foresters; chemical manufacturers; railroad workers	Phenoxys, 2,4D, 2,4,5T, amitrol, MCPA	Soft tissue, immune system, ovary, blood	2–6x
Asphalt, coal tar, and pitch workers; coke oven workers; gashouse workers; miners; still cleaners; chimney sweeps	Coal soot, coal tar, other products of coal combustion	Lung, larynx, skin, scrotum, bladder	2–6x
Explosives, benzene, or rubber cement workers; distillers; dye users; painters; shoemakers	Benzene	Bone marrow	2–3x

certain commonly used garden herbicides.[33] At present, no one really knows whether Agent Orange actually has caused cancer among Vietnam veterans, or whether routine use of garden herbicides poses a significant health risk.

The first known relationship between a chemical carcinogen and a cancer was that of arylamines and urinary tract cancer. Arylamines are typically encountered by workers in the dye-production or textile industries. The carcinogenic effect of arylamines on the bladder is strikingly similar to the effect of cigarette smoking on the bladder; apparently the chemicals used in dye production that induce bladder cancer are similar to the chemicals in tobacco smoke that induce bladder cancer. Thus, these chemicals can have a damaging effect no matter what the means of exposure.

The effect of arylamines on the bladder was first recognized at the turn of the century. The aniline dye industry was established and grew rapidly after the mid-nineteenth century, but within 30 years it became clear that workers who handled aniline were suffering a dramatically higher incidence of bladder cancer.[34] Early studies indicated that bladder cancer risk was increased 50- to 60-fold compared to persons not exposed to the dyes, and some cases of bladder cancer were induced in as little as one year. A recent study suggests that the bladder cancer risk associated with dye manufacture is lower now, presumably because of increased safety precautions in the workplace, but the level of risk is still about five-fold higher than normal.[35] As it turns out, aniline itself is probably not carcinogenic, but early processes of chemical manufacture may have resulted in significant contamination of the aniline with 4-aminobiphenyl and 2-naphthylamine. Both of these chemicals are also present in tobacco smoke and both are highly carcinogenic in laboratory animal experiments, although the mechanism by which they have their effect is largely unknown.

Given that organic dyes have been identified as significant human carcinogens, concern has been expressed that hair dye use could be a significant cause of cancer in women.[36] Since about one-third of adult women in the United States use hair dye, and since hair dye often contains arylamine compounds known to be carcinogenic, hair dye is potentially an important risk factor for cancer. This risk was evaluated prospectively in a group of 573,369 women who were enrolled in a Cancer Prevention Study begun by the American Cancer Society in 1982. At enrollment, each woman answered an extensive series of questions on potential cancer risk factors, including hair dye use. The mortality from cancer among this group of women was tracked until 1989, so there were more than four million person-years of follow-up involved in this study. At the end of the study, cancer mortality among the 180,458 women who used hair dye was compared to cancer mortality among the 392,911 women who did not use hair dye. It was found that, among hair dye users, the overall death rate from cancer was actually somewhat lower than normal and, in particular, there was a 35% lower risk of cancers of the urinary tract. While this probably does not mean that hair dye actually protects from urinary tract cancer, it does indicate fairly conclusively that hair dye is not a risk factor. However, women who used black hair dye for 20 years or more had a roughly four-fold higher risk of non-Hodgkin's lymphoma and multiple myeloma. This finding was based on a very small number of cases, because only 4% of women who dye their hair use black hair dye, so there is a chance that these results are a statistical artifact. The most common hair dye colors are brown (39% of users) and blond (33% of users), and these colors were not associated with any increases in cancer, even among 20-year users. In contrast with several other smaller studies, this study found that hair dye use led to no increase in risk of cancers of the mouth, breast, lung, bladder, or cervix. Overall, women using permanent hair dyes are not generally at an increased risk of fatal cancer.[37]

Apparently the urinary tract, including the bladder, is particularly vulnerable to the effects of chemical carcinogens, since a number of different carcinogens have an effect on these organs. For example, one study of 187 cases of cancer of the renal pelvis or ureter found that cigarette use was generally the strongest risk factor.[38] However, it was also found that heavy use of over-the-counter pain killers was associated with a significant elevation of risk for these cancers. Most of the major ingredients of over-the-counter pain killers were implicated, including aspirin, caffeine, acetaminophen, phenacetin, or a combination of acetaminophen and phenacetin. Subjects who used any of these medications more than 30 days a year at any point in their life were more at risk of urinary tract cancer, and if these pain medications were used for more than 30 consecutive days, risk was still higher. In fact, risk of cancer of the renal pelvis and ureter was elevated about two-fold with respect to a population who did not use pain medications.[39] In addition, renal cell cancer, or cancer of the kidney, seems to be associated with use of diuretics, which are commonly used to reduce water retention during menstruation. Renal cell cancer risk was increased about 4.5-fold among women who used diuretics.[40] These several findings suggest that the urinary tract (including the kidney) may be especially vulnerable to the carcinogenic effect of several seemingly innocuous chemicals we encounter in our daily life.

Bladder cancer can also be caused by several chemicals that are typically encountered in high concentration only during occupational exposures. For example, exposure to very high levels of fluoride has been implicated in causing bladder cancer.[41] Scientists studied cancer risk in a group of 523

Danish factory workers who were involved in processing cryolite ore. Since cryolite ore is composed of about 50% fluoride, workers were typically exposed to a large amount of fluoride in dust form, which can be inhaled. Old medical records were examined, so that workers could be evaluated for cancer incidence over a period of more than 30 years; the period of risk factor exposure was thus greater than 12,000 years in total. These factory workers suffered a higher risk of lung and laryngeal cancer with respect to other Danish adults; relative risk of lung cancer was elevated about 1.4-fold, while risk of laryngeal cancer was elevated 2.3-fold. Surprisingly, the factory workers' relative risk of bladder cancer was also elevated about 1.8-fold with respect to other Danes. Since exposure to cryolite dust can result in fluoride absorption, fluoride is concentrated in urine within the bladder prior to excretion. However, this study, while interesting, failed to control for the effects of smoking, even though the rate of smoking among the factory workers was apparently higher than normal. This is a major flaw, since smoking could account for the elevated incidence of lung and laryngeal cancer, and it could also account for the elevated incidence of bladder cancer. Since bladder cancer risk was elevated only 1.8-fold among these workers, risk was not elevated above what could be explained as a result of smoking alone. Yet the connection between fluoride and bladder cancer is alarming, since 260 million people worldwide drink fluoridated water to promote oral hygiene. But the level of fluoride in drinking water is typically 1 milligram per liter, whereas industrial exposures were as high as 35 milligrams a day.[42] Therefore, to be exposed to an equivalent amount of fluoride as the cryolite workers, one would have to drink 35 liters (more than nine gallons) of water every day. This is roughly 10 times more water than most people drink in a day, so it is likely that fluoride is not a significant carcinogen in drinking water.

Another potential occupational exposure that has received a great deal more attention recently, perhaps as a result of the litigation involving Agent Orange, is exposure to herbicides and pesticides. Herbicides and pesticides are used in farming virtually every crop in the United States, and residues from these chemicals find their way into our water supply and our foods. Herbicides and pesticides are a diverse group of chemicals, but most recent research has focused on the phenoxy herbicides, a group that includes 2,4D (2,4-dichlorophenoxyacetic acid), 2,4,5T (2,4,5-trichloro-phenoxyacetic acid), and the related chlorophenols.[43] Recently, a review examined the data from about 60 separate studies, many of which contradicted each other, to determine whether there was good evidence that herbicides and pesticides cause cancer. Each of the different studies typically looked at a single type of cancer and tried to link an elevated incidence of the cancer with exposure to one or a few types of chemicals.

Many of these separate studies had one or two major flaws; the most common flaws were either that a relatively small group of people was studied or that no way was found to accurately determine each patient's exposure to herbicides and pesticides. For these reasons, many of the findings of the separate studies are equivocal, weak, or open to criticism. But, when taken on balance, the weight of separate studies suggests that exposure to herbicides and pesticides is indeed linked to an increased incidence of several cancers.

The strongest evidence linking herbicide or pesticide exposure to cancer is seen for non-Hodgkin's lymphoma (NHL), a cancer affecting the immune system. An increased risk of NHL has been reported among farmers from the United States, Australia, and New Zealand.[44] Relative risk was elevated between one- and six-fold in the various studies, and some of the strongest studies were actually able to show a dose-response relationship between herbicide exposure and cancer risk. For example, a study that compared NHL cases in eastern Nebraska with a control group of farmers from the same area showed that men who reported mixing or applying 2,4D had a relative risk of NHL that was 1.5-fold higher than normal. Among men who reported exposures lasting more than 20 days a year, the risk of NHL increased to 3.1-fold higher than a control group of Nebraska farmers.[45]

A case-control study of the link between pesticide exposure and NHL was completed very recently in Sweden.[46] This study examined the pesticide exposure of a case group of 105 patients with NHL, and compared their exposure to that of a control group of 335 healthy persons. Cases and controls were matched for age, sex, place of residence, and general state of health, as well as for exposure to suspected carcinogens for NHL, such as tobacco and asbestos. Exposure to pesticides was assessed retrospectively, by asking each respondent about the pesticide exposure that they could remember, and by obtaining a complete working history for each person and determining the level of pesticide exposure typical for each occupation. Exposure to phenoxyacetic acids (such as 2,4D and 2,4,5T) was found to increase the risk of NHL more than five-fold, by comparison with controls who were not exposed to these chemicals. Exposure to chlorophenols (particularly pentachlorophenol) increased the risk of NHL more than four-fold with respect to control individuals. However, several problems with this study necessarily limit the confidence that can be placed in the results. The approach of assessing pesticide exposure retrospectively has the major drawback that pesticide exposure cannot be measured with real accuracy, especially when considering exposures that may have occurred two decades in the past. Exposures were thus calculated largely on the basis of the exposure thought to be typical for a particular occupation. While it is fair to assume that a miner will generally have a lower cumulative exposure to pesticides than a farmer, miners were actually found to be more likely to develop NHL than farmers. This is hard to rationalize, and argues against occupation being a risk factor for NHL. Nevertheless, this study did find a fairly strong relationship between NHL and exposure to certain chemicals found in pesticides, so it is imperative that scientists replicate and extend this study to find the truth.

While the evidence is relatively clear that herbicides can cause NHL, the evidence linking these chemicals to other types of cancer is much weaker. Nevertheless, at least some data suggest that herbicide or pesticide exposure can increase the incidence of cancers of the immune system, soft tissues, and ovary.[47] In an effort to overcome some of the weaknesses in the studies that have already been done, the International Agency for Research on Cancer recently established a registry of over 18,000 workers exposed to either phenoxy herbicides or chlorophenols, and these individuals will be followed over time to determine whether they have an unusually high incidence of cancer. This forward-thinking approach to cancer epidemiology should perhaps serve as a model for what can be done to maintain public health. Increasingly widespread use of computer databases by health care providers should make it increasingly easy to establish cancer registries. This will make it more feasible to track cancer incidence and epidemiology through large numbers of people, so that trends and associations can be identified before they become full-scale disasters.

Very recently, a new connection was identified between pesticide use and cancer; DDT is now thought to lead to an increased risk of breast cancer.[48] DDT is an example of an organochlorine which is widely used as a pesticide. The organochlorines, including PCB, are persistent environmental contaminants that can also act as animal carcinogens. These chemicals are found as residues on fruits and vegetables, and when consumed, the chemicals are not broken down, but rather are stored in adipose (fatty) tissue for very long periods of time. A reasonable estimate of a person's exposure to DDT can be obtained by measuring the amount of a DDT metabolite (called DDE) that binds to fats in the bloodstream. This assay permits researchers to screen large numbers of people for DDT exposure, since it is much easier to collect a blood sample than a sample of adipose tissue. Blood samples, collected from 14,290 women who entered a study of hormones, diet, and cancer between 1985 and 1991, were analyzed for DDE and PCB content. In this large group of women, 58 subjects were diagnosed with breast cancer shortly after entry into the study. Content of DDE and PCB in blood from breast cancer patients was compared with levels of these chemicals in blood from matched control subjects who did not develop cancer during the course of the study. Average blood concentration of DDE was significantly higher in cases than in controls, although the levels of PCB were not significantly different. Thus DDE appears to be linked to a diagnosis of cancer, although a number of other possible factors must be considered. When results were adjusted to take into account the family history of breast cancer, the age at first full-term pregnancy, and the total amount of time spent nursing, it was found that DDE was still associated with breast cancer risk. Women at the 90th percentile of DDE concentration in the blood were nearly four-fold more likely to get breast cancer than women at the 10th percentile of DDE concentration. Thus, breast cancer incidence appears to be strongly associated with exposure to DDT, but not associated with exposure to PCB. These findings are very alarming because environmental accumulation of DDT has been documented for at least 30 years; although DDT concentration in the environment has been declining since the late 1970s, exposure to DDT is still very common. Elimination of DDE from the body is very slow, and can take several decades, so cancer risks from DDT may continue for years to come.[49] This study really must be corroborated before being fully accepted, but the results are nevertheless very compelling. It is a particularly strong study because it involved a large number of women, because it followed them for a reasonable period of time, and because measurement of DDE in the bloodstream is an objective and probably reliable way to characterize DDT exposure.

These results recently received some confirmation from a very small study that found a link between breast cancer risk and the concentration of DDE in breast tissue.[50] A control group of 17 women with benign breast disease was compared to a case group of 18 breast cancer patients, half of whom were diagnosed with estrogen receptor (ER)-positive tumors and half of whom were diagnosed with ER-negative tumors. Since DDE was measured in a tissue that acts as a depot (because it has a very slow turnover rate), this probably is an accurate reflection of DDT exposure over long periods. No significant differences in DDE concentration were found between the control women and those women with ER-negative tumors, but women with ER-positive tumors had a level of DDE in their tissue that was nearly three-fold higher than the control women. These results can be explained because DDE is believed to have chemical properties that mimic estrogen, so DDE may be able to induce growth of ER-positive breast tumors. Unfortunately, this study was so small that the relative risk of breast cancer could not be accurately estimated for women exposed to DDT.[51]

EFFECTS OF CHEMICAL CARCINOGENS ON CELLS

The process of induction of cancer by many different chemicals tends to be similar, in that induction is usually associated with some mechanism that increases the normal rate of cell growth.[52] A dividing cell seems to be more at risk of mutating than a quiescent cell, perhaps because cellular DNA is not as well protected during cell growth. Studies in which a chemical carcinogen is painted onto the skin of a mouse or rat clearly show that induction of an increased rate of cell division is the basic mechanism of chemical carcinogenesis. Typically, if the dose level of the chemical is increased, so that cell growth rate is enhanced, then the time period before appearance of a tumor is shortened. Thus the rate of tumor progression is increased if the rate of cell growth is increased. This finding suggests that cell growth increases the risk of those mutations that result in cancer.[53] Carcinogens may also cause cancer by interfering with the ability of cells to repair mutated DNA. But these effects on cellular DNA cannot produce a tumor in the absence of cell growth because the toxic effects of a carcinogen on a cell are limited to a single cell unless that cell continues to grow.

MULTIPLICATIVE RISK IN CHEMICAL CARCINOGENESIS

Multiplicative risk is the term used to describe a condition in which two separate risks interact with each other to increase total risk in a more-than-additive fashion. These separate risks can arise as a result of many different processes, including the inheritance of a particular set of genes that makes the inheritor relatively vulnerable to another risk factor. But the classic example of multiplicative risk involves smoking and alcohol consumption.

When smoking, bad enough in itself, is combined with consumption of alcohol, laryngeal cancer risk is dramatically increased, even with respect to a heavy smoker.[54] In one study, the relative risk from smoking more than 20 cigarettes a day was 37-fold higher than in non-smokers, while the relative risk from drinking vodka regularly for more than 15 years was nine-fold higher than among non-drinkers. But if this amount of smoking and drinking were combined, the relative risk of laryngeal cancer was increased 330-fold, so that smoking and drinking together was nine-fold worse than smoking alone. Alcohol is not a carcinogen in most animal studies, so it is unknown how it induces cancer in humans or how it can potentiate the effect of exposure to other carcinogens. Some scientists speculate that alcohol can act as a solvent, dissolving carcinogens so that they have better access to cells.

Another multiplicative risk is the interaction between smoking and asbestos exposure, which together increase the risk of lung cancer. Asbestos exposure is not truly a chemical exposure; it is probably more similar to a chronic injury, and asbestos as a cause of cancer will be discussed more fully in Chapter 9. Nevertheless, the interaction between asbestos exposure and smoking is a good example of a multiplicative risk. Inhalation of asbestos dust or air-borne asbestos fibers can cause a type of lung scarring known as asbestosis. Asbestosis itself can be fatal, but asbestosis patients are also at an elevated risk of lung cancer. Autopsy studies of persons who died of asbestosis have shown that between 20% and 50% of them also have lung cancer, often in a form too early to be diagnosed.[53] An early study of lung cancer deaths among insulation workers showed that lung cancer risk was elevated five-fold from asbestos exposure alone, was elevated 10-fold from smoking alone, but that when asbestos exposure and smoking were combined, relative risk of lung cancer was elevated 50-fold.[56] More recent estimates are more conservative though, as the incidence of lung cancer is now thought to be roughly two-fold higher among workers exposed to asbestos fibers than among men who do not suffer asbestos fiber exposure.[57]

Another type of multiplicative risk is the potential interaction between genes and other risk factors (first discussed in Chapter 4). A recent study indicates that there may be a strong genetic predisposition to lung cancer, which is not expressed unless the person with that predisposition is also exposed to a lung carcinogen such as tobacco smoke, radon gas, or radioactivity.[58] One study identified 337 people who had died of lung cancer during a four-year period (1976–1979) in southern Louisiana, and obtained full medical histories of all male and female relatives of the deceased over three generations. The pattern of cancer occurrence within these families was then analyzed to determine whether lung cancer patients came from families more prone to cancer generally, and to determine what proportion of lung cancers could be related to a genetic predisposition to cancer. Virtually all lung cancer cases were found to occur among people identified as carriers of a lung cancer-susceptibility gene. The incidence of this lung cancer-susceptibility gene is quite high, since at least 60% of the general population is genetically susceptible. The cumulative probability of lung cancer by age 80 for people who do not carry the gene, even when they are heavy smokers, is close to zero. It should be emphasized that these data do not argue that lung cancer is a genetic disease. The cumulative risk of lung cancer by age 80 for gene carriers who smoke was 42-fold higher than for gene carriers who do not smoke. In other words, for the lung cancer susceptible, smoking is almost always lethal. This implies that lung cancer is the result of a gene-environment interaction, but that lung cancer will only affect those who smoke.[59] If individuals at high risk could be identified, strenuous efforts might be undertaken to induce smoking cessation.

Genes determine, among many other things, the quantity and activity of enzymes within the body, so that some people have a greater ability than other people to metabolize certain chemicals. If carcinogenic risk is determined by the extent of metabolization of a chemical, then some individuals' risk of cancer may be higher or lower simply because of inheritance of a gene that may seem unrelated to cancer. For example, an enzyme called P-450 is involved in the metabolization of many different chemicals within the liver. Usually this enzyme is used to make toxic chemicals less toxic, but sometimes the same enzyme will metabolize a compound to a more toxic form.

Recent results suggest that the type and activity of the P-450 enzyme can have an effect on lung cancer risk among smokers.[60] A drug called debrisoquine is often prescribed to control high blood pressure. This drug is metabolized by the P-450 enzyme to form a single product that is excreted in the urine. Therefore, the activity of the P-450 enzyme can be characterized by measuring the amount of metabolized debrisoquine in a urine sample. One study compared debrisoquine metabolism in 104 smokers who developed lung cancer and 104 smokers of the same age, who smoked as much for as long, but who did not develop lung cancer. It was found that nearly 9% of healthy smokers had a very poor ability to metabolize debrisoquine, which suggests that their P-450 enzyme was slow. Among smokers who developed lung cancer, only about 2% had a similarly poor ability to metabolize debrisoquine. On average, the rate of debrisoquine metabolism was about 30% higher among cancer patients than among healthy smokers. This may mean that smokers who developed lung cancer were, in a sense, victims of their own genes. Their ability to efficiently metabolize some chemical into a more toxic form may have resulted in their exposure to a potent carcinogen that other people were able to avoid because of their inefficient metabolisms.

REDUCING EXPOSURE TO CHEMICAL CARCINOGENS

Clearly, tobacco smoke is the most important chemical carcinogen and the greatest single preventable cause of cancer. Yet smoking cessation is not easy: less than 8% of smokers are successful when they try to quit, and many smokers have tried to quit again and again without success. More

TABLE 5-3
WEIGHTED RISK CALCULATIONS FOR CHEMICAL RISK FACTORS

CHEMICAL RISK FACTOR	RELATED CANCER	RELATIVE RISK	RELATIVE FREQUENCY	WEIGHTED RISK
Tobacco × alcohol	Larynx	330	2	660c
Tobacco smoke	Lung	81 (≥2 pks/day, 10 yrs)	5	406a
Tobacco × asbestos	Lung	50	5	250c
Tobacco smoke	Larynx	59.7 (>30 cigs/dy)	2	119b
Tobacco × alcohol	Oral	38 (40 cigs + 5 drinks/dy)	3	114b
Tobacco smoke	Lung	22.4 (men, any use)	5	112a
Tobacco smoke	Oral	8.9 (10 yr smoker)	3	27b
Tobacco smoke	Larynx	10.3	2	21a
DDT in pesticides	Breast	3.5	5	18c
Arylamines	Bladder	4.6	4	18c
Phenoxyacetic acid in pesticides	Lymphoma	5.5	3	17b
Tobacco smoke	Urinary tract	4.5 (for 25 yrs)	3	14a
Chlorophenols in pesticides	Lymphoma	4.8	3	14b
Diuretic use	Kidney	4.5 (regular use)	3	14c
Use of black hair dye	Lymphoma	4.4	3	13a

CHEMICAL RISK FACTOR	RELATED CANCER	RELATIVE RISK	RELATIVE FREQUENCY	WEIGHTED RISK
Tobacco smoke	Bladder	2.9 (current smoker)	4	12b
Second-hand smoke	Lung	2.4 (>22 years)	5	12b
Tobacco smoke	Cervix	3.4 (smokers only)	3	10b
Tobacco use	Colorectal	1.7 (>35 years)	5	9a
Use of black hair dye	Multiple myeloma	4.4	2	9a
Second-hand smoke	Cervix	3.0 (non-smokers)	3	9c
Pain killers	Kidney	2.1 (regular use)	4	8a
Tobacco smoke	Prostate	1.8	4	7a
Tobacco smoke	ALL	3.4	2	7b
Tobacco smoke	Esophagus	3.6	2	7b
Organic solvent exposure	Lymphoma	2.4	3	7b
Tobacco smoke	Kidney	2.4 (men only)	3	7c
Fluoride	Bladder	1.8 (35 mg/day)	4	7c
Herbicide exposure	Lymphoma	1.9	3	6b
Tobacco smoke	AML	2.0	2	4b
Maternal smoking in pregnancy	ALL in offspring	2.2 (10 cigs/day)	2	4c

The relative importance of a risk factor is quantified by considering three factors: the relative risk associated with the risk factor; the relative frequency of the related cancer; and the statistical power of the study which linked the risk factor with the cancer.

than 80% of smokers say that they would like to quit but are unable to do so. In fact, smoking is such an addictive habit that many smokers find it easier to lie about their habit than to change it: one survey of 1,369 women found that 2–3% of the subjects were active smokers who denied that they smoked.[61] The long lag time between smoke exposure and cancer death is a major factor that stymies the effort to get people to quit. It would be far easier to motivate people to quit if lung cancer affected younger people or people who had smoked for less time.

From a public health standpoint, ensuring that young people never start smoking is just as important as helping confirmed smokers to quit. About one million teenagers begin smoking every year, and more than 90% of all smokers report that they became addicted before the age of 21. It is simply appalling that cigarette companies are permitted to direct advertisements specifically to young people and to portray smoking as being somehow glamorous.

Among all the bad news about smoking, there is some good news. The Centers for Disease Control recently reported that the proportion of adults who smoke is declining: in 1965, 42% of all adults smoked, while in 1993, only 25% of all adults smoked. About 43 million Americans have successfully quit smoking.[62] Several new techniques for smoking cessation appear to be effective, at least for helping motivated people to quit. However, most people who succeed at smoking cessation do so by quitting "cold turkey."

In the future it may become possible to predict which chemicals are most likely to cause cancer before these chemicals are released into the environment. Recent research has demonstrated that is is possible to predict the type of damage that might be caused by a particular type of chemical.[63] The logical extension of this work is that it may become possible to predict which chemicals cause cancer and which are relatively harmless. Furthermore, it may become possible to determine, on the basis of theory alone, what type of carcinogen is responsible for a particular type of cancer.[64] This may sound farfetched, but it really amounts to a new type of medical forensics. For many years, experts in forensics have been able to determine the cause of death of an individual using medical data gathered during an autopsy. It is now known that particular types of carcinogens leave characteristic patterns of DNA damage. Therefore, if the DNA of cancerous cells is studied, it may become possible to determine the chemical cause of cancer, much as an expert in medical forensics can determine the cause of death of a body. However, major obstacles must be overcome before this is feasible. One of the more challenging problems is that carcinogens are often present in the environment as long-lived, stable chemicals that are not in themselves carcinogenic. However, these inactive chemicals, called procarcinogens, can be metabolized into an active and carcinogenic form after they enter the body. Since the procarcinogen is both stable and noncarcinogenic, it is only dangeous to the extent that it is metabolically activated to be a carcinogen. The extent of metabolic activation may differ from one person to the next, so this would make it difficult to predict which procarcinogens are most dangerous.

SUMMARY

This chapter can be summarized very simply: stop smoking. Desire for a long and healthy life can be a very strong motivator, but it is often not enough. Part of the problem is that a long-term smoker doesn't know what clear lungs feel like anymore and has forgotten what it is like to wake up without a scratchy throat. About a month after quitting, smokers will begin to feel the benefits; they will notice that their wind and endurance has improved, that they no longer feel chest congestion, and that there is a general feeling of greater energy and health.

One of the most powerful motivators for some people is the realization that not only are they hurting themselves, they are also hurting the ones they love. Second-hand smoke is a real risk, and evidence that women who smoke may even harm their unborn children has come to light. But these risks are still relatively small and may be dismissed by some. More difficult to dismiss are the effects of smoking on the smoker. If a smoker dies prematurely of cancer, then the family of that smoker is deprived of all the benefits of an intact family. Premature death of a parent is a very difficult burden for children to bear, especially if the children feel that the death was preventable. Smoking is the most common, and one of the most easily prevented, causes of cancer. We need to find ways, on a personal and societal level, to make sure that smoking stops with our generation.

NOTES TO CHAPTER 5

1. B.R. Henderson, R.K. Ross, M.C. Pike, "Toward the primary prevention of cancer," *Science* 254 (1991): 1131–1138.
2. J.H. Holbrook, "Tobacco," in *Harrison's principles of internal medicine*, E. Braunwald, et al., editors (New York: McGraw-Hill Book Co., 1987), 855–859.
3. H.B. Simon, *Staying well: your complete guide to disease prevention*, (New York: Houghton Mifflin Co., 1992), p. 319.
4. D.R. Shopland, H.J. Eyre, T.F. Pechacek, "Smoking-attributable

cancer mortality in 1991: is lung cancer now the leading cause of death among smokers in the United States?," *J. Natl. Cancer Instit.* 83 (1991): 1142–1148.

5. Simon, *Staying well,* p. 316.

6. *Ibid.*

7. *Ibid.*

8. K.E. Osann, "Lung cancer in women: the importance of smoking, family history of cancer, and medical history of respiratory disease," *Cancer Res.* 51 (1991): 4893–4897.

9. M.T. Halpern, B.W. Gillespie, K.E. Warner, "Patterns of absolute risk of lung cancer mortality in former smokers," *J. Natl. Cancer Instit.* 85 (1993): 457–464.

10. *Ibid.*

11. E.T.H. Fontham, P. Correa, A. Wu-Williams, P. Reynolds, R.S. Greenberg, et al., "Lung cancer in nonsmoking women: a multi-center case-control study," *Cancer Epidemiol. Biomarkers Prev.* 1 (1991): 35–43.

12. H.G. Stockwell, A.L. Goldman, G.H. Lyman, C.I. Noss, A.W. Armstrong, et al., "Environmental tobacco smoke and lung cancer risk in nonsmoking women," *J. Natl. Cancer Instit.* 84 (1992): 1417–1422.

13. W. Zatonski, H. Becher, J. Lissowska, J. Wahrendorf, "Tobacco, alcohol, and diet in the etiology of laryngeal cancer: a population-based case-control study," *Cancer Causes Control* 2 (1991): 3–10.

14. W.J. Blot, J.K. McLaughlin, D.M. Winn, D.F. Austin, R.S. Greenberg, et al., "Smoking and drinking in relation to oral and pharyngeal cancer," *Cancer Res.* 48 (1988): 3282–3287.

15. *Ibid.*

16. E. Giovannucci, E.B. Rimm, M.J. Stampfer, G.A. Colditz, A. Ascherio, et al., "A prospective study of cigarette smoking and risk of colorectal adenoma and colorectal cancer in U. S. men," *J. Natl. Cancer Inst.* 86 (1994): 183–191.

17. *Ibid.*

18. E. Giovannucci, G.A. Colditz, M.J. Stampfer, D. Hunter, B.A. Rosner, et al., "A prospective study of cigarette smoking and risk of colorectal adenoma and colorectal cancer in U. S. women," *J. Natl. Cancer Instit.* 86 (1994): 192–199.

19. *Ibid.*

20. M.C. Yu, T.M. Mack, R. Hanisch, C. Cicioni, B.E. Henderson, "Cigarette smoking, obesity, diuretic use, and coffee consumption as risk factors for renal cell carcinoma," *J. Natl. Cancer Instit.* 77 (1986): 351–356.

21. R.K. Ross, A. Paganini-Hill, J. Landolph, V. Gerkins, B.E. Hen-

derson, "Analgesics, cigarette smoking, and other risk factors for cancer of the renal pelvis and ureter," *Cancer Res.*, 49 (1989): 1045–1048.

22. P.B. Burns, G.M. Swanson, "Risk of urinary bladder cancer among Blacks and Whites: the role of cigarette use and occupation," *Cancer Causes Control* 2 (1991): 371–379.

23. P. Vineis, "Epidemiological models of carcinogenesis: the example of bladder cancer," *Cancer Epidemiol. Biomarkers Prev.* 1 (1992): 149–153.

24. *Ibid.*

25. A.W. Hsing, J.K. McLaughlin, L.M. Schuman, E. Bjelke, G. Gridley, et al., "Diet, tobacco use, and fatal prostate cancer: results from the Lutheran Brotherhood Cohort Study," *Cancer Res.* 50 (1990): 6836–6840.

26. M.L. Slattery, L.M. Robison, K.L. Schuman, T.K. French, T.M. Abbott, et al., "Cigarette smoking and exposure to passive smoke are risk factors for cervical cancer," *J. Amer. Med. Assoc.* 261 (1989): 1593–1598.

27. *Ibid.*

28. M.F. McCann, D.E. Irwin, L.A. Walton, B.S. Hulka, J.L. Morton, C.M. Axelrad, "Nicotine and cotinine in the cervical mucus of smokers, passive smokers, and nonsmokers," *Cancer Epidem. Biom. Prev.* 1 (1992): 125–129.

29. D.P. Sandler, D.L. Shore, J.R. Anderson, F.R. Davey, D. Arthur, et al., "Cigarette smoking and risk of acute leukemia: associations with morphology and cytogenetic abnormalities in bone marrow," *J. Natl. Cancer Instit.* 85 (1993): 1994–2002.

30. M. Stjernfeldt, K. Berglund, J. Lindsten, J. Ludvigsson, "Maternal smoking and irradiation during pregnancy as risk factors for child leukemia," *Cancer Detect. Prevent.* 16 (1992): 129–135.

31. *Ibid.*

32. E. Marshall, "Toxicology goes molecular," *Science* 259 (1993): 1394–1398.

33. *Ibid.*

34. C.D. Sherman, et al., "Aetiology," in *Manual of clincial oncology* (New York: Springer-Verlag, 1987), 13–29.

35. C. La Vecchia, E. Negri, B. D'Avanzo, S. Franceschi, "Occupation and the risk of bladder cancer," *Int. J. Epidemiol.* 19 (1990): 264–268.

36. M.J. Thun, S.F. Altekruse, M.M. Namboodiri, E.E. Calle, D.G. Myers, C.W. Heath, "Hair dye use and risk of fatal cancers in U. S. women," *J. Natl. Cancer Instit.* 86 (1994): 210–215.

37. *Ibid.*

38. Ross, "Analgesics, cigarette smoking, and other risk factors," 1045–1048.
39. Ibid.
40. Yu, "Cigarette smoking, obesity, diuretic use, and coffee consumption," 351–356.
41. P. Grandjean, J.H. Olsen, O.M. Jensen, K. Juel, "Cancer incidence and mortality in workers exposed to fluoride," J. Natl. Cancer Instit. 84 (1992): 1903–1909.
42. Ibid.
43. H.I. Morrison, K. Wilkins, R. Semenciw, Y. Mao, D. Wigle, "Herbicides and cancer," J. Natl. Cancer Instit. 84 (1992): 1866–1874.
44. Ibid.
45. S. Hoar-Zahm, D.D. Weisenburger, P. Babbitt, et al., "A case-control study of non-Hodgkin's lymphoma and the herbicide 2,4-dichlorophenoxyacetic acid (2,4-D) in eastern Nebraska," Epidemiol. 1 (1990): 349–356.
46. L. Hardell, M. Eriksson, A. Degerman, "Exposure to phenoxyacetic acids, chlorophenols, or organic solvents in relation to histopathology, stage, and anatomical locatization of non-Hodgkin's lymphoma," Cancer Res. 54 (1994): 2386–2389.
47. Morrison, "Herbicides and cancer," 1866–1874.
48. M.S. Wolff, P.G. Toniolo, E.W. Lee, M. Rivera, N. Dubin, "Blood levels of organochlorine residues and risk of breast cancer," J. Natl. Cancer Instit. 85 (1993): 648–652.
49. Ibid.
50. E. Dewailly, S. Dodin, R. Verreault, P. Ayotte, L. Sauve, et al., "High organochlorine body burden in women with estrogen receptor-positive breast cancer," J. Natl. Cancer Instit. 86 (1994): 232–233.
51. Ibid.
52. B.N. Ames, L.S. Gold, "Too many rat carcinogens: mitogenesis increases mutagenesis," Science 249 (1990): 970–971.
53. C.W. Boone, G.J. Kelloff, V.E. Steele, "Natural history of intra-epithelial neoplasia in humans with implications for cancer chemo-prevention strategy," Cancer Res. 52 (1992): 1651–1659.
54. Zatonski, "Tobacco, alcohol, and diet in the etiology of laryngeal cancer," 3–10.
55. Sherman, "Aetiology," 13–29.
56. E.C. Hammond, I.J. Selikoff, H. Seidman, "Asbestos exposure, cigarette smoking, and death rates," Ann. N. Y. Acad. Sci. 330 (1979): 473–490.
57. B.T. Mossman, J.B. Gee, "Asbestos-related diseases," New Engl. J. Med. 320 (1989): 1721–1730.

58. T.A. Sellers, L.H. Kushi, J.D. Potter, S.A. Kaye, C.L. Nelson, et al., "Effect of family history, body-fat distribution, and reproductive factors on the risk of post-menopausal breast cancer," *N. Engl. J. Med.* 326 (1992): 1323–1329.
59. *Ibid.*
60. M.R. Law, M.R. Hetzel, J.R. Idle, "Debrisoquine metabolism and genetic predisposition to lung cancer," *Br. J. Cancer* 59 (1989): 686–687.
61. E. Riboli, S. Preston-Martin, R. Saracci, N.J. Haley, D. Trichopoulos, et al., "Exposure of nonsmoking women to environmental tobacco smoke: a 10-country collaborative study," *Cancer Causes Control* 1 (1990): 243–252.
62. Simon, *Staying well*, p. 321.
63. J.N. Weinstein, K.W. Kohn, M.R. Grever, V.N. Viswanadhan, L.V. Rubinstein, et al., "Neural computing in cancer drug development: predicting mechanism of action," *Science* 258 (1992): 447–451.
64. Henderson, "Toward the primary prevention of cancer," 1131–1138.
65. Simon, *Staying well*, p. 317.
66. Sherman, "Aetiology," 13–29.

6

. . . .

DIET AND CANCER

For many years now, health advocates and the popular press have been telling us that diet is a major risk factor for many kinds of cancer. This implies that anyone who is careful about his or her diet has a greatly reduced chance of developing any of a variety of cancers. People have been very receptive to this message, and there has been a proliferation of health food stores stocking dietary supplements of questionable worth, self-professed diet experts selling their wares on late-night television, and cookbooks filled with recipes for a healthful lifestyle. The fascination with diet as a key to cancer causation probably arose because of the strong relationship between diet and heart disease; if diet is, in part, responsible for the leading cause of death, it is possible that diet could also contribute to the second leading cause of death. Furthermore, since it is well-accepted that exposure to many different chemicals in the environment can cause cancer, it is reasonable to expect that exposure to certain chemicals in food might also be carcinogenic. But, plausible as these ideas seem, relatively little scientific evidence supported them until fairly recently. Now however, many recent scientific studies have shown clearly that an improper diet can be carcinogenic, and that a well-balanced diet can be preventive of cancer.

DIET AS A MAJOR CANCER RISK FACTOR

It is now believed that diet is responsible for between 17% and 35% of all human cancers. The major cancers of the gastrointestinal tract— stomach, colon, and rectum—are all caused, at least in part, by dietary factors. Since these cancers together accounted for 17% of all new cancers in the United States in 1990,[1] this accounts for the minimum estimate above. However, this estimate is likely to be conservative; dietary factors appear to play a major or minor role in many other cancers, including cancer of the esophagus, lung, breast, prostate, cervix, and bladder, so that diet may actually be responsible for nearly one-third of all cancers. In fact, one group of scientists has even claimed that diet is responsible for about 40% of the cancer incidence in men, and about 60% of the incidence in women,[2] but this estimate frankly seems excessive.

CALORIES AS CARCINOGENS

It has been known for some time that caloric restriction of rats, or what amounts to chronic semi-starvation, can reduce the incidence of colon tumors. But it was not known whether a similar effect is present in humans. However, a recent study of dietary effects on colon cancer incidence suggests that the total intake of calories may be related to colon cancer risk, such that the higher the caloric intake, the greater the risk.[3] This is something of a surprise because, in the past, attention has been directed toward specific components of the diet, rather than to the total dietary intake.

In this new study, scientists matched a group of 746 colon cancer patients from Los Angeles County with an equal number of men and women free of cancer. The control population of healthy individuals was matched to the case population on the basis of age, sex, race, and neighborhood, in order to eliminate these potential confounding variables. A detailed questionnaire about frequency of consumption of various foods was answered by both case and control subjects, in order to obtain information about food preferences. Statistical adjustments were made to eliminate the effects of weight, physical activity, family history, and, for women, the history of pregnancy. It was found that, in both men and women, higher total caloric intake was associated with a higher risk of cancer.

In men, additional calories in the diet tended to be derived from alcohol and dietary fat, both of which are known carcinogens. Therefore, an increased incidence of colon cancer in men consuming more calories could be explained simply on the basis of more exposure to these known carcinogens. However, in women, no individual calorie sources could be identified as contributing to cancer risk. While high intake of meats, poultry, breads, and sweets was associated with a higher risk of colon cancer, analysis suggested that it was actually the caloric content of these foods that was to blame.[4] What this implies is that the source of calories may be irrelevant; what is important is the actual quantity of calories.

There has been some recent confirmation that caloric restriction in humans can reduce the risk of colon cancer.[5] The rate of growth of cells in the colon is often taken as a "biomarker" of colon cancer risk, since rapidly growing cells in the colon are associated with an increased risk of colon cancer. The effect of caloric restriction on colon cell growth rate was examined in a small group of volunteers, all of whom were obese. The rate of colon cell growth in these volunteers was measured prior to caloric restriction, then again at several points during a 16-week weight reduction program. At the end of the weight reduction program, volunteers had lost an average of about 9% of their initial weight, and their caloric intake had decreased by 34%. At the same time, the rate of growth of cells in the colon decreased about 39%. If this decline in growth rate of cells reflects a similar decline in colon cancer risk, caloric restriction could become an important cancer preventive measure. However, these results need to be confirmed in a larger prospective study that follows volunteers long enough to know whether there is a real reduction in colon cancer incidence, or merely a reduction in some biomarker that poorly predicts colon cancer risk.

The conclusion that limiting caloric intake can lead to a reduction in colon cancer risk must be regarded as tentative. What is especially troubling is that scientists do not have a clear understanding of how calories could increase the risk of colon cancer. It is possible that nutrients in a high-calorie diet directly stimulate the rate of growth of colon cells. However, it is also possible that carcinogenic contaminants are present in certain foods, so that a high calorie diet might lead to a high intake of those contaminants. The cause, therefore, might not be the calories themselves, but rather some chemical contaminant consumed with the calories. Alternatively, obesity is widely accepted as a contributing factor in a number of cancers, including cancer of the breast, ovary, cervix, and colon. The simplest interpretation of the data might be that obesity itself (rather than caloric intake) led to the increased cancer risk.

MEAT CONSUMPTION, DIETARY FAT, AND COLON CANCER

One of the strongest cases for a relationship between diet and cancer is the case of meat consumption and colon cancer risk.[6] Nutritional factors have long been suspected to be causative of colon cancer because disease incidence differs so sharply between different countries and between different ethnic groups in the same country. The incidence of colon cancer is generally low in developing nations and in cultures where meat consumption is low, while in Europe and North America, where meat consumption is high, colon cancer incidence is also high. Colorectal cancers are unusual in countries such as Mexico, Poland, Greece, and Egypt, while the incidence is three- to seven-fold higher in the United

States, Australia, Great Britain, Germany, and Switzerland. The highest incidence in the world is found in Scotland and New Zealand, where colon cancer is four- to eight-fold more common than in the developing nations.

People who move from a low incidence area, such as Japan, to a high incidence area, such as the United States, tend to acquire the high colon cancer incidence rate of the adopted country. This shows conclusively that genetic or racial differences alone cannot account for the difference in cancer incidence and suggests instead that diet is critical. Studies of the incidence of colorectal cancer in various ethnic groups with different diets have identified a link between incidence of colorectal cancer and consumption of animal fat. But diets that are high in animal fats also tend to be high in total fat, saturated fat, and even refined sugar, so it has been difficult to separate out these variables to determine which is most important in cancer causation.

One of the best studies of the relationship between dietary fat and colon cancer is known as the Nurses' Health Study, because it involved many female registered nurses who were each studied for up to six years.[7] Subjects were initially contacted in 1976, when they were sent a questionnaire on known and suspected risk factors for cancer. Every two years thereafter subjects were sent a follow-up questionnaire, to update information on risk factors and to identify newly diagnosed cases of cancer. At the beginning of this prospective study, 121,700 women were identified and surveyed while they were healthy and free of symptoms, then all of these women were followed over time. Women were eliminated from the study if they did not properly complete the dietary questionnaire, or if they had implausibly high or low scores for dietary intake, or if they had previously had cancer or other bowel disease. This left a group of 88,751 women who were closely followed until 1986—yielding a total of more than half a million person-years of follow-up. During the course of the study 150 women developed colon cancer, and this small group of patients was then compared to the other women in the study who did not develop cancer.

It was found that dietary consumption of animal fat was associated with an 89% increase in colon cancer risk (i.e., relative risk = 1.89).[8] This figure was computed by comparing colon cancer incidence in the 20% of women with the highest consumption of dietary fat, versus the 20% of women with the lowest consumption of dietary fat. This particular comparison should obviously show the clearest difference in cancer incidence if animal fat is indeed carcinogenic, because the two extremes are being directly compared. But these results could be a bit misleading, since the majority of women fall somewhere in the middle in terms of fat consumption. However, colon cancer incidence was found to increase progressively with a progressive increase in fat consumption. The results were so strong that a high degree of statistical certainty is associated with the conclusion that fat consumption is related to colon cancer.

These results provide strong support for the recommendation that fish and chicken be substituted for red meat whenever possible. The relative risk of colon cancer was 2.5-fold higher in women who ate beef, pork, or lamb as a main dish every day, compared to women who reported eating these foods less than once a month. Processed meats (e.g., sausage, hot dogs, bacon, and sandwich meats) and liver were also associated with an increase in colon cancer risk, but consumption of chicken without skin was actually protective from colon cancer. Women who reported eating chicken without skin two or more times a week had half the risk of colon cancer of women who ate it less than once a month. A similar protective effect was seen for fish, but this trend did not reach statistical significance (i.e., the trend may not be real).

Overall, the ratio of red to white meat in the diet was highly predictive of colon cancer risk. This was by far the strongest relationship identified in the study: women for whom this ratio was greater than 5.2 had a relative risk 2.5-fold higher than women for whom this ratio was less than 1.2. This means that women who consumed red meat six or more times a week were more than twice as likely to get colon cancer as women who had a more balanced consumption of red and white meat. Therefore, some component of red meat, whether it be animal fat or something else, seems to lead to an elevation of colon cancer risk.[9] These findings translate very easily into a specific dietary recommendation: since the evening meal is usually the major source of meat in the diet, it would be wise to have chicken or fish at least three times a week.

The findings of the Nurses' Health Study have been confirmed, at least in part, by results from a study known as the Health Professionals Follow-up Study.[10] This study examined the colon cancer risk of 47,949 male health professionals, all free of cancer, who were enrolled in the study in 1986. At enrollment, each participant completed a food-frequency questionnaire and provided information on age, weight, height, personal medical history, family history of cancer, smoking history, physical activity, and use of common medications. Participants were followed for a period of six years, during which a total of 205 new cases of colon cancer were diagnosed. Even though the Health Professionals Follow-up Study was smaller than the Nurses' Health Study, in terms of the total number of participants, more cases of colon cancer were diagnosed among the participants of the Health Professionals study. This means that a comparison of cases to controls in the Health Professionals study may actually have a better chance of detecting subtle risk factors, and a smaller chance of being led astray by false risk factors, than the Nurses' Health Study. When men in the highest quintile of red meat consumption were compared to men in the lowest quintile, it was found that red meat eaters were 1.7-fold more likely to get colon cancer than were vegetarians. The ratio of red meat to white meat consumption was also related to colon cancer risk, and men who ate beef, pork, or lamb as a main dish more than four times a week were 3.6-fold more prone to colon cancer than those who never ate meat. In fact, red meat protein was closely related to colon cancer risk, while animal protein other than red meat protein was unrelated to colon cancer risk.[11] Together, the Nurses' Health Study and the Health Professionals Follow-up Study make a very convincing argument that it is worthwhile to reduce red meat consumption.

There is now evidence that dietary fat can also cause a condition thought to be a precursor to colon cancer. The majority of colon cancers begin as small, mushroom-like growths on the inner surface of the large intestine; these growths are called polyps. It has been estimated that the time required for progression from polyp to cancer averages about 10 to 15 years, and often does not occur at all in a normal life span.[12] Fortunately, polyps can often be identified before they become cancerous, using a medical device called a colonoscope or a sigmoidoscope to inspect the inner surface of the colon.

The Health Professionals Follow-up Study has shown that a diet high in saturated fat increases the risk of colon polyps.[13] A group of 7,284 male health care professionals were given a food-frequency questionnaire in 1986, then the men were followed until 1988. These men were physically examined (by colonoscopy or sigmoidoscopy) during the study, and 170 men with colon polyps were identified. The food-frequency questionnaire was then used to determine what particular foods were associated with an increased risk of colon polyps. A high dietary intake of saturated fat was found to lead to an increased risk of colon polyps. Comparing the 20% of men with the greatest consumption of dietary fat to the 20% of men with the lowest intake of fat, the risk of colon polyps was elevated two-fold by saturated fat consumption. This study also confirmed that the ratio of red to white meat consumption is an important predictor of risk for bowel malignancy. These findings are important because, by providing a kind of continuum of tumor development, they make it easier to accept the idea that a diet high in animal fat can increase colon cancer risk.

From a scientific standpoint, the link between dietary fat and colon cancer is now quite compelling because the mechanism by which fat has its effect is at least partly understood. Several experimental studies (using mice and rats) have shown that a high intake of dietary fat increases the odds of contracting colon cancer and that inflammation of the bowel is often related to a large amount of saturated fat in the diet. A series of experiments has shown that when colon tissues of mice are exposed to chemicals derived from fat, the tissues become inflamed.[14] Fatty acids even caused the surface layer of cells lining the colon to slough off, so that the remaining cells in the colon were stimulated to grow to replace those cells. Thus, chemicals commonly found in dietary fat can indirectly cause an increased rate of growth of cells lining the colon. The increased rate of cell growth that occurs when the colon is exposed to fatty acids can apparently make cells more vulnerable to mutation, or it can enhance the growth of cells that are already mutated. Thus measures that reduce the concentration of fatty acids within the colon also reduce the carcinogenic potential of these chemicals.

However, some contradictory results have been found. The most recent report of the Health Professionals Study[15] was unable to confirm that total fat intake, saturated fat intake, or animal fat intake is related to colon cancer risk. Furthermore, a recent and very large prospective study in the Netherlands was unable to find any increase in risk of colon cancer associated with the consumption of dietary fat.[16] This study enrolled 120,852 men and women between the ages of 55 and 69 in 1986, and followed them for about three years. All these people answered a set of questions that measured the frequency of consumption of 150 different food items and beverages. During the follow-up period, a total of 215 cases of colon cancer were diagnosed. These case individuals were compared to a group of 3,123 healthy control individuals who did not develop cancer during the study. No significant differences were found between cases and controls in the total amount of calories consumed, nor were there any differences in consumption of fat, saturated fat, protein, total fresh meat, beef, pork, minced meat (e.g., hamburger), chicken, or fish. However, processed meats were associated with a fairly strong increase in risk of colon cancer; for each 15 gram increment of bacon consumption, the relative risk of colon cancer increased 1.25-fold, or 25%. Similarly, for each 15 gram increment of sausage consumption, the relative risk of colon cancer increased by 27%, while dried and cured meats were associated with a 14% increase in colon cancer risk. Perhaps this difference in risk between fresh and processed meats arises because processed meats are usually cured with the addition of preservatives such as salt, nitrite, smoke, or other additives. Furthermore, in the Netherlands, fresh meat is a part of the hot meal taken once a day, while processed meats are used in sandwiches for one or two meals per day. Generally, the hot meal is consumed with vegetables and fruit, whereas the cold meals tend not to be supplemented with vegetables, perhaps suggesting that the circumstance in which meats are eaten has an effect on colon cancer risk. However, this study should not be accepted without caution: the study enrolled a large number of individuals, but the follow-up period was rather short. Therefore, this study has less ability to identify small risk factors and may also be more prone to error in identifying what appear to be large risk factors. The only sure way to resolve the question of whether dietary fat increases the risk of colon cancer is to continue to study this and other populations until clearer answers emerge.[17]

DIETARY FAT AND BREAST CANCER

The connection between dietary fat and breast cancer risk is much more problematic than the connection between dietary fat and colon cancer risk.[18] Marked international differences in breast cancer incidence had suggested that environmental factors are important in breast cancer causation. Diet immediately came under suspicion because there appeared to be a correlation between the national average of fat consumption and the national average rate of breast cancer incidence. The Nurses' Health Study, which was discussed in connection with colon cancer, enrolled 89,538 women who were questioned on food consumption and followed for a total of four years. During the four years of the study, a total of 601 women developed breast cancer, and the relative incidence of breast cancer was studied to determine whether it was related to intake of dietary fat.

It was found that dietary fat intake did not significantly affect the relative risk of breast cancer.[19] In fact, women in the highest quintile (20%) of total fat intake actually had an 18% lower risk of breast cancer, compared to women in the lowest quintile of fat intake, although this difference was not significant. Even when fat intake was broken down into the various types of fat consumed (e.g., saturated fat, cholesterol, linoleic acid), no significant difference in breast cancer incidence was found between women with a high fat intake and those with a low fat intake.

These surprising results are based on a rather limited period of follow-up (four years), so the findings cannot be regarded as definitive. If fat intake does have an effect, possibly that effect is manifested in younger women than were followed in this study, since this study was limited to women between 34 and 59 years of age. Therefore, eventual breast cancer risk may be determined by fat consumption in young adulthood, or even in childhood. Furthermore, this study cannot exclude the possiblity that very low levels of fat consumption (fat forming less than 30% of dietary calories, which is lower than the lowest level reported in this study) would reduce the risk of breast cancer. Nevertheless, this study is the largest study yet reported that examines the relationship between fat intake and breast cancer and the methods used were adequate to address the question. We are forced to conclude that a moderate reduction in fat intake by adult women is unlikely to result in a reduction in the incidence of breast cancer, despite our expectations to the contrary, and that dietary fat is probably not responsible for the high incidence of breast cancer in the United States.[20]

These results have been confirmed by several smaller but more recent studies. The Adventist Health Study followed 20,341 women for six years and concluded that dietary consumption of animal fat is not associated with an increased risk of breast cancer.[21] Even consumption of a purely vegetarian diet was not protective from breast cancer, although these results are not very strong. The Adventist study confirmed that a number of other major factors that are related to an increased risk of breast cancer, including maternal history of breast cancer, obesity, early menarche, late menopause, or bearing children at an advanced age. However, all of these risk factors have been known for a long time. The only relationships found between diet and risk of breast cancer were that frequent consumption of fish or cheese seemed to increase breast cancer risk.[22] It is ironic that increasing the dietary intake of fish seems to reduce the relative risk of colon cancer, but may increase the risk of developing breast cancer.

An even more recent study done in the Netherlands offers further confirmation that dietary fat intake is not a risk factor for breast cancer.[23] A total of 62,573 women were followed for 3.5 years; all of these women were post-menopausal, aged between 55 and 69 years of age. Therefore, all of these women were in a high-risk group, as the incidence of breast cancer increases strongly with age. Yet even within this high-risk group no major causative role was found for dietary fat in the development of breast cancer.

As clearcut as the preceding studies seem, two recent studies contradict them. The Canadian National Breast Cancer Screening Study followed a total of 56,837 women for five years, so this is a moderately large number of person-years.[24] This study found that very large increments of total fat intake (about 77 grams) elevated the relative risk of breast cancer by about 35%. Thus, dietary fat is much less important than family history, menstrual history, childbearing history, or obesity as a cause of breast cancer. Furthermore, this study was unable to show a significant dose-response relationship between fat intake and breast cancer risk,[25] so the results must be viewed with suspicion. The Iowa Cohort Study followed 34,388 post-menopausal Iowa women for four years.[26] This study concluded that the relative breast cancer risk was 1.5-fold higher for the highest quartile (25%) of intake of polyunsaturated fat, as compared to the lowest quartile of intake. Again, a dose-response relationship between fat intake and cancer risk could not be demonstrated, so the results are not terribly convincing.

Taken on balance, these studies suggest that the relationship between fat intake and breast cancer risk is weak at best, and that there is likely to be no significant relationship between dietary fat and breast cancer. In science random chance can suggest a relationship where none really exists and data can conspire to lead researchers astray; the only way to overcome such aspects of research is to study very large groups of patients for as long as possible. The two studies purporting to show a relationship between dietary fat intake and breast cancer are simply too small to produce very compelling data, especially in comparison with the larger studies that were unable to show such a relationship.

Although no strong relationship can be found between dietary fat intake and breast cancer, an important relationship exists between obesity and breast cancer. Since a large proportion of the caloric intake of Americans comes from fat, one of the easier ways to lose weight is to reduce the total dietary intake of fat. Reduction of fat consumption will have a major effect on the risk of developing heart disease, diabetes, and colon cancer, and it may have a minor impact on breast cancer risk as well. Thus the prudent course would be to avoid dietary fat and other empty calories and to keep body weight close to a reasonable level.

DIETARY FAT AND PROSTATE CANCER

As we have seen, dietary fat has been the focus of a large number of studies that sought to determine whether this common dietary component is actually a culprit in cancer causation. Recently, attention has been focused on a potential relationship between dietary fat intake and prostate cancer risk.[27] The data used in the Adventist Health Study, which was discussed in connection with breast cancer, have been analyzed to determine whether a high dietary intake of fat increases the risk of prostate cancer. Approximately 14,000 Seventh-Day Adventist men, who had completed a dietary survey form in 1976, were monitored for cancer incidence until 1982. During this six-year monitoring period, which involved 78,000 person-years of follow-up, 180 cases of prostate cancer were confirmed. Although initially the data seemed to show a relationship between meat consumption and increased risk, more thorough analysis showed that animal products were not a risk factor. Instead, a diet including a variety of beans and fruits lessened the risk of prostate cancer, and once this protective effect was factored in, the apparent increase in risk from animal products disappeared.[28] These results have been partly confirmed by a more recent study, which found that meat, poultry, eggs, and dairy products are not significant risk factors for prostate cancer.[29] The latter study is fairly convincing because it followed a cohort of 17,633 men prospectively for a total of 20 years and because it evaluated many different sources of dietary fat. These two studies provide a good example of the complexity that can be found in dietary data; there is every reason to expect that different components of the diet will interact with one another to increase or decrease cancer risk. These complexities are difficult to discern from the relatively simple data that can be obtained in a dietary survey form. It is quite probable that many otherwise good studies have been marred by an inadequate dietary survey form that did not solicit information detailed enough to explore all possible dietary interactions.

These results, showing no association between dietary fat and risk of prostate cancer, are directly contradicted by several new studies that find dietary fat to be a risk factor for prostate cancer. A prospective study of dietary fat intake and prostate cancer risk followed a group of 47,855 men, aged 40 to 75, who were enrolled in the Health Professionals Follow-up Study.[30] These men completed a food-frequency questionnaire in 1986, then were re-surveyed in 1988 and 1990 to update exposure information and to document new cancer cases. During the four-year follow-up period, a total of 126 men were diagnosed with advanced prostate cancer, and these men were compared to men in the study who remained healthy. The risk of advanced prostate cancer was closely correlated with dietary fat consumption, such that risk was 1.8-fold higher for men in the highest quintile (20%) of intake, compared to the lowest quintile of intake. Risk was primarily associated with intake of animal fat, and red meat had the greatest impact on risk; men in the highest quintile of red meat intake were 2.6-fold more likely to be diagnosed with advanced prostate cancer. Fat from dairy products or fish was generally unrelated to prostate cancer risk, with the exception of butter, which did lead to an increased risk. When the various types of fats and fatty acids were analyzed, it was found that α-linolenic acid, which is present in red meat, was associated with the greatest increase in prostate cancer risk. High intake of α-linolenic acid led to a 3.4-fold higher risk of advanced prostate cancer. These results are consistent with the interpretation that animal fat, especially fat from red meat, is associated with an increased risk of advanced prostate cancer.[31]

Another prospective study examined the risk of prostate cancer as a function of the quantity of fatty acids in the bloodstream.[32] At the start of the Physicians' Health Study, a group of 14,916 male physicians answered a food-frequency questionnaire and provided a blood sample, which was frozen and stored. Among these men, a total of 120 cases of prostate cancer were diagnosed, and these men were compared to 120 men who remained healthy. The quantity of individual fatty acids in the blood were measured for each case and control. It was found that case men tended to have higher levels of fatty acids, including α-linolenic acid, in the bloodstream, and that men in the highest quartile of α-linolenic acid had about twice the risk of prostate cancer. The relative risk of prostate cancer was 2.5-fold higher in men who ate red meat at least five times per week, compared with men who ate red meat less than once a week. These results suggest that high levels of α-linolenic acid in the bloodstream are associated with a high risk of prostate cancer, even if the α-linolenic acid does not come from red meat.[33]

Still another study matched 358 confirmed prostate cancer cases with 679 healthy men to determine (retrospectively) whether there was a difference between cases and controls in terms of dietary consumption.[34] This study was well designed, in that the dietary survey form was adequate to assess intake of total energy, protein, and a range of vitamins and trace nutrients, as well as dietary fat. However, retrospective studies all have the flaw that they rely upon a person's memory to ascertain eating habits, not only over the last day or week, but over the last several years. This can be a particular problem if subjects have deliberately changed their diet, since remembering what one had for dinner last night can be difficult, let alone last year. In any case, this study found that dietary fat was the greatest single risk factor for prostate cancer, with an overall relative risk of 2.9. This means that (at least in the context of this study) a subject with a high-fat diet is nearly three times more likely to develop prostate cancer than a subject with a low-fat diet. Risk was highest for monounsaturated fats (relative risk RR=3.6) and next highest for total fat (RR=2.9), followed by polyunsaturated fat (RR=2.7) and saturated fat (RR=2.2). As convincing as these numbers may seem, statistical analysis showed that the significance of the findings was not high; many of the results barely achieved statistical significance, so the findings are not particularly compelling.

Finally, another study of prostate cancer risk factors found a trend toward increasing prostate cancer risk with increasing fat intake, but this trend was not significant.[35] However, above-average reported consumption of high-fat milk was associated with a two-fold increase in prostate cancer risk (RR=1.92). Men who reported drinking three or more glasses of whole milk daily had a relative risk 2.5-fold higher than men who reported never drinking whole milk.[36] This suggests that there may be something unique about milk that elevates prostate cancer risk. Since many carcinogenic chemicals dissolve well in fat, it is possible that the carcinogenic component of milk is not milk fat, but rather something dissolved in the milk fat.

The connection between dietary fat intake and prostate cancer remains problematic, because there are so much conflicting data. It is very worrisome that different studies should produce such strikingly different results; the only way to resolve this discordance is to undertake larger, more thorough prospective studies. However, the balance of results seems to suggest that dietary fat is at least a weak risk factor for prostate cancer. Therefore, it would be a very good idea to generally minimize the consumption of dietary fat and to specifically reduce consumption of red meat.

DIETARY FAT AND OTHER CANCERS

Very recently some findings have suggested that saturated fat intake in the diet can be a surprisingly strong risk factor for lung cancer.[37] While the vast majority of lung cancers affect smokers, between 9% and 20% of lung cancers in women affect non-smokers. Almost certainly some of these cases are caused by second-hand smoke, but a disturbing number of lung cancers cannot be attributed to smoking at all. In an effort to identify the risk factors that specifically affect non-smoking women, a large study was undertaken in Missouri. A total of 429 non-smoking women, all of whom had been diagnosed with lung cancer between 1986 and 1991, were identified from the Missouri Cancer Registry. These women were compared to 1,021 healthy non-smoking women using a food-frequency questionnaire that measured consumption of a wide range of dietary components. Lung cancer risk increased strongly with consumption of saturated fat, such that women in the highest quintile of saturated fat consumption were more than six-fold more likely to have lung cancer. The major drawback of this study was that the effect of past smoking may not have been adequately controlled: the proportion of former smokers among case subjects was about twice as high as among control subjects. However, the relationship between saturated fat intake and lung cancer was strongest specifically for adenocarcinoma of the lung, the type of lung cancer least closely related to smoking. This implies that while past smoking may have been a factor in the non-adenocarcinoma lung cancers, smoking is less likely to be a cause of adenocarcinomas. Since nearly half of the women in the study had been diagnosed with adenocarcinoma (the non-smokers' lung cancer), it was possible to calculate the risk of adenocarcinoma for women in the highest quintile of saturated fat consumption. High dietary consumption of saturated fat was found to increase the risk of lung adenocarcinoma 11-fold over women in the lowest quintile of fat consumption. This clearly suggests that saturated fat somehow increases the risk of lung cancer, although the mechanism of this relationship is unknown. Possibly saturated fat increases the risk of cancer at many sites, and this relationship may be easier to define in the lung, which is a common site of cancer. In any case, this study found a clear association between saturated fat consumption and lung cancer by looking specifically at non-smoking women; this association may have been masked in earlier studies that included a large proportion of women who were smokers.[38]

In reviewing the studies relating cancer incidence to dietary fat intake, it becomes clear that, for cancers other than colon cancer, there is a weak association between fat intake and cancer risk. Yet the differences in cancer incidence between various countries would seem to suggest that the relationship between dietary fat intake and cancer risk should be a strong one. An attempt was made to resolve this apparent discrepancy by re-analyzing the international incidence of cancers of the breast, colon, rectum, prostate, ovary, and endometrium.[39] Subjects were divided into younger and older age groups (30–44 and 55–69), thus effectively separating women into pre-menopausal and post-menopausal populations. Disease incidence in each of several countries was then analyzed as a function of the average national fat intake. In addition, changes in disease incidence within a single country over time were analyzed as a function of changes in the national diet. The biggest surprise of this study was the claim that fat consumption is as strongly linked to cancers of the breast, prostate, ovary, and endometrium as it is to cancers of the colon and rectum. This conclusion is not yet well-supported by case-control or cohort studies, so one must maintain a skeptical stance. Nevertheless, dietary fat may indeed play a role in causation of several cancers in addition to colon cancer, suggesting that a reduction in fat intake could lead to a reduction in overall cancer incidence.[40]

Several scientists have attempted to estimate the extent of the reduction in cancer incidence that might be achieved if dietary fat consumption was reduced. Since there is disagreement about the importance of fat as a carcinogen, it should come as no surprise that there is also disagreement about the extent to which cancer incidence could be reduced by reducing dietary fat intake. One group of scientists has estimated that a 50% decrease in dietary fat consumption could lead to a 50% decrease in colon cancer risk.[41] This estimate is somewhat problematic because it assumes that dietary fat is really the only major colon carcinogen. Furthermore, it is probably unrealistic to think that the fat consumption of the average person could be halved, because this would have a dramatic impact on palatability of the diet. Convincing the average person that a trade-off between palatability and cancer risk was worthwhile would be very difficult—unless that person was highly motivated by a personal experience with cancer. A second group of scientists has estimated that there would only be a 10–20% reduction in risk for cancers of the breast, prostate, and lung, following a reduction in fat consumption equivalent to approximately 25%.[42] A third group of scientists has estimated that only a 2% reduction in cancer deaths would result if fat consumption decreased by 20%.[43] This 2% reduction is equivalent to an increase in average life expectancy of only three to four months, and this benefit would accrue principally to those who had already reached the age of 65. But it was also calculated that a 20% reduction in fat consumption could result in a 5% to 20% reduction in heart disease mortality.[44]

Clearly, alarming discrepancies are present among the various estimates of benefit from reducing fat consumption. These discrepancies suggest that it is perhaps too soon to indulge in such mathematical speculations. It is generally wise to reduce the consumption of foods, such as potato chips and ice cream, that are not really nourishing yet are often a major source of dietary fat. But it is probably too soon to radically revise all of our eating habits to eliminate dietary fat because of a perceived benefit that, in fact, may not be real. The best advice, at this point, may be to practice moderation in all things (including moderation).

FOOD PRESERVATION PRACTICES AND CANCER

Epidemiological studies have suggested that food preservation practices, particularly the salting and pickling of food, can play a major role in cancer causation. Early evidence for this was the very striking regional variation in the incidence of stomach cancer; stomach cancer is more than seven times as common in Japan, where food is commonly salted or pickled, as it is in the United States. In China, stomach cancer is the leading cause of cancer death, while in the United States stomach cancer accounts for only 2% of all new cancer diagnoses. Yet, at the turn of this century, stomach cancer was the leading cause of cancer death in the United States too, and the decline in stomach cancer deaths in the United States has paralleled a sharp decline in the use of salt as a food preservative.[45]

The incidence of stomach cancer is very high in China, but even here incidence varies 70-fold from one region to another.[46] A survey of diet and lifestyle was conducted, involving nearly 13,000 Chinese men and women from 65 different provinces across China. The findings from this survey were correlated with the stomach cancer death rate for each of these provinces, to identify correlations between diet and death rate. A high incidence of stomach cancer was found to generally correlate with a high consumption of salted vegetables, but fresh green vegetables were actually protective from this cancer. The findings of this study are particularly noteworthy because of the clear indication that the salt itself causes stomach cancer. However, salted vegetables also contain nitrosamines and other compounds that may be carcinogenic. In general, stomach cancer incidence is lower in the southern parts of China, where fresh vegetables are easily grown. This cancer is much more prevalent in the north, where pickling is an important means of preserving vegetables for winter and spring consumption.[47] The conclusion that salt is an important risk factor for gastric cancer has been confirmed by a recent study of diet and cancer incidence in Italy.[48] The Italian study found that the risk of gastric cancer grew with increasing consumption of salted or dried fish. Experimental animal studies have shown that dietary salt is corrosive to the lining of the stomach, and that excessive salt intake can lead to sloughing of cells from the stomach.[49]

Stomach cancer may also be associated with an entirely different technique of food preservation.[50] Nitrites are currently permitted as preservatives in processed meats, although their use has been banned in vegetable products. Nitrites themselves are not harmful and are quite effective in stopping the growth of bacteria in meat. But these chemicals can be metabolized to chemicals (called nitrosamines) that are implicated in cancer causation. This type of chemical change is not limited to nitrites from preserved meats but can also involve nitrates that occur naturally in certain foods, including spinach, lettuce, carrots, and beets.[51] Nitrosamines are known to induce cancer at high doses in experimental animals, but it is unclear whether they also have significant risk for humans, who are usually exposed to much lower doses of the chemicals. The chemical reactions that result in production of nitrosamines can apparently be inhibited by ascorbic acid,[52] which may explain in part why fruit consumption is often found to be protective from gastrointestinal cancers.[53]

Another cancer that appears to be caused by food preservation practices is nasopharyngeal cancer, a cancer affecting the passages connecting the nose, mouth, and pharynx. This is a very rare cancer in Europe and North America, but one of the most common cancers in China; in parts of China the incidence rate in males is 50-fold higher than in the West. The incidence rate of this cancer is much lower among Chinese who have moved to the West, suggesting that some environmental factor causes the extraordinarily high rate of this disease in southern China. The first thought was that indoor cooking fires might be causative since cooking fires had already been linked to an increased risk of lung cancer, but several large studies were unable to confirm this idea. Suspicion then fell on diet as a causative agent, since the usual diet in southern China is different from diets in other parts of China where disease incidence is lower. Several studies have now implicated the consumption of Cantonese-style salted fish as causative of nasopharyngeal cancer.[54]

The pickling process involved in making Cantonese-style salted fish allows ample opportunity for novel and potentially carcinogenic chemicals to be inadvertently introduced into the fish.[55] A study in Hong Kong involved 250 young patients (under 35 years of age) with nasopharyngeal cancer who were matched to an equal number of persons, of the same age and sex, who did not have the disease. All individuals were interviewed as to their current dietary preferences and, whenever possible, the mothers of the subjects were also interviewed to establish dietary intake of the subjects as children. It was found that consumption of Cantonese-style salted fish by adults was associated with a three-fold increase in risk of nasopharyngeal cancer. But if an adult's salted fish consumption occurred during childhood the risks were dramatically higher. Since salted fish is commonly one of the first solid foods fed to infants in southern China, this is an important risk factor. It was found that if a child was weaned directly to salted fish, the relative risk of nasopharyngeal cancer was elevated nearly eight-fold. The relative risk for consuming salted fish at least once a week at age 10, as compared to less than once a month, was 37.7 for men and women together. Considering adult men only, the relative risk from childhood consumption of salted fish was 57-fold higher than for men who rarely ate this food at age 10. All possible sources of domestic exposure to smoke, dust, and chemical fumes were also considered, but none of these potential exposures led to a significant increase in relative risk. In fact, it was estimated that consumption of salted fish during childhood could explain 90% of all nasopharyngeal cancers among young adults in Hong Kong.[56]

An entirely new source of potential cancer risk was introduced several years ago, when radiation sterilization was first used for food preservation.[57] The principle behind this practice is that bacteria, parasites, and insects are responsible for food decomposition and spoilage, and all of these agents can be killed very effectively by radiation. The very compelling reason for eliminating these pests is that nearly 25% of the annual worldwide food production is lost to spoilage. The potential risk is not that food will become radioactive, but rather that high-energy radiation will induce chemical changes within the food, resulting in the production of carcinogenic chemicals absent before irradiation. In essence, irradiation could possibly result in production of the same carcinogens that can be produced by cooking. Early indications are that, under strictly controlled conditions, no unhealthful changes are induced by irradiation of food.[58] Meaningful epidemiological studies cannot be undertaken in the United States because so few Americans have been exposed to irradiated food, but it is not too early to initiate such studies in Europe, where the average citizen has been exposed to irradiated food for several years now.

FOOD PREPARATION PRACTICES AND CANCER

When food is heated during cooking, the added energy can cause changes to occur in those chemicals that occur naturally in foods. Studies have shown that such changes can produce carcinogenic chemicals that were not present in the food before it was cooked. Chemical changes are particularly likely to occur in foods that are high in protein, such as meat, fish, or eggs, although foods high in sugar can also undergo carcinogenic changes. In particular, risk is associated with heterocyclic amines, chemicals that are produced when raw meat or fish is exposed to the high heat used in frying, grilling, or broiling.[59] The burnt, browned material that results from cooking protein-rich foods, or that results from the carmelization of sugars, contains a wide variety of chemicals that may be human carcinogens.[60]

Most of these food carcinogens have only been identified and studied in the laboratory, and there is still very little evidence about whether or not these chemicals are actually associated with an increased risk of cancer in people. But in several cases the laboratory evidence is persuasive, even though it would be difficult ever to conduct a meaningful population study, because a proper control group would be almost impossible to find. Why? Cooking induces carcinogen formation in foods that do not have these carcinogens before they are cooked, thus a control group would have to be studied that eats the same foods without cooking them. While it is not hard to find a vegetarian control group, finding a control group that eats uncooked meat is essentially impossible. Any group of people that eats uncooked meat is likely to have a much higher incidence of parasite infestation, so their health would be compromised in ways that would not be seen in people who cook their meat. Nevertheless, epidemiological studies have implied that consumption of cooked meat and fish can lead to a slight increase in risk for cancer of the stomach and colon.[61]

ACCIDENTAL CHEMICAL CONTAMINANTS AS FOOD CARCINOGENS

Many different herbicides, fungicides, and insecticides (collectively called pesticides) are used in the farming of food plants. Because pesticide residues left on plants could conceivably be carcinogenic, the public exposure to these pesticides has been regulated since 1958. The maximum levels of pesticide residue that can legally be tolerated in unprocessed plant products was originally determined by laboratory experiments with rodents. Generally this limit is set by testing for carcinogenicity in animals, which are acutely exposed to huge doses of the suspected carcinogen, and then extrapolating to humans, who may be chronically exposed to tiny doses of carcinogen. The goal of regulation is to assure that individuals consuming a particular foodstuff for 70 years will have less than one chance in a million of getting cancer from a potential carcinogen. In fact, the actual risk of getting cancer from a regulated pesticide may effectively be nil, since extrapolating from high-dose acute rodent exposures to low-dose chronic human exposures is very problematic. While no one wants to do these experiments on humans, rodents may not be an adequate surrogate for humans in this sort of experiment. Furthermore, an excess cancer risk of one in a million may be an unrealistic goal, since the excess cancer risk of an improper diet is about 70,000 in a million.[62]

In 1991, 19,082 samples of domestic and imported food were analyzed by the Food and Drug Administration (FDA) to assure that farmers were in compliance with federally mandated standards for pesticide residue.[63] There is a very strong impetus for both growers and importers of food to comply, since the FDA has the authority to seize any produce found to be in violation of standards. Substantially less than 1% of all of samples from domestic food sources were found to be in violation of the standards; in fact, 64% of all domestic samples had no detectable pesticide residues whatsoever. Thus, by stringent current standards, consumption of agricultural products presents no reasonable threat to human health. Yet controversy remains as to whether the Delaney Clause (legislation that is responsible for regulating pesticide exposure) should be more rigidly enforced than at present. Rigid enforcement of the Clause could result in banning many pesticides, with the result that crop losses would increase, farm productivity would decrease, and soil erosion would increase (because of increased tilling of soil). Given that we now have no better yardstick than is already employed by the Delaney Clause, and given that more rigid enforcement would lead to negligible gains in public health at the cost of considerable economic burden, stricter enforcement of the Delaney Clause does not seem warranted. However, there are problems with enforcement that need to be corrected. The FDA currently tests for pesticides in less than 1% of the fresh fruits and vegetables that are sold, and the tests fail to detect nearly half the pesticides in use.[64] Furthermore, food safety testing usually takes nearly a month, by which time the tested food may have been sold and eaten. Rather than stricter enforcement, what may be necessary is more rapid and effective testing, so that the spirit of the Delaney Clause can be honored, without imposing an onerous burden on farmers.

NATURAL PRODUCTS IN PLANTS AS CARCINOGENS

During the course of evolution many plants developed natural pesticides, as a defense against the vast number of bacteria, insects, and fungi that prey upon them. Certain plants even developed chemical defenses to deter animals from consuming them. Natural pesticides are thus abundant in food plants; with every meal, we are exposed to a wide range of plant natural products that may be carcinogenic. In fact, it has been calculated that humans ingest 10,000 times more natural than artifical pesticides in their diet. About 82% of the chemicals that have been adequately tested for carcinogenicity are man-made, meaning that less than 18% of the tests conducted have analyzed the carcinogenic potential of plant natural products.[65] Of those plant natural products that have been tested, nearly half are carcinogenic. The range of potential carcinogens in common food plants seems truly alarming.

Probably the clearest example of a natural product that acts as a dietary carcinogen in humans is aflatoxin in peanuts.[66] Aflatoxin is actually made by a fungus that infests peanuts, but the important point is that human exposure occurs during consumption of plant material. Peanuts are a dietary staple in parts of Africa and Asia, where refrigeration of food is less common than in the West, and aflatoxin can be present in large quantity in contaminated foods. Since the liver is the major organ of chemical detoxification, it is exposed to any toxins eaten inadvertently. Individuals may be continuously exposed to high concentrations of aflatoxin, which may account for the fact that liver cancer is about 20-fold more common in West Africa than in the United States. There is some evidence that aflatoxin exposure may act in conjunction with hepatitis B viral exposure to further increase the risk of liver cancer. In addition, malnutrition may play a role in increasing the carcinogenicity of aflatoxin.

In the West, aflatoxin poisoning is not a major problem, but we are nonetheless exposed to a range of potential dietary carcinogens. For example, there are approximately 826 different naturally occurring chemicals that have been identified in roasted coffee beans, of which only 21 have been tested for carcinogenicity.[67] Of those few chemicals that have been tested, nearly 80% were found to be rodent carcinogens. A single cup of brewed coffee contains at least 10 mg of rodent carcinogens.[68] Yet the actual risk of cancer from coffee consumption does not appear to be high.

TABLE 6-1 NATURAL PRODUCTS AND CANCER CAUSING POTENTIAL		
CHEMICAL	NATURAL SOURCE	POWER AS A CARCINOGEN
1. Nitrates (metabolized to nitrosamines)	lettuce celery beets carrots spinach radishes rhubard	Induces tumors (carcinogenic)
2. Furocoumarins (psoralens)	celery parsnips figs parsley	Damages cell DNA (mutagenic)
3. Hydrazines	mushrooms morels	Carcinogenic
4. Glycoalkaloids	potatoes	Induces birth defects (teratogenic)
5. Flavonoids (quercetin)	very widespread in vegetables	Carcinogenic
6. Quinones	widespread rhubarb food mold	Causes cell damage Mutagenic
7. Safrole and Estragole	black pepper oil of sassafras	Carcinogenic
8. Theobromine	chocolate tea	Mutagenic
9. Pyrrolizidine (alkaloids)	very widespread herbs herbal teas honey	Carcinogenic Mutagenic Teratogenic
10. Vicine and Convicine	Fava beans	Causes cell damage Mutagenic
11. Gossypol	cottonseed oil	Sterility Causes cell damage Carcinogenic Teratogenic
12. Cyclopropenoids (sterculic acid, malvalic acid)	widespread cottonseed oil meat, eggs from animals fed cottonseed	Causes cell damage Carcinogenic
13. Methylglyoxal	coffee	Mutagenic Carcinogenic

TABLE 6-1
NATURAL PRODUCTS AND CANCER CAUSING POTENTIAL

CHEMICAL	NATURAL SOURCE	POWER AS A CARCINOGEN
14. Caffeic acid	coffee	Carcinogenic
15. Isothiocyanate	mustard	Mutagenic
	horse radish	Carcinogenic
16. Canavanine	alfalfa sprouts	Mutagenic
17. Anagyrine	milk from animals eating lupine	Teratogenic
18. Lactones (sesquiterpenes)	folk remedies	Mutagenic
19. Phorbol esters	folk remedies herb teas	Carcinogenic
20. Aflatoxin Mold toxins	mold on peanuts, nuts, corn, grain, bread, peanut butter, cheese, fruit, fruit juice	Mutagenic Carcinogenic

Plant natural products that are commonly consumed in the diet, with an indication of their potential to cause damage that may lead to cancer in humans.[75,77] In virtually every case where a chemical is shown as mutagenic, teratogenic, or carcinogenic, this determination was made from laboratory studies rather than epidemiological studies. Therefore, it is unknown to what extent these chemicals actually cause cancer in humans.

One study compared a group of 187 patients with kidney cancer (cancer of the renal pelvis and ureter) to a control group in order to determine risk factors for this cancer.[69] The control group was matched to the patient group for sex, age, race, and neighborhood to eliminate these variables. It was found that people who drank more than seven cups of coffee per day had an 80% higher risk of cancer of the renal pelvis (relative risk = 1.8). However, kidney cancer risk did not increase with increasing coffee dose, so the association between coffee consumption and cancer risk is somewhat suspect. Furthermore, it was found that smoking increased the risk of renal pelvis cancer by 4.5-fold. When risk associated with heavy coffee consumption was corrected for the risk due to smoking, the risk from coffee consumption declined to 1.3.[70] What this means is that, in the context of this study, coffee is not an important risk factor for kidney cancer, even though coffee supposedly contains at least 16 different carcinogens.

The effect of coffee consumption on cancer risk at a variety of other tumor sites has also been analyzed.[71] One study examined 1,771 patients with primary cancer at any of a number of sites (mouth, pharynx, esophagus, stomach, colon, rectum, liver, or pancreas) and compared their coffee consumption with that of 1,944 control subjects. No association was found between caffeinated coffee consumption and risk for cancers of the mouth, pharynx, esophagus, stomach, liver, or pancreas. This finding is reassuring, because previous studies had suggested that coffee consumption led to an increased risk of pancreatic cancer. Moreover, coffee consumption was found to be actually protective for cancers of the colon and rectum. In fact, when comparing the cancer risk of people who drank one or fewer cups of coffee per day, with those who drank two cups, and those who drank three or more cups per day, the relative risk of colon cancer declined by 36% for those in the highest category of coffee consumption. Relative risk of rectal cancer was reduced by 34% in those people who drank three or more cups of coffee per day. Both of these trends showed a dose-response relationship, and both were statistically significant. Since colorectal cancer is one of the most common of all cancers, the finding that coffee reduces risk is potentially important.[72] Certainly it is far more forceful to say that coffee reduces the risk of a common cancer than it is to say that coffee slightly increases the risk of a rare cancer. Even if coffee doesn't actually protect one from colorectal cancer, the evidence that it does any harm is so weak that there is probably no reason to worry about it.

The finding that cancer risk is not elevated by coffee consumption may be instructive. On the basis of the fact that coffee has 16 known carcinogens, the prediction would be that coffee is strongly carcinogenic. Yet several studies have shown that coffee is, at worst, only weakly carcinogenic. Therefore, avoiding exposure to plant natural products may not be as important as the laboratory data would imply. One of the most widely used tests for carcinogenicity seems to consistently over-estimate the human cancer risk from chemical exposures.[73] This is because human beings usually endure long-term exposure to a chemical at extremely low concentrations. But their cancer risk is predicted from what happens to rats who suffer short-term exposures to the same chemical at extremely high concentrations. In fact, the doses used on rats are maximum tolerated doses, so that the chemical acts as an irritant as well as a potential carcinogen. Chronic cell damage is known to be carcinogenic, so the rat exposed to a maximum tolerated dose of a chemical may, in effect, be experiencing two carcinogens at the same time (i.e., cell damage and chemical exposure). The fact that a chemical is carcinogenic under these circumstances may not provide any information as to whether it is a cancer risk to humans at low doses.[74]

It is simply impossible to avoid exposure to plant natural products and, in fact, avoiding such exposures may not be important. Over the course of the millions of years that plants evolved natural pesticides, those organisms that eat plants were busily evolving mechanisms to detoxify plant natural products. Thus the interaction between plants and the organisms that eat plants amounts to a kind of evolutionary arms race. The result of this evolutionary process is that humans may be well protected from the toxic effect of most plant natural products. It may be that most plant natural products are rather innocuous, although there are several examples of natural products that are known to cause large increases in the risk of human cancer (e.g., those chemicals in tobacco that make smoking so dangerous). In general, more research is needed, to determine how best to predict human cancer risk and also to determine whether plant natural products do, in fact, pose a major human cancer risk.

SUMMARY

Diet is a major cancer risk factor, in terms both of what is eaten and of how much is eaten. High food intake can lead to obesity, which is a major risk factor for many cancers, so excessive consumption of calories should be avoided. This is true even though the evidence linking total caloric intake to colon cancer risk is very weak; although calories probably are not in themselves carcinogenic, obesity is a major risk factor for disease. Therefore, it is a good idea to reduce food consumption to achieve an "ideal weight." This should be done in consultation with a physician, since the ideal weight for an individual is affected by age, sex, and physical build.

Specific recommendations as to what foods should be eaten are made in the next chapter; here the focus is more on what foods should not be eaten. In general, it is a good idea to reduce fat consumption as much as possible without affecting food palatibility. This can be accomplished by the substitution of cooking oils for butter, a reduction in consumption of red meat, and the substitution of grilling or broiling for frying. Since the evening meal is usually the major source of meat in the diet, it would be wise to eat red meat at the evening meal no more than four nights a week. This may mean increasing the consumption of chicken or fish, or it may mean an increased reliance on vegetable main courses. The National Academy of Sciences has estimated that Americans consume about 40% of total calories as fat and has recommended that total fat intake be reduced, so that fat is no more than 30% of the diet. This is a fairly stringent recommendation, since fat is often responsible for food palatibility and

	TABLE 6-2			
	WEIGHTED RISK CALCULATIONS FOR DIETARY RISK FACTORS			
RISK FACTOR	**RELATED CANCER**	**RELATIVE RISK**	**RELATIVE FREQUENCY**	**RISK WEIGHT**
Salted fish consumption	Nasopharynx	38	1	38b
Saturated fat	Lung	6.1	5	31a
Frequent meat consumption	Colon	3.6	5	18a
High ratio of red: white meat	Colon	2.5	5	13a
Low intake raw fruits and vegs	Lung	2.5	5	13b
Dietary fat	Colon	1.9	5	10a
Red meat consumption	Prostate	2.6	4	10b
Low fiber intake	Colorectal	1.9	5	10c
Total caloric intake	Prostate	2.5	4	10c
Red meat consumption	Colon	1.7	5	9a
Processed meat consumption	Colon	1.7	5	9a
Aflatoxin	Liver	3.8	2	8b
High-fat milk consumption	Prostate	1.9	4	8c
Dietary fat	Prostate	1.8	4	7a
Dietary fat	Breast	1.2	5	7c

In most studies, dietary fat is not a significant risk factor for breast cancer, yet a relationship has been found between fat consumption and breast cancer risk in some studies. To be conservative, this relationship is shown in the table, although the weight of evidence suggests that dietary fat is not really a risk factor for breast cancer.

for the feeling of satiation after eating. Nevertheless, this is a reasonable goal.

Finally, certain elements of the diet should be minimized as much as possible, or perhaps even eliminated. This includes salt-cured, smoked, or nitrite-cured foods, such as smoked or salted hams, bacons, sausage, and fish. Yet Americans generally eat less of these foods than is consumed in countries where refrigeration is less common, and a further reduction may not be necessary. It is probably more important to eat a balanced diet, including a wide range of fruits, vegetables, and grains, than it is to reduce consumption of one or a few specific foods.

NOTES TO CHAPTER 6

1. B.E. Henderson, R.K. Ross, M.C. Pike, "Toward the primary prevention of cancer," *Science* 254 (1991): 1131–1138.
2. J.H. Hankin, L.P. Zhao, L.R. Wilkens, L.N. Kolonel, "Attributable risk of breast, prostate, and lung cancer in Hawaii due to saturated fat," *Cancer Causes Cont.* 3 (1992): 17–23.
3. R.K. Peters, M.C. Pike, D. Garabrant, "Diet and colon cancer in Los Angeles County, California," *Cancer Causes Cont.* 3 (1992): 457–473.
4. *Ibid.*
4. G. Steinbach, S. Heymsfield, N.E. Olansen, A. Tighe, P.R. Holt, "Effect of caloric restriction on colonic proliferation in obese persons: implications for colon cancer prevention," *Cancer Res.* 54 (1994): 1194–1197.
6. Henderson, "Toward the primary prevention of cancer," 1131–1138.
7. W. Willett, M.J. Stampfer, G.A. Colditz, B.A. Rosner, F.E. Speizer, "Relation of meat, fat, and fiber intake to the risk of colon cancer in a prospective study among women," *N. Engl. J. Med.* 323 (1990): 1664–1672.
8. *Ibid.*
9. *Ibid.*
10. E. Giovannucci, E.B. Rimm, M.J. Stampfer, G.A. Colditz, A. Ascherio, W.C. Willett, "Intake of fat, meat, and fiber in relation to risk of colon cancer in men," *Cancer Res.* 54(1994): 2390–2397.
11. *Ibid.*
12. D.E. Beck, D.R. Welling, *Patient care in colorectal surgery* (Boston: Little, Brown and Co., 1991), 23.
13. E. Giovannucci, M.J. Stampfer, G. Colditz, E.B. Rimm, W.C. Willett, "Relationship of diet to risk of colorectal adenoma in men," *J. Natl. Cancer Instit.* 84 (1992): 91–98.
14. M.J. Wargovich, V.W.S. Eng, H.L. Newmark, "Calcium inhibits the damaging and compensatory proliferative effects of fatty acids on mouse colon epithelium," *Cancer Lett.* 23(1984): 253–258.
15. Giovannucci, "Intake of fat, meat, and fiber in relation to risk of colon cancer in men," 2390–2397.
16. R.A. Goldbohm, P. van den Brandt, P. van't Veer, H.A.M. Brants, E. Dorant, et al., "A prospective cohort study on the relation between meat consumption and the risk of colon cancer," *Cancer Res.* 54 (1994): 718–723.
17. *Ibid.*

18. W.C. Willett, M.J. Stampfer, G.A. Colditz, B.A. Rosner, C.H. Hennekens, F.E. Speizer, "Dietary fat and the risk of breast cancer." *N. Engl. J. Med.* 316 (1987): 22–28.
19. *Ibid.*
20. *Ibid.*
21. P.K. Mills, W.L. Beeson, R.L. Phillips, G.E. Fraser, "Dietary habits and breast cancer incidence among Seventh-day Adventists," *Cancer* 64 (1989): 582–590.
22. *Ibid.*
23. P. van den Brandt, P. van't Veer, R.A. Goldbohm, E. Dorant, A. Volovics, et al., "A prospective cohort study on dietary fat and the risk of postmenopausal breast cancer," *Cancer Res.* 53 (1993): 75–82.
24. G.R. Howe, C.M. Friedenreich, M. Jain, A.B. Miller, "A cohort study of fat intake and risk of breast cancer," *J. Natl. Cancer Instit.* 83 (1991): 336–340.
25. *Ibid.*
26. L.H. Kushi, K. Yamaguchi, K. Inagasaki, C. Hayashi, A. Suzaki, et al., "Dietary fat and postmenopausal breast cancer," *J. Natl. Cancer Instit.* 84 (1992): 1092–1099.
27. P.K. Mills, W.L. Beeson, R.L. Phillips, G.E. Fraser, "Cohort study of diet, lifestyle, and prostate cancer in Adventist men," *Cancer* 64 (1989): 598–604.
28. *Ibid.*
29. A.W. Hsing, J.K. McLaughlin, L.M. Schuman, E. Bjelke, G. Gridley, et al., "Diet, tobacco use, and fatal prostate cancer: results from the Lutheran Brotherhood Cohort Study," *Cancer Res.* 50 (1990): 6836–6840.
30. E. Giovannucci, E.B. Rimm, G.A. Colditz, M.J. Stampfer, A. Ascherio, et al., "A prospective study of dietary fat and risk of prostate cancer," *J. Natl. Cancer Institl.* 85 (1993): 1571–1579.
31. *Ibid.*
32. P.H. Gann, C.H. Hennekens, F.M. Sacks, F. Grodstein, E.L. Giovannucci, M.J. Stampfer, "Prospective study of plasma fatty acids and risk of prostate cancer," *J. Natl. Cancer Instit.* 86 (1994): 281–286.
33. *Ibid.*
34. D.W. West, M.L. Slattery, L.M. Robison, T.K. French, A.W. Mahoney, "Adult dietary intake and prostate cancer risk in Utah: a case-control study with special emphasis on aggressive tumors," *Cancer Causes Control* 2 (1991): 85–94.
35. C. Mettlin, S. Selenskas, N. Natarajan, R. Huben, "Beta-carotene and animal fats and their relationship to prostate cancer risk: a

case-control study," *Cancer* 64(1989): 605–612.
36. *Ibid.*
37. M.C.R. Alavanja, C.C. Brown, C. Swanson, R.C. Brownson, "Saturated fat intake and lung cancer risk among nonsmoking women in Missouri," *J. Natl. Cancer Instit.* 85(1993): 1906–1916.
38. *Ibid.*
39. R.L. Prentice, L. Sheppard, "Dietary fat and cancer: consistency of the epidemiologic data, and disease prevention that may follow from a practical reduction in fat consumption," *Cancer Causes Control* 1 (1991): 81–97.
40. *Ibid.*
41. Henderson, "Toward the primary prevention of cancer," 1131–1138.
42. Hankin, "Attributable risk of breast, prostate, and lung cancer in Hawaii," 17–23.
43. W.S. Browner, J. Westenhouse, J.A. Tice, "What if Americans ate less fat? A quantitative estimate of the effect on mortality," *J. Amer. Med. Assoc.* 265 (1991): 3285–3291.
44. *Ibid.*
45. S. Preston-Martin, M.C. Pike, R.K. Ross, P.A. Jones, B.E. Henderson, "Increased cell division as a cause of human cancer," *Cancer Res.* 50 (1990): 7415–7421.
46. R.W. Kneller, W-D. Guo, A.W. Hsing, J-S. Chen, W.J. Blot, et al., "Risk factors for stomach cancer in sixty-five Chinese counties," *Cancer Epidemiol. Biomarkers Prev.* 1 (1992): 113–118.
47. *Ibid.*
48. D. Palli, A. Decarli, F. Cipriani, D. Forman, D. Amadori, et al., "Plasma pepsinogens, nutrients and diet in areas of Italy at varying gastric cancer risk," Cancer Epidemiol. Biomarkers Prev. (1991): 45–50.
49. Preston-Martin, "Increased cell division as a cause of human cancer," 7415–7421.
50. P. Correa, "Human gastric carcinogenesis: a multistep and mutifactorial process," *Cancer Res.* 52 (1992): 6735–6740.
51. H.B. Simon, *Staying well: your complete guide to disease prevention* (New York: Houghton Mifflin Co., 1992), 409.
52. S.R. Tannenbaum, J.S. Wishnok, C.D. Leaf, "Inhibition of nitrosamine formation by ascorbic acid," *Am. J. Clin. Nutr.* 53 (1991): 247S–250S.
53. G. Block, "Vitamin C and cancer prevention: the epidemiological evidence," *Am. J. Clin. Nutr.* 53 (1991): 270S–282S.
54. M.C. Yu, J.H.C. Ho, S.H. Lai, B.E. Henderson, "Cantonese-style

salted fish as a cause of nasopharyngeal carcinoma: results of a case-control study in Hong Kong," *Cancer Res.* 46 (1986): 956–961.

55. *Ibid.*

56. *Ibid.*

57. A. Olszyna-Marzys, "Radioactivity and food preservation," *Nutr. Rev.* 50 (1992): 162–165.

58. *Ibid.*

59. T. Sugimura, "Multistage carcinogenesis: a 1992 perspective," *Science* 258(1992): 603–607.

60. B.N. Ames, L.S. Gold, "Mitogenesis increases mutagenesis," *Science* 249 (1990): 970–971.

61. Sugimura, "Multistage carcinogenesis," 603–607.

62. P.H. Abelson, "Pesticides and food,," *Science* 259 (1993): 1235.

63. *Ibid.*

64. Simon, *Staying Well,* 469.

65. Ames, "Mitogenesis increases mutagenesis," 970–971.

66. B.N. Ames, "Dietary carcinogens and anticarcinogens: oxygen radicals and degenerative diseases," *Science* 221 (1983): 1256–1264.

67. Ames, "Mitogenesis increases mutagenesis," 970–971.

68. *Ibid.*

69. R.K. Ross, A. Paganini-Hill, J. Landolph, V. Gerkins, B.E. Henderson, "Analgesics, cigarette smoking, and other risk factors for cancer of the renal pelvis and ureter," *Cancer Res.* 49 (1989): 1045–1048.

70. *Ibid.*

71. C. La Vecchia, M. Ferraroni, E. Negri, B. D'Avanzo, A. Decarli, et al., "Coffee consumption and digestive tract cancers," *Cancer Res.* 49 (1989): 1049–1051.

72. *Ibid.*

73. Ames, "Mitogenesis increases mutagenesis," 970–971.

74. *Ibid.*

75. *Ibid.*

76. Ames, "Dietary carcinogens and anticarcinogens," 1256–1264.

7

NUTRITION AND CANCER

In the preceding chapter, we discussed evidence that specific dietary elements can be harmful or can cause cancer. In this chapter we will shift our focus somewhat, to discuss specific dietary components that can be beneficial and that are implicated in cancer prevention. The American public has grown accustomed to hearing that an improper diet plays a major role in cancer causation and that good nutrition can prevent cancer. Yet most Americans are confused by what appear to be conflicting or even outright contradictory messages in the media. In fact, many people are so exasperated with arguments about diet that they have simply stopped listening.

It is unfortunate that many people now ignore the scientific dialogue about diet. Several dietary truths are emerging, and a consensus appears to be growing among scientists about certain simple measures that can prevent cancer. This chapter will attempt to present a balanced summary of the present state of scientific knowledge; nevertheless, the reader should be warned that nutrition and cancer prevention is a field in flux, so that some ideas presented here may soon prove to be false.

GOOD NUTRITION AS A CANCER PREVENTION STRATEGY

For literally thousands of years, physicians have believed that certain foods have curative or restorative powers, and much of early medicine involved the prescription of certain foods to cure medical conditions. For example, in ancient Egypt, Pliny believed that consumption of cabbage could cure 87 diseases, that onions in the diet could cure another 28 illnesses, and that garlic was a holy plant with many important uses.[1] The last few decades of research in cancer prevention have shown us that these beliefs are not far wrong, and we now have hard evidence to support many of the early dietary traditions and beliefs. We can now say with confidence that the consumption of fruits and vegetables generally reduces cancer risk. Yet this general statement alone is not very satisfying. We need to consider in greater depth which fruits and vegetables are protective from which cancers, while trying to develop a feel for the strength of the evidence. Only with a balanced and detailed assessment of evidence can we hope to separate fact from fiction and achieve a clearer understanding of cancer prevention.

Recently several scientists reviewed the massive literature about dietary influences on cancer to clarify the role of good nutrition as a cancer prevention strategy. These scientists undertook what is called a meta-analysis, or a formal re-analysis of data presented by a large number of other scientists. Approximately 200 different studies were re-analyzed, each of which examined the relationship between fruit and vegetable consumption and a major cancer.[2] Of these 200 separate studies, which discussed cancers of the lung, breast, esophagus, oral cavity, stomach, colon, bladder, pancreas, cervix, and ovary, 156 studies expressed results in terms of the effect of fruits and vegetables on the relative risk of cancer. A significant protective effect was found in 82% of all these studies (128 of 156), which strongly suggests that fruits and vegetables can prevent cancer. For most types of cancer, persons in the lowest quartile (lowest 25%) of fruit or vegetable intake were at a two-fold higher risk of developing cancer, compared to persons in the highest quartile of intake. For lung cancer, significant protection was found in 96% of all studies (24 of 25), even after the effects of smoking were controlled. Fruits were protective from cancers of the esophagus, oral cavity, and larynx in 97% of all studies (28 of 29). For cancers of the pancreas and stomach, 87% of all studies (26 of 30) found that fruit and vegetable consumption was protective, while for cancers of the colon, rectum, and bladder, 61% of studies (23 of 38) found fruits and vegetables to be protective. For cancers of the cervix, endometrium, and ovary, a significant protective effect was shown in 85% of studies (11 of 13). This meta-analysis concluded that major public health benefits could be achieved by a general increase in the consumption of fruits and vegetables.[3]

A similar meta-analysis, which reviewed the results from 137 studies, also concluded that high consumption of fruits and vegetables is protective from cancer.[4] Consumption of fruits and vegetables was especially protective from epithelial cancers, or those cancers that affect the cells lining the lungs and digestive tract, while little or no protective effect was found for the hormone-related cancers, such as breast cancer or prostate cancer. A very wide variety of fruits and vegetables as found to be protective, and some evidence suggested that raw vegetables are superior to cooked vegetables in their protective effect. Overall, the weight of evidence clearly supported the idea that fruits and vegetables of any kind are protective.[5]

Fruit and vegetable intake can apparently reduce the risk of cancers of the mouth, pharynx, larynx, esophagus, lung, stomach, colon, rectum, cervix, prostate, and bladder. Some evidence even shows that fruit and vegetable consumption can have an effect on hormone-related cancers. For example, prostate cancer incidence was followed among 14,000 Adventist men over the course of six years, for a total of 78,000 person-years of follow-up. It was found that an increasing consumption of fruits and vegetables, especially beans, lentils, peas, tomatoes, dates, raisins, and other dried fruits, was associated with a reduced risk of prostate cancer.[6] Consumption of dark yellow-orange vegetables is related to a significantly reduced incidence of early cervical cancer.[7] The only recent contradictory evidence is that a high intake of citrus fruits and juices may increase the risk of lung cancer about two-fold in non-smoking women.[8] This same study found that non-citrus fruits were protective from lung cancer, as were certain vegetables. Thus, for unknown reasons, risk of lung cancer may attach specifically to citrus fruits.

MACRONUTRIENTS AND CANCER PREVENTION

Macronutrients are those broad categories of nutrients that comprise foods, such as protein, carbohydrates (starches), and fats. Some of the clearest evidence that macronutrients have a major effect on cancer incidence has come from the study of colon cancer. As we noted in the previous chapter, diets high in saturated fats increase the risk of colorectal cancer. Now strong evidence has surfaced that certain macronutrients can reduce colorectal cancer risk. For example, Seventh-Day Adventists have a high consumption of fruits, vegetables, milk, and eggs, but no meat in their diet, and they have a colorectal cancer rate 40% lower than the average in the United States. Mormons, who consume meat and fat at a level comparable to the average in the United States but who also consume large amounts of fruits and vegetables, have an incidence rate of colorectal cancer similar to Seventh-Day Adventists.[9] This implies that fruit and vegetable consumption itself is somehow protective from colorectal cancer.

Recently macronutrient intake was found to affect the incidence of a medical condition known to be a precursor to colorectal cancer. Adenomas (polyps) are wart-like or stalked growths that arise from the lining of the colon or rectum and which can slowly grow into large masses. Initially, these growths are not cancerous, but they can eventually transform into cancers if they are not surgically removed. Many physicians screen older individuals for the presence of colorectal polyps, because if a polyp is removed before it has transformed to a cancerous state, then the individual is at a greatly reduced risk of cancer. Recently a study compared the diets of 236 case patients treated for colorectal adenomas, with the diets of 409 control subjects who did not have adenomas.[10] The cases and controls were carefully matched so that they were similar with respect to gender, body mass, race, marital status, education, and clinical symptoms of disease. A food-frequency questionnaire was given to both cases and controls to profile the diet of each group. The diet of men and women differed significantly, so all subsequent analyses were conducted separately for men and women. In women, a greater intake of carbohydrates resulted in a lesser risk of adenomas. Women in the highest quintile (20%) of carbohydrate consumption were 60% less likely to develop adenomas than women in the lowest quintile of carbohydrate consumption.[11]

High carbohydrate consumption protects women from adenomas because individuals with a high intake of carbohydrate tend to have a lower intake of protein and saturated fat. This indicates that, among the protected women, carbohydrates simply replaced some of the protein and saturated fat in the average diet. Since saturated fat is known to be harmful, a proportionate increase in consumption of carbohydrates is protective. It was also found that intake of fruit or dietary fiber (primarily derived from fruit) was protective from adenomas in women. Conversely, a high intake of total fat was harmful, as women in the highest quintile of fat consumption were 2.7-fold more likely to develop colorectal adenomas than women in the lowest quintile of total fat intake. Generally, the trends in men were similar in direction and magnitude to those in women, but they were not statistically significant. Nevertheless, the study concludes that a diet high in fat and low in carbohydrates, fruits, and fibers increases risk not only for colorectal cancer, but also for the precursor condition of colorectal adenomas.[12]

DIETARY FIBER AS A PROTECTIVE AGENT

Over the last decade a great deal of research has been done on the effects of dietary fiber on colorectal cancer incidence. This research has been hampered by lack of consensus on a precise definition of dietary fiber and by lack of a well-accepted and consistent way to measure fiber in the diet.[13] The U.S. Expert Panel on Dietary Fiber recently defined fiber as those "components of plant materials in the diet which are resistant to digestion by [digestive] enzymes produced by humans." Thus fiber is composed of those woody materials that give a fruit or vegetable its texture and that form a pulpy material if plant material is pureed in a blender. Dietary fiber is found in most plants, but particularly rich sources of fiber include the bran (outer) layer of grains, fruit skins, seeds, nuts, berries, and legumes such as peas and pea pods.

One of the best studies of the relationship between diet and colon cancer is the Nurses' Health Study, discussed at length in the previous chapter because it found definitive evidence that dietary fat is a risk factor for colorectal cancer.[14] This study involved 88,751 female registered nurses who were each followed for up to six years, so that total follow-up was 512,488 person-years. During this time a total of 150 women developed colon cancer, and this small group was then compared to other women in the study who did not develop colon cancer. Unfortunately, this study was unable to clearly determine whether dietary fiber was protective from colon cancer. These researchers concluded that a low intake of fiber from fruit appeared to increase the risk of colon cancer, but the relationship was weak and risk was increased by consumption of dietary fat. Even in the subgroup having the highest consumption of fruit fiber, the reduction in colon cancer risk was not significant. The study found that women who consumed diets high in animal fat tended to consume less dietary fiber. If the risk of colon cancer was calculated for women who were simultaneously in the highest category of animal fat intake and the lowest category of dietary fiber intake, their relative risk of colon cancer was 2.5-fold higher than normal.[15] However, since animal fat is clearly established as a risk factor for colon cancer, it is not surprising that women in the highest category of fat consumption are at an increased risk for colon cancer. Ultimately, this study did not provide a satisfying answer about whether intake of dietary fiber offers much protection against colon cancer.

The Health Professionals Follow-up Study, discussed in the preceding chapter in connection with dietary fat as a risk factor for colon cancer, also examined fiber intake in relation to colon cancer.[16] This study followed a cohort of 47,949 male health professionals, all of whom were initially free of cancer, for a total of six years. Although this study clearly implicated red meat as a risk factor for colon cancer, it was unable to find any relationship between dietary fiber and colon cancer risk. Finding no relationship between a cancer and a particular risk factor could mean either that there really is no relationship or that scientists were simply unable to uncover an existing relationship. Nevertheless, the findings of the Health Professionals Study are convincing because a large number of individuals were involved in the study and because fiber from a wide range of sources was included in the analysis. In fact, researchers scored total dietary fiber, total crude fiber, fruit fiber, vegetable fiber, and cereal fiber separately, so that even if only one source of fiber was protective, that source could have been identified. Fiber was very weakly related to colon cancer risk until the effects of red meat consumption and physical activity were eliminated, then all relationship between fiber consumption and risk disappeared. Therefore, both red meat consumption and physical activity are important in determining colon cancer risk, while fiber consumption is probably not related to risk.

However, contrary results have come from a large meta-analysis of already published data, which involved combining the results of 13 different case-control studies.[17] By combining these separate studies, scientists were able to compare the diets of 5,287 case subjects with colorectal cancer and 10,470 control subjects without cancer. The risk of colorectal cancer was found to decrease progressively as the dietary intake of fiber increased. Individuals in the highest quintile (20%) of fiber intake were at roughly half the risk of developing colorectal cancer as individuals in the lowest quintile of fiber intake. Increasing dietary fiber even by a relatively small amount was found to provide some protection against colorectal cancer, since relative risk for the five quintiles was as follows (from lowest to highest fiber intake): 100%, 79%, 69%, 63%, and 53%. Thus, if an individual increased dietary fiber consumption enough to move from the lowest quintile to the next lowest quintile, the risk of colorectal cancer would be reduced by roughly 21%. If this individual moved from the lowest quintile to the middle quintile, the risk of colorectal cancer would be reduced by roughly 31%. This inverse relationship between fiber consumption and colorectal cancer risk was seen in 12 of the 13 studies analyzed, and was true for men and women, for young and old, and for cancers of the left and right colon. After adjusting for fiber intake, it was found that dietary intake of vitamin C and beta-carotene played a relatively minor role in protecting from colorectal cancer. It was concluded that if the average person increased fiber consumption by only 13 grams a day, the incidence of colorectal cancer in the United States would be reduced by 31% overall. Since this amounts to roughly 50,000 fewer deaths from colorectal cancer each year, this is a stunning drop in mortality for a relatively small change in diet.[18] Nevertheless, a skeptical attitude must be maintained about the relationship between dietary fiber intake and colorectal cancer, since most of the 13 individual studies combined in the meta-analysis failed to find a significant relationship between fiber and cancer. Furthermore, the definition of dietary fiber used in the 13 separate studies varied somewhat, so there is a possibility that the trends observed are artifactual.[19] In general, the results of one strong study should take precedence over a combination of results from several weak studies, since the act of combining studies can introduce more errors than were present in any of the studies originally.

Evidence to corroborate the relationship between dietary fiber and colorectal cancer incidence has come from several studies of the diet of patients with colorectal adenoma. This type of study is worthwhile because adenomas are thought to be precursors to colorectal cancer; because a great many people have adenomas, it is relatively easy to accrue a large number of adenoma patients. In one study, a total of 170 case men, each of whom had completed a food-frequency questionnaire and had a colonoscopic examination that found an adenoma, were compared to 7,114 men who had undergone similar exams but who did not have adenomas.[20] The relative risk of adenoma was found to decrease with increasing dietary fiber consumption. Men in the lowest quintile of fiber consumption were at a 2.8-fold higher risk of adenoma than men in the highest quintile of fiber consumption. All sources of fiber, whether vegetables, fruits, or grains, were associated with a reduction in adenoma risk. For subjects on a high-fat, low-fiber diet, the relative risk of adenoma was 3.7-fold higher than those on a low-fat, high-fiber diet. A second study, which compared 236 case subjects with adenomas to 409 adenoma-free control subjects, provides strong corroboration for the earlier study.[21] Intake of fruit and intake of fiber derived from fruit and vegetables were both correlated with a significantly reduced risk of adenoma.

A very recent study has turned up evidence that dietary fiber may also be protective from lung cancer.[22] The connection between fiber and lung cancer is much harder to understand than the connection between fiber and colon cancer, but the evidence is still intriguing. A case group of 429 non-smoking Missouri women who had been diagnosed with lung cancer was compared with a control group of 1,021 healthy non-smoking women to determine the major risk factors for lung cancer (besides smoking). It was found that saturated fat in the diet caused a fairly substantial increase in risk of lung cancer, but it was also found that dietary fiber was protective. In fact, women in the highest quintile of fiber consumption were 24% less likely to get lung cancer than women in the lowest quintile. The protective effect was strongest for fiber derived from peas and beans, which reduced lung cancer risk by 55% for women in the highest quintile of consumption of these foods. There was a clear dose-response relationship, so that the greater the consumption of peas and beans, the greater the protective effect. The protective effect of fiber remained, even when age, smoking history, previous medical history, and total dietary calories consumed were factored in. There seemed to be an interaction between dietary fiber and dietary saturated fat, in that the protective effect of fiber was lessened in those subjects with a low intake of fat.[23] While it is difficult to understand how fiber could protect one from lung cancer, our inability to understand the relationship does not disprove it.

Many key questions about dietary fiber remain unanswered.[24] Is fiber truly responsible for the protective effect of fruit and vegetable consumption, or is some micronutrient in these foods actually the protective agent? If fiber is protective, which type of fiber is most effective? In animal experiments, only wheat bran provides consistent protection against colon tumors; is this also true for humans? How does dietary fiber actually reduce risk of colorectal cancer? There is some indication that dietary fiber decreases the transit time of food through the bowel and increases the water content of feces, so that carcinogens may remain in a diluted state. However, no one can really be sure of the mechanism by which dietary fiber has an effect on colorectal cancer, so we cannot yet have confidence that this effect is real. Finally, if fiber is effective in reducing colorectal cancer risk, what quantity of fiber intake is advisable? As yet, none of these questions has a satisfactory answer.[25]

MICRONUTRIENTS AND NATURAL PRODUCTS AS CHEMOPREVENTIVE AGENTS

Many different mechanisms have been proposed for the protective effects of fruit and vegetable consumption. It is probably fair to assume that these foods are protective because they are a major source of various micronutrients, and that it is the micronutrients (*e.g.,* vitamins and minerals) that are protective. However, a problem arises when attributing the protective effects of fruits and vegetables to a particular micronutrient. A large number of micronutrients have been identified in foods, and there is evidence that many of these micronutrients are potentially capable of preventing human cancers.[26] Since fruits and vegetables are sources of a whole constellation of micronutrients, discerning which of these nutrients is active in preventing a specific cancer is difficult. The most important micronutrients so far identified include a large family of chemicals known as carotenoids, certain minerals such as selenium, and the vitamins, including A, B, C, and E. Each of these micronutrients is present in certain fruits or vegetables, and each appears to be important in the prevention of at least one type of cancer. There is apparently no single substance responsible for a generalized protective effect. Instead, all of these micronutrients seem to be required, in order to be maximally protected from the effects of cancer. This implies that humans evolved as omnivores, adapted to a high intake of plant foods of all kinds, as well as animal foods, and that we move away from this heritage at our own peril. A whole range of plant substances are required for a healthful life and, thus far, only some of these substances have been identified as "essential nutrients." Essential nutrients may function by inhibiting carcinogen formation in the body, or by inducing systems to detoxify carcinogens, or by binding and inactivating carcinogens, or by providing substrates required for the synthesis of anti-carcinogens, or by some as-yet-unknown mechanism.[27] What is clear is that fruits and vegetables are a readily available source of a vast range of micronutrients (Table 7-1). While we do not yet understand how many of these micronutrients work, it is apparent that we cannot live long or well without them.

CAROTENOIDS IN CANCER PREVENTION

Some of the most widely studied food micronutrients are the carotenoids, of which more than 500 different types have been described.[28] Carotenoids are found in all yellow and orange fruits and vegetables, and in dark-green leafy vegetables. The best known carotenoid is β-carotene (beta-carotene), which is not generally the most abundant carotenoid but which is present in abundance in sweet potatoes, carrots, and red palm oil. Beta-carotene is also present in spinach, kale, broccoli, Brussel sprouts, and cabbage, although all of the latter vegetables tend to have more of a second carotenoid, called xanthophyll. The other major carotenoids present in food are lutein, lycopene, and α-carotene, all of which are destroyed to a certain extent by cooking. All of the carotenoids apparently can be converted within the human body to vitamin A, although less than a third of one's store of vitamin A is thought to come from the carotenoids. The remaining two-thirds of the total vitamin A comes from retinol, which is derived from animal sources. Vitamin A is thought generally to play a role in regulating cell growth rate and may also protect the body from certain damaging chemicals known as free radicals.[29]

High dietary intake of carotenoids is known to result in high concentrations of carotenes in the bloodstream. Therefore it is possible to correlate cancer incidence with carotenoid consumption simply by measuring blood plasma levels of the carotenoids. This has the advantage of being a far more accurate and objective measure of diet than can be obtained by simply asking someone to recall what he or she has eaten. A very large prospective study of the effect of plasma beta-carotene on cancer incidence was recently reported, which found clear evidence of a protective effect of beta-carotene.[30] More than 22,000 English men between the ages of 35 and 64 years were enrolled in the study, and a blood sample and a medical history were taken at the time of enrollment. Blood was frozen and stored over a seven-year follow-up period, during which time 271 men were diagnosed with cancer. These cases were compared to a sample of

TABLE 7-1
NATURAL PRODUCTS AND CANCER PREVENTION

NATURAL PRODUCT	SOURCE	PROTECTS FROM
1. Carotenoids (α- and beta-carotene, lutein, lycopene)	sweet potatoes carrots tomatoes red palm oil spinach kale broccoli Brussels sprouts parsley mustard greens yellow and orange vegetables yellow and orange fruits dark-green leafy vegetables	Lung cancer Breast cancer Stomach cancer Pancreatic cancer(?) Bladder cancer(?) Rectal cancer(?)
2. Vitamin C (L-ascorbic acid, dehydroascorbic acid)	citrus fruits citrus juices broccoli green peppers tomatoes strawberries melon cabbage leafy green vegetables	Oral cancer Esophageal cancer Laryngeal cancer Stomach cancer Pancreatic cancer Rectal cancer Breast cancer(?) Cervical cancer(?) Lung cancer(?)
3. Vitamin E (α-tocopherol)	vegetable oils margarines whole grains nuts and seeds wheat germ asparagus lettuce	Colorectal cancer Oral cancers(?) Breast cancer(?) Lung cancer(?)
4. Folic acid	asparagus leafy green vegetables lima and other beans broccoli beets oranges and orange juice	Cervical cancer(?) Lung cancer(?)
5. Selenium	many plants grown in selenium-rich soil	Lung cancer Stomach cancer(?) Bladder cancer(?) Skin cancer(?) Liver cancer(?) Colon cancer(?) Breast cancer(?)

TABLE 7-1 (CONTINUED)
NATURAL PRODUCTS AND CANCER PREVENTION

NATURAL PRODUCT	SOURCE	PROTECTS FROM
6. Dietary fiber (cellulose, hemicellulose, pectin, gums)	many vegetables and fruits nuts and seeds unrefined grains	Colorectal cancer Breast cancer(?)
7. Dithiolthiones	cruciferous vegetables (cabbage, broccoli, kohlrabi, Brussels sprouts, cauliflower, turnips, mustard, radishes)	Stomach cancer(?) Liver cancer(?) Kidney cancer(?) Lung cancer(?)
8. Glucosinolates and indoles (glucobrassicin, sinigrin)	cruciferous vegetables, especially: Brussels sprouts rutabaga mustard greens dried horseradish	Estrogen-related cancers(?)
9. Isothiocyanates and thiocyanates	cruciferous vegetables	Lung cancer(?) Stomach cancer(?)
10. Coumarins	most vegetables citrus fruits	Breast cancer(?) Stomach cancer(?) Liver cancer(?) Colon cancer(?)
11. Flavonoids (quercetin, kaempferol, myricetin, chrysin)	most vegetables citrus fruits berries tomatoes potatoes broad (fava) beans pea pods onions radishes horseradish	Estrogen-related cancers(?) Ovarian cancer(?) Uterine cancer(?) Breast cancer(?) Lung cancer(?) Colon cancer(?)
12. Phenols (caffeic, ferulic, ellagic, and quinic acids)	freshly harvested fruits and vegetables	Lung cancer(?) Skin cancer(?)
13. Protease inhibitors (trypsin, chymo-trypsin, plasmin, thrombin, elastase)	seeds and legumes soybeans kidney beans chick peas grains (barley, wheat, oats, rye) potatoes sweet corn spinach broccoli cucumbers Brussels sprouts	Lung cancer(?) Stomach cancer(?)

TABLE 7-1 (CONTINUED)
NATURAL PRODUCTS AND CANCER PREVENTION

NATURAL PRODUCT	SOURCE	PROTECTS FROM
14. Plant sterols (β-sitosterol, campesterol, stigmasterol)	most vegetables	Colon cancer(?)
15. Isoflavones (genistein, daidzein)	most vegetables	Breast cancer(?) Estrogen-related cancers(?) Prostate cancer(?)
16. Saponins	soybeans	Colorectal cancer(?)
17. Inositol hexaphospate	soybeans cereal grains	Colon cancer(?)
18. Allium compounds (diallyl sulfide, allyl methyl trisulfide)	onions garlic garlic oil chives	Stomach cancer(?)
19. Limonene (D-limonene)	citrus fruits	Stomach cancer(?) Lung cancer(?) Breast cancer(?)

Plant natural products that are commonly consumed in the diet, with an indication of their potential to protect from cancer in humans.[95,96] Question marks indicate that the relationship between the natural product and the cancer has not been established in humans, but that research with animals or with cultured cells suggests a plausible relationship. It is usually very difficult to prove that a given natural product has a specific effect on human cancer, because the sources of the specific natural product often contain many other natural products.

normal control men, who were carefully matched for age, smoking habits, and previous medical history. Care was even taken to compare cases and controls from whom blood was drawn at about the same time, in case there were subtle changes in chemistry of the frozen blood. The serum level of β-carotene was found to be more than 10% lower in cases than controls, suggesting that beta-carotene is protective from cancer. Since plasma carotene levels reflect dietary carotene intake, this suggests that dietary sources of carotene are protective from cancer. The protective effect of beta-carotene was strongest for stomach and lung cancer, although a slight protective effect appeared for colorectal cancer and cancers of the central nervous system. Men in the lowest quintile (20%) of serum beta-carotene had a cancer risk two-fold higher than normal, while men in the highest quintile of serum beta-carotene had a cancer risk 18% lower than normal. However, as strong as this study is, it does not prove that beta-carotene actually prevents cancer. While beta-carotene may reduce risk directly, it is also possible that some other component of vegetables reduces risk and that plasma beta-carotene is simply a good indicator of the availability of this unknown component.[31] To a certain extent, this type of argument is only of academic interest, since vegetable consumption would be protective from cancer in either case. Nevertheless, it is important eventually to determine the active protective ingredient of vegetables, since this may give us some insight into a general mechanism of cancer prevention.

In 1971, a study of the relationship between cancer risk and plasma levels of vitamins and carotenes was initiated in Basel, Switzerland.[32] This study, which has become known as the Basel Study, followed a total of 2,974 men for up to 12 years. During the 12-year observation period, 553 of these men died, with 204 of the deaths caused by cancer. When plasma levels of carotene in the cancer patients were compared to plasma carotene levels in the healthy study participants, cancer patients were found to have had a significantly lower concentration of plasma carotene than did the 2,421 survivors. Low levels of plasma carotene resulted in a significant elevation of risk for lung cancer. If levels of carotene and retinol were both low, then there was a significantly higher risk of all cancers.[33]

Recently a prospective study of the effect of beta-carotene consumption on lung cancer was undertaken.[34] A group of 5,080 men living in a retirement community in California, all of whom were free from lung cancer at the beginning of the study, were followed for more tha.. eight years. At the beginning of the study, each participant completed a questionnaire on medical history, cigarette use, and consumption of 44 vegetables and fruits during the preceding 12 months. Men who had never smoked had the highest average daily intake of beta-carotene (at 8.5 mg), followed by past smokers (7.8 mg), and current smokers (6.2 mg). During 31,477 person-years of follow-up, 125 cases of lung cancer were diagnosed in this cohort of 5,080 men. The relative risk of lung cancer was lower for men with a greater dietary consumption of beta-carotene, or of all vegetables and fruits, or of yellow vegetables alone. However, when these relative risks were adjusted for personal smoking, the protective effect of beta-carotene consumption seemed to vanish. This means either that beta-carotene had no significant effect on lung cancer risk in this study, or that people who consume a healthy diet are less likely to indulge in unhealthy habits like smoking, or that beta-carotene intake somehow suppresses the urge to smoke. While the last possibility seems remote, it cannot be dismissed entirely. In fact, among married couples, a person's dietary intake of beta-carotene is very closely correlated with the smoking habit of the spouse.[35] This implies that, for a given household, there is an inverse relationship between intake of beta-carotene and total cigarette consumption. Nevertheless, the comparison between cases and controls was not definitive in this study, and we cannot determine with certainty whether there is a relationship between beta-carotene consumption and lower risk of lung cancer.

However, another larger prospective study of the effect of beta-carotene consumption on lung cancer was reported recently. This study involved more subjects and followed the subjects for a longer time, thus the results are more likely to be correct. In this study, serum samples were collected from 25,802 volunteers in rural Washington County, Maryland.[36] The volunteers represented about 30% of the population of the whole county, so this is a thorough sampling of the study group. Serum samples were kept frozen during a follow-up period of more than 10 years, and a total of 436 people developed cancer in this interval. The cancer cases were carefully matched to 765 controls of the same age, then all of the case and control serum samples were analyzed. The relationship between serum carotenoids and nine different cancers was analyzed, with a focus on cancers of the colon, rectum, pancreas, lung, skin, breast, prostate, and bladder. High serum beta-carotene levels showed a strong protective effect for lung cancer, and a somewhat weaker protective effect for melanoma and bladder cancer. High levels of serum lycopene, another major carotenoid, were strongly associated with a reduced risk of pancreatic cancer and less strongly associated with protection from bladder and rectal cancer. This study is particularly convincing since blood samples were drawn well before diagnosis, during the time when the cancers were presumably just developing.[37] This and several other studies show a reduced risk of epithelial cancers, particularly lung cancer, with increasing consumption of beta-carotene.[38]

Very recently a study tested the relationship between beta-carotene consumption and lung cancer risk specifically in non-smokers.[39] A case-control approach was taken, in which 413 non-smoking case patients newly diagnosed with lung cancer were compared with 413 healthy control individuals. Controls were selected to match cases, in terms of age, sex, smoking history (former or never-smoker), ethnicity, education, and so on. Cases and controls completed a questionnaire about consumption of dietary items such as fruits and vegetables, which are common sources of beta-carotene. Consumption of greens, raw fruit, and cheese was found to reduce the risk of lung cancer, while consumption of whole milk actually increased the risk. In particular, persons in the highest quartile of consumption of raw and cooked greens (except lettuce) were 2.4-fold less likely to develop lung cancer than those in the lowest quartile of consumption. Similarly, those in the highest quartile of consumption of fresh fruit were 2.3-fold less likely to develop lung cancer. However, those in the highest quartile of consumption of whole milk were 1.6-fold more likely to develop lung cancer. These results show convincingly that dietary beta-carotene consumption is protective from lung cancer, although retinol was not protective. In addition, there was evidence that vitamin E supplements are protective, as persons who took such supplements were half as likely to develop lung cancer.[40]

Evidence is also beginning to accumulate that beta-carotene is protective from several cancers beyond lung cancer. For example, a recent case-control study examined the carotene consumption of 371 prostate cancer patients and a comparable number of control subjects in Buffalo, New York.[41] Dietary data were obtained from routine questionnaires administered to all patients upon admission, and an index of beta-carotene intake was computed from a food frequency checklist that included 27 common fruits and vegetables. A significant protective effect was found for high levels of β-carotene intake, such that men with a high intake of beta-carotene reduced their prostate cancer risk about 40%. The protective effect was particularly evident among men 68 years old or younger, in whom prostate cancer risk was reduced by 70%. However, no significant protective effect was found among men older than 68 years, the age group in which prostate cancer risk is highest.[42] However, a more recent study also found a protective effect of beta-carotene even in men older than 75 years of age.[43]

The relationship between cancer and dietary carotenoid is by no means established for most cancers. Clearly, something is protective about consumption of fruits and vegetables, and it has been widely assumed that the protective agent is beta-carotene. But, as yet, no definitive proof has been found showing beta-carotene is critical. To add to the confusion, although both beta-carotene and retinol in the diet are thought to be metabolized into vitamin A, beta-carotene is generally thought to be protective, while retinol in some studies is associated with a higher incidence of cancer.[44] This just highlights the difficulty in determining which of the many components of a particular food are actually protective, which are neutral, and which may lead to an increased risk of cancer. Even if a particular foodstuff is eventually proven beyond shadow of a doubt to be protective, it will be very difficult to determine which particular component of that food is actively protective. But note that this uncertainty does not argue against eating fruits and vegetables; perhaps the best approach is to eat the fruits and vegetables without worrying about the protective agent. In fact, it may not even be necessary to increase vegetable consumption by very much, since a single carrot a day may supply enough beta-carotene to roughly halve the risk of lung cancer.[45]

MINERALS IN CANCER PREVENTION

Numerous other components of food have been credited with reducing the incidence of cancer. One of the protective agents that has been studied recently is selenium, a mineral that is a part of the diet because it is taken up and retained by plants and by the animals that consume plants. Studies of global cancer incidence have shown that areas of the world with selenium-rich soil tend to have a lower incidence of several cancers, including lung cancer. This suggests that selenium may play a protective role, and since lung cancer is such a common and devastating cancer, this clue has been vigorously pursued. A prospective study in the Netherlands characterized dietary intake of selenium by measuring the quantity of selenium present in toenail clippings from 120,852 Dutch men and women.[46] These people were followed for more than three years, during which time 550 cases of lung cancer were diagnosed. Toenail selenium data were available for 370 lung cancer cases and for 2,459 members of the control group. When a direct comparison was made between these two groups, mean levels of selenium were found to be nearly 5% lower in cases than in controls, implying that the long-term dietary intake of selenium was also 5% lower in cases. People in the highest quintile (20%) of selenium consumption were less than half as likely to get lung cancer as people in the lowest quintile, even after age, gender, smoking, and other variables had been controlled. The protective effect of selenium was seen most clearly in subjects whose dietary intake of vitamin C and beta-carotene was low. Thus dietary selenium gives a strong protective effect, and this effect is strongest in those who are most at risk because of low consumption of vitamin C and beta-carotene.[47]

Selenium has also been shown to be protective from stomach cancer.[48] In China, stomach cancer incidence is more than four times higher than in the United States, and stomach cancer is the leading cause of cancer mortality. However, the stomach cancer incidence within China varies dramatically by county, from a rate that is only slightly higher than in the United States, to a rate that is more than 22-fold higher than that of the United States. By examining diet and stomach cancer incidence within China, it should be possible to determine whether there are dietary risk factors or protective factors for stomach cancer. A massive study examined dietary and biochemical data from 65 Chinese counties and compared this data to the incidence of stomach cancer within each county. Intake of fresh leafy green vegetables was found to be protective from stomach cancer and both beta-carotene and selenium reduced the risk of this cancer. Selenium was by far the most significant protective factor, as selenium intake was the single best predictor of stomach cancer risk.[49] However, this type of ecological study, in which population-level risks are studied but individual risks are not, is inherently unsatisfying. It is impossible to determine from such a study the degree of protection conferred by selenium or the relative risk of cancer in individuals with a low selenium intake. Nevertheless, the study clearly indicates that high selenium intake reduces the incidence of stomach cancer.

There is also fairly strong evidence that selenium in the diet is a protective agent from bladder cancer.[50] The Washington County Study, which was discussed in connection with the effect of beta-carotene consumption on lung cancer, correlated data on cancer incidence with levels of micronutrients in frozen serum samples. In a 12-year follow-up period, a total of 35 cases of bladder cancer were diagnosed among the 25,802 study participants. When these cases were compared to a matched set of controls, it was found that serum levels of selenium were slightly lower in cases than in controls, although the serum levels of retinol, beta-carotene, lycopene, and α-tocopherol did not differ between cases and controls. Persons in the lowest third of serum selenium content were twice as likely to have bladder cancer as persons in the highest third of serum selenium. Although a relatively small number of cases and controls were included in this study, the results are still relatively convincing, especially since care was taken to control for the effects of smoking.[51]

VITAMINS A AND B IN CANCER PREVENTION

The human supply of vitamin A is derived from two major dietary sources. The most important dietary source, at least in the United States, is meat, since roughly two-thirds of the total vitamin A is derived from retinol in animal products.[52] The other major dietary source of vitamin A is beta-carotene, which has already been discussed. Both retinol and beta-carotene are metabolized into vitamin A within the human body. There is some controversy as to whether retinol is actually harmful or helpful, but this argument will be very difficult to resolve since both retinol and beta-carotene are metabolized to vitamin A, and vitamin A seems to be at least moderately protective from cancer.[53]

Vitamin A and vitamins C and E are considered to be anti-oxidants, meaning that they are capable of quenching the damaging effects of activated oxygen. It is somewhat ironic that oxygen is one of the few things absolutely required for life, yet it can damage a cell or organism if too much is present. The class of chemicals known as antioxidants oppose the damaging and carcinogenic effects that oxygen can have if it is over-abundant. Therefore, large intake of these antioxidants in the diet is thought to be protective.

A large prospective study recently reported on the effect of antioxidant vitamins on risk of breast cancer.[54] A total of 89,494 women between the ages of 34 and 59 years were enrolled in the Nurses' Health Study in 1980, at a time when none of these women had been diagnosed with cancer. Dietary intake of vitamins A, C, and E was assessed with a questionnaire at enrollment and again in 1984. Over the course of an eight-year follow-up, a total of 1,439 women were diagnosed with breast cancer, and these cases were compared to the control group of women who did not develop breast cancer. The most significant link between vitamin intake and breast cancer risk was found for intake of vitamin A. The foods that contributed most to intake of vitamin A were spinach, carrots, liver, and sweet potatoes. Women in the highest quintile (20%) of intake of these foods and other foods rich in vitamin A precursors were about 16% less likely to get breast cancer as women in the lowest quintile of intake. Vitamin A was also protective when it was obtained from the diet in the form of carotenoids from plants, but the protective effect was less pronounced. The protective effect of vitamin A was generally stronger when vitamin A was obtained from the diet than when preformed vitamin A was obtained from multivitamin pills. Overall, these results clearly suggest that intake of foods rich in vitamin A can offer significant protection from breast cancer, and that women would be well served by increasing their vegetable consumption.[55]

As clear as the relationship between vitamin A consumption and lower incidence of breast cancer seems to be, there is relatively little evidence that vitamin A protects from other cancers. Lack of clear evidence for a protective effect for vitamin A may arise in part from a fundamental lack of understanding about whether retinol and beta-carotene are equivalent. Both are ultimately metabolized to vitamin A, so the simple interpretation is that both are equivalent to vitamin A, and that, if one has a protective effect, then both will have a protective effect. But such may not be the case. While beta-carotene is clearly protective from lung cancer, retinol is not.[56] In fact, retinol may be a risk factor for cancer of the oral cavity, esophagus, pharynx, larynx, stomach, colon, rectum, and prostate.[57] But this finding could be an artifact, since retinol is found in meat, and meat is strongly linked to cancer of the digestive tract. Nevertheless, it has been suggested that beta-carotene is protective through a mechanism that does not require conversion to vitamin A, meaning that beta-carotene could function independently of retinol in cancer protection.[58]

Recent evidence suggests a possible link between maternal intake of vitamins during pregnancy and the risk of cancer in offspring.[59] It has been proposed that dietary intake of nitrates and nitrites is a risk factor for brain tumors. These chemicals are metabolized to nitrosamines, which are potential risk factors for brain cancer, but the metabolism of nitrates and nitrites to nitrosamines can be partly blocked by vitamins. Because of this possible connection between vitamin intake and brain cancer, a study was undertaken examining the effect of maternal diet during pregnancy on the risk of the two most common brain tumors in children. A total of 166 children who developed brain tumors (astrocytoma or primitive neuroec-todermal tumor) before the age of six were compared to 166 children from similar backgrounds who did not develop tumors. Telephone interviews were conducted with the mothers of these children, and interviews included questions on the frequency of consumption of alcohol, vitamin and mineral supplements, and 53 different food items. Maternal diet had a strong protective effect on development of brain cancer in offspring, particularly if the mother consumed canned, dried, or frozen peaches or apricots, hot cereal, or fresh fish. In general, a maternal diet of cured meats, especially bacon and sausage, increased the risk of brain cancer in offspring, while fruits and vegetables were protective. A maternal diet high in fruits and fruit juices reduced childhood brain cancer risk by 72%, while a maternal diet high in vegetables reduced risk 63%. Vitamin A was protective, lowering the risk of childhood brain cancer by 41%, while folate (B-group vitamin) reduced risk 62%. The use of multivitamins during the first six weeks of pregnancy, or the use of iron, calcium, or vitamin C supplements at any time during pregnancy, was associated with decreased risk of cancer in offspring. The overall conclusion of this study was that maternal diet can strongly influence the risk of cancer in offspring. However, no evidence could be obtained that nitrosamines were a risk factor for brain cancer in children.[60] The counter-intuitive connection between maternal diet during pregnancy and brain cancer in children may arise because of the rapid development of the nervous system of infants in the uterus. It is possible that there is a phase during which vitamins are absolutely required for normal development of the infant nervous system. If vitamins are unavailable from the mother during this critical time, then aberrant cell growth may occur that predisposes an infant to brain cancer at some time after birth.

Relatively little is known about the relationship between cancer and vitamin B. Folate (or folic acid), a B-group vitamin, is necessary for normal cell growth, and there is some indication that folate deficiency can lead to cancer. Perhaps the strongest evidence for a protective effect of B-group vitamins is found for the relationship between folic acid and risk of early stage cervical cancer.[61] A total of 102 women between the ages of 18 and 49, all diagnosed with early stage cervical cancer, were compared to a similar number of women free of cancer. Each woman completed a food-frequency questionnaire and donated a blood sample, which was analyzed for folate content. An effort was made to control for variables such as income, obesity, smoking habits, number of sexual partners, contraceptive use, history of venereal disease, and frequency of Pap smears. The strongest risk factor for cervical cancer was a reported history of genital warts, which increased the risk of cancer more than three-fold. However, folate concentration in the bloodstream was closely linked to risk of cervical cancer, so that a woman in the lowest quartile (25%) of blood folate had about 10 times the risk of cervical cancer as a woman in the highest quartile, even after controlling for all other variables. Similarly, a woman in the lowest quartile (25%) of dietary folate intake had more than twice the risk of cervical cancer as a woman in the highest quartile of intake, after controlling for other variables. Vitamin C intake, which was also examined in this study, had a less striking effect on risk of cervical cancer. These findings argue strongly for increasing the consumption of vegetables rich in folates, such as legumes and whole grains.[62]

Dietary folate deficiency has also been linked to an increased risk of colorectal adenoma, a pre-malignant condition of the colon and rectum.[63] A massive prospective study evaluated the diet of a large group of people over the course of one year, then examined these people using an endoscope to determine the incidence of adenoma. A total of 15,984 women and 9,490 men were examined, and adenomas were found in 564 women and 331 men. Scientists then determined the relationship between ademona risk and dietary intake of folate and methionine. A high dietary intake of folate was found to reduce the risk of colorectal adenoma by about 35% in men and women, even after eliminating the effects of age, obesity, family and medical history, and dietary intake of fat and fiber. Dietary intake of methionine also reduced the risk of adenoma, as subjects with a high intake reduced their adenoma risk by about 38%. The involvement of B-group vitamins in preventing cancer of the gastrointestinal tract may be more important than is generally recognized, since deficiencies of B vitamins are also a risk factor for stomach cancer. Patients with pernicious anemia, a progressive wasting disease of older adults associated with chronic shortage of vitamin B12, are 18 times more likely to get gastric cancer than normal adults.[64]

VITAMINS C AND D IN CANCER PREVENTION

Vitamin C, also known as ascorbate or ascorbic acid, appears to be involved in protection from a fairly wide range of cancers. Generally, vitamin C protects from cancers that are not related to hormone stimulation, although recent evidence shows that vitamin C may also be protective from breast cancer.[65] Vitamin C is largely obtained from vegetables and fruits, particularly in citrus fruits, cantaloupe, and certain vegetables such as broccoli, Brussels sprouts, and peppers. A meta-analysis of many different studies in which dietary vitamin C was measured showed that vitamin C reduces the risk of several cancers roughly two-fold. Vitamin C was particularly important in reducing the incidence of cancers of the oral cavity, larynx, esophagus, and pancreas, but there was also evidence that vitamin C could protect from cancers of the lung, stomach, rectum, breast, and cervix. Again, it is essentially impossible to determine whether Vitamin C or some other component of fruits and vegetables is actually protective, and it is even possible that vitamin C, carotenoids, and other factors must all be present in order to be protective.[66]

Recently, evidence was obtained that Vitamin C may be protective from breast cancer.[67] A meta-analysis of 12 different studies of diet and breast cancer examined a total of 4,427 women with breast cancer (cases) and 6,095 women without evidence of disease (controls). This study showed there was relatively little impact of any dietary intake on pre-menopausal breast cancer, which is consistent with the idea that pre-menopausal breast cancer is largely a result of hereditary susceptibility. However, examining post-menopausal women only, diet had a profound impact on breast cancer incidence. A significant protective effect was identified for dietary fiber, beta-carotene, and vitamins A and C, with vitamin C providing the most powerful protective effect. Comparing women in the highest and the lowest quintiles of intake, dietary fiber reduced breast cancer risk by 17% in post-menopausal women, while vitamin A reduced breast cancer risk by 18%, and beta-carotene reduced breast cancer risk by 19%. However, vitamin C reduced breast cancer incidence in post-menopausal women by a startling 37%. If the effect of vitamin C on breast cancer incidence is calculated for all women, not just post-menopausal women, then women in the highest quintile are 31% less likely to develop breast cancer than women in the lowest quintile of vitamin C intake. The usual caveat must be repeated that vitamin C should simply be regarded as a marker for fruit and vegetable consumption and that it may actually be some other ingredient of these foods that is protective. However, if we assume that the protective effect is actually due to vitamin C, then about 24% of all post-menopausal breast cancer cases could be prevented by increasing the dietary intake of vitamin C.[68]

However, this meta-analysis is not as strong as one would wish, because it combined the results of 12 different studies, and it is not certain that all of these studies should be combined. The separate studies were performed in Argentina, Canada, China, Greece, Israel, Italy, and the United States, and the diets of women in these countries differ radically. Dietary assessment was done using food-frequency questionnaires, and it is not clear that these separate questionnaires are comparable. Furthermore, the separate studies were conducted over the course of 13 years, during which time many variables could have changed, including the techniques for food-frequency assessment. The follow-up periods for these studies were all short, usually ranging from one to three years, and only two studies had a five-year follow-up. In summary, there are problems with every meta-analysis and this type of study should not be completely trusted unless it can be confirmed in a large prospective study where all cases and all controls are handled in an identical manner. Unfortunately, the most recent large prospective study[69] was unable to confirm the results of the earlier meta-analysis.

The Nurses' Health Study has already been mentioned in connection with assessing the importance of vitamin A in prevention of breast cancer.[70] This study also offers the latest word on whether vitamin C has an impact on breast cancer prevention. In this study, a total of 89,494 women between 34 and 59 years of age were followed for eight years, during which 1,439 women developed breast cancer. In contrasting the vitamin C intake of these cases with the vitamin C intake of controls, who did not develop breast cancer, no significant difference was found between the groups in vitamin C intake. While this study cannot exclude the possibility that very low intakes of vitamin C are associated with an increased risk of breast cancer, the results show clearly that high levels of intake are not protective. However, this same study found an important protective effect for vitamin A: among women in the highest quintile for intake of vitamin A, the relative risk of breast cancer was reduced 16%.[71] Since this study was prospective, involved a larger group of women, followed those women for a long period, and used a food-frequency questionnaire that has been well validated, its results are more likely to be correct than the meta-analysis previously discussed. Therefore, we can conclude, at least for the time being, that vitamin C in high doses is not protective from breast cancer, although very low levels of intake may be a risk factor.

A recent study of the risk of early stage cervical cancer has shown a very clearcut reduction in risk with increasing consumption of dietary sources of vitamin C.[72] A total of 102 women diagnosed with cervical cancer were compared to 100 healthy women, using a food-frequency questionnaire. Women in the lowest quartile of dietary vitamin C consumption were found to be at a five-fold higher risk of cervical cancer than were women in the highest quartile of vitamin C consumption. Risk increased with declining vitamin C consumption in a dose-dependent fashion, which argues strongly that vitamin C acts as an anticarcinogen. Even when a mathematical approach was used to eliminate variables such as smoking status, number of sexual partners, frequency of Pap smear examination, use of spermicidal contraceptive foams, or past history of venereal disease, the relationship between vitamin C intake and cervical cancer risk remained. However, this same study also found that dietary folate also offers significant protection from cervical cancer. Since folate and vitamin C tend to be present in the same foods (*e.g.,* legumes), it is not really possible to determine whether both these chemicals are active in prevention of cervical cancer, or whether perhaps one is active and the other is simply a marker for the active chemical.[73]

Finally, there is some evidence that maternal intake of vitamin C during pregnancy protects young children from brain tumors after birth.[74] Children of mothers in the highest quartile (25%) of dietary vitamin C intake had a risk of brain cancer that was 58% lower than children of mothers in the lowest quartile of vitamin C intake. Vitamin C supplements, in the form of multivitamin pills, effectively reduced cancer risk; a comparison of highest to lowest quartile shows that vitamin C supplements reduced brain tumor risk by 65%. This protective effect probably arose because the fetus in the uterus develops very rapidly, and shortage of a particular vitamin at this critical juncture may set the stage for later development of cancer.

Relatively little is known about the effect of vitamin D on cancer incidence. Vitamin D is obtained in the diet, but it remains in a relatively inactive form until activated in the skin by sunlight. High concentrations of vitamin D in the bloodstream appear to be at least moderately protective from colon cancer. Studies of cancer incidence among populations of people throughout the world show that colon cancer incidence is higher in parts of the world that get relatively little sunshine. Furthermore, incidence of breast cancer is lower in sunny parts of the country and in women who are regularly exposed to sunlight, suggesting that vitamin D may play a protective role for breast cancer as well.[75]

VITAMIN E IN CANCER PREVENTION

Vitamin E, also known as α-tocopherol, is another vitamin that has been credited with protection from cancer, but for this vitamin the evidence seems stronger. A very large study in Finland measured the serum concentration of α-tocopherol in 36,265 adults, then followed these adults for up to eight years.[76] During the follow-up period, a total of 766 persons developed cancer, and these case individuals were compared to 1,419 control individuals who did not develop cancer. Individuals with low serum levels of α-tocopherol were about 1.5-fold more likely to develop cancer, compared to persons with a high blood level of vitamin E. The strength of the association between serum vitamin E and cancer varied for different cancers, as would be expected if vitamin E was protective from some cancers, but not all. Vitamin E provided the strongest protection from cancers of the gastrointestinal tract and from the group of cancers unrelated to smoking. The protective effect of vitamin E was strongest in men who did not smoke and among women with low serum levels of selenium. These findings suggest that vitamin E protects from certain cancers, most notably colorectal cancer.[77]

Recently, a very large study confirmed that high dietary intake of vitamin E has a strong impact on colon cancer risk.[78] This study was prospective, meaning that the relevant variables were measured before the subjects were diagnosed with cancer, and a huge number of subjects were involved. For both these reasons, this study should be regarded as a very powerful indicator of colon cancer risk. A total of 35,216 Iowa women, all free from cancer and all between the ages of 55 and 69, filled out a dietary questionnaire and donated a blood sample in 1986. Over a four-year period, involving 167,447 person-years of follow-up, a total of 212 cases of colon cancer were diagnosed in this cohort of women. Cancer cases were compared to the remaining 35,004 women, who did not develop colon cancer. Interestingly, total intake of calories did not differ between cases and controls, which argues against energy intake being a risk factor for colon cancer (as was suggested in a study discussed in the previous chapter). There was also no difference between cases and controls in intake of total beta-carotene, dietary vitamin A, or total vitamin C. However controls were found to be substantially more likely to have a high dietary intake of vitamin E; in fact, intake of vitamin E by cases was found to be 45% lower than intake by controls. This difference was due to use of vitamin E supplements by control women, since the dietary intake of vitamin E was essentially equal in cases and controls. Use of vitamin E supplements caused a very significant decrease in colon cancer risk. Generally, users of vitamin supplements were marginally healthier than nonusers by a number of different measures. Although vitamin users did not differ from nonusers in terms of age or alcohol use, users were slightly slimmer, and they consumed three grams less total fat per day, two grams less animal fat per day, and about a gram more dietary fiber each day. These differences are so small that they arguably did not contribute to a reduction of colon cancer risk. The biggest difference between cases and controls was clearly in the total intake of vitamin E.[79]

The relative risk of colon cancer in those women with the highest consumption of vitamin E was 68% lower than those women with the lowest consumption of vitamin E.[80] The effect of vitamin E was so strong that when the effects of age, total energy intake, intake of dietary fat or nitrites, or consumption of other vitamins were removed, the protective effect of vitamin E was still strong. When the effect of vitamin E consumption was examined more closely, it was found that the protective effect was strongest in younger women. For women in the highest quintile (20%) of vitamin E consumption, relative risk of colon cancer varied with age as follows: for women aged 55 to 59, relative risk was reduced 84% by vitamin E consumption; for women aged 60 to 64, relative risk was reduced 73%; and for women aged 65 to 69, relative risk was only reduced 7%. The vitamin E effect on colon cancer risk was stronger and more significant than any other dietary effect, especially in women under the age of 65.[81]

The Iowa Women's Study also confirms several earlier studies showing that colorectal cancer incidence is reduced among persons with high intake of vitamin E. For example, an earlier meta-analysis had combined five separate studies of serum α-tocopherol and colorectal cancer incidence.[82] The major difference between the meta-analysis and the Iowa Women's study was that the meta-analysis measured serum levels of α-tocopherol rather than dietary intake of vitamin E, and the meta-analysis examined the impact of α-tocopherol on cancers of both colon and rectum. By combining the results of five separate studies, the meta-analysis was able to compare a total of 289 cases of colorectal cancer with 1,267 matched control individuals who did not have cancer. Individuals in the highest quartile (25%) of serum α-tocopherol had a risk of colorectal cancer 40% lower than individuals in the lowest quartile of α-tocopherol. Although this would seem to make a strong case for a reduction in colorectal cancer risk by serum α-tocopherol, the meta-analysis was flawed in several ways. Despite achieving a relatively large sample of cases by lumping cases together from different studies, the results were still unclear. The relative risk associated with low serum α-tocopherol was rather small, and the protective effects reported were not statistically significant.[83] While the meta-analysis was able to suggest some interesting connections between vitamin E intake and colorectal cancer risk, it is fortunate that this study has been confirmed and strengthened by the later study of Iowa Women.

Another study of a large group of people in Maryland has provided confirmation for the idea that vitamin E protects from cancer. However this study is different from previous studies in that it concluded that vitamin E protects from lung cancer.[84] This study, which was already discussed in connection with carotenoids and cancer risk, examined levels of vitamin E in serum drawn from 25,802 volunteers in Washington County, Maryland. Serum vitamin E was found to have a slightly protective effect from lung cancer, but the effect of vitamin E on lung cancer risk was not all that strong.[85] An earlier study of the same Washington County residents had reported that persons with serum levels of vitamin E in the lowest quintile (20%) had a risk of lung cancer nearly three-fold higher than persons in the highest quintile.[86] However, while a three-fold difference may seem very convincing, the difference barely achieved statistical significance. Therefore, the last word has not been heard about the relationship between vitamin E and lung cancer.

Similarly, the relationship between vitamin E intake and breast cancer risk is not definitive. A recent study examined serum levels of retinol, α-carotene, β-carotene, lycopene, α-tocopherol, and γ-tocopherol, as well as dietary intakes of retinol, carotene, and vitamin E, as risk factors for breast cancer.[37] Serum from 377 women with breast cancer, and from 173 women with a non-malignant form of breast disease, was compared with serum from 403 women free of breast disease. No significant relationship was found between breast disease and serum levels of any of these vitamins and micronutrients. However, women in the highest quintile of intake of vitamin E from food sources only were at a reduced risk of breast cancer. Dietary intake of vitamin E put women in the highest quintile of intake at a level of risk 60% lower than women in the lowest quintile. Vitamin E obtained from dietary supplements was not as effective at reducing breast cancer risk, as women in the highest quintile of supplementary vitamin E intake were only 30% less likely to suffer breast cancer.[88] It is not at all clear why dietary intake of vitamin E should be protective from breast cancer in the absence of a protective effect of vitamin E in the bloodstream. This paradoxical result must call the whole study into question, since there is no easy explanation as to why this paradox should exist.

Nevertheless, the evidence linking vitamin E intake to protection from cancer is strong, at least in the case of colon cancer. It may also have a protective effect from other cancers, but whether there is or not, the advice would be the same. A diet rich in vegetables and fruits will also be rich in all of the vitamins and minerals we have discussed. Therefore, no matter which agent is having a protective effect for which cancer, increasing consumption of fruits and vegetables is an easy and pleasant way to reduce the risk of cancer. In this light, an argument about whether vitamin E (or some other vitamin) protects women from breast cancer (or some other cancer) is somewhat less relevant. The gist is the same: to minimize the chances of getting a wide range of cancers, one should eat less meat and more fruits and vegetables.

NUTRITIONAL DEFICITS AS AN INTERACTIVE RISK FACTOR

Nutritional deficits may act as an interactive risk. Thus people who are chronically deprived of certain micronutrients may be more vulnerable to other agents that cause cancer. For example, chronic malnutrition increases the carcinogenic effect of aflatoxin, with the result that liver cancer is strikingly more common in those parts of the world where malnutrition is common.

Alternatively, people who are chronically exposed to some carcinogen may be more likely to have a nutritionally inadequate diet. This latter possibility certainly sounds strange, but there is actually some evidence that people exposed to environmental tobacco smoke are likely to have a diet low in beta-carotene.[89] A study examined the diet of 82 women who were themselves non-smokers, but who were married to heavy smokers. The extent of exposure to environmental tobacco smoke was objectively assessed by measuring the quantity of a nicotine breakdown product in urine. Diet was assessed by the now familiar dietary questionnaire, and other variables were also measured, including age, ethnicity, education, and alcohol intake. It was found that intake of beta-carotene and cholesterol were both reduced in women exposed to high levels of environmental tobacco smoke. Since high beta-carotene intake reduces the risk of lung cancer, this means that women exposed to environmental tobacco smoke are often exposed to the interactive risks of tobacco and low intake of beta-carotene.[90] While this interactive risk is likely to be small, it is potentially important, albeit difficult to rationalize. Smokers are generally known to have a diet low in fruits and vegetables and high in dietary fat. Perhaps smoking simply depresses the appetite or perhaps smokers, who are to some extent self-destructive, are more likely to eat a nutritionally inadequate diet. The alternative, that smoking somehow specifically depresses the intake of fruits and vegetables, frankly seems unlikely.

These unusual findings have been confirmed by another more recent study. A cohort of 5,080 men living in a retirement community in California were followed over eight years, to determine the relationship between dietary beta-carotene intake, cigarette smoking, and lung cancer risk.[91] While this study was unable to demonstrate a clearcut reduction in lung cancer risk with increased dietary intake of beta-carotene, there were several other interesting findings. Men who had never smoked had the

TABLE 7-2
WEIGHTED RISK CALCULATIONS FOR NUTRITIONAL RISK FACTORS

NUTRITIONAL RISK FACTOR	RELATED CANCER	RELATIVE RISK	RELATIVE FREQUENCY	WEIGHTED RISK
Low intake of folate	Cervical	10	3	30b
Low intake of vitamin E	Colon	3.1	5	16a
Low intake of vitamin C	Cervical	5	3	15c
Low intake of vitamin E	Breast	2.5	5	13b
Low carbohydrate intake	Colorectal	2.5	5	12a
Low fruit and vegetable intake	All cancers	2	5	10a
Low intake of selenium	Lung	2	5	10a
Low intake of peas and beans	Lung	1.9	5	10b
Low fiber intake	Colorectal	1.9	5	10b
High intake of citrus juices	Lung	1.7	5	9b
Low intake of vitamin E	Lung	1.8	5	9c
Low intake of vitamin A	Colon	1.6	5	8a

NUTRITIONAL RISK FACTOR	RELATED CANCER	RELATIVE RISK	RELATIVE FREQUENCY	WEIGHTED RISK
Low intake of methionine	Colon	1.6	5	8a
Low intake of folate	Colon	1.5	5	8a
Low intake of vitamin E	All cancers	1.5	5	8a
Low intake of selenium	Bladder	2	4	8b
Low intake of beta-carotene	Lung	1.4	5	7a
Low intake of beta-carotene	Prostate	1.7	4	7b
Low intake of vitamin A	Breast	1.2	5	6a
Low intake of vitamin C	Colon	1.2	5	6b
Maternal diet low in produce	Brain (in offspring)	3.6	1	4a
Maternal diet low in folate	Brain (in offspring)	2.6	1	3a
Maternal diet low in vitamin C	Brain (in offspring)	2.4	1	2a
Maternal diet low in vitamin A	Brain (in offspring)	1.7	1	2a

The relative importance of a risk factor is quantified by considering three factors: the relative risk associated with the risk factor; the relative frequency of the related cancer; 'nd the statistical power of the study that linked the risk factor with the cancer. Weighted risk is rounded upward in every case.

highest dietary intake of beta-carotene, followed by men who had quit smoking, while men who were current smokers had an average intake of beta-carotene that was 27% lower than non-smokers. When a comparison was made between the diets of men and the diets of women to whom they were married, it was found that the diets of spouse pairs were highly correlated. This means that a smoker's wife is likely to have a low intake of beta-carotene, thereby potentially increasing her risk of lung cancer from environmental tobacco smoke. Furthermore, when a comparison was made between men with similar smoking habits, it was found that men's dietary intake of beta-carotene declined as the smoking habit of their wives increased.[92] Thus, the cumulative intake of fruits and vegetables in a household decreases as the cumulative intake of cigarettes increases. This is probably a consequence of the well-known fact that smoking acts as a powerful appetite suppressant.

SUMMARY

Specific recommendations about diet are relatively easy to make; basically, your mother was right. The American Cancer Society has recommended that everyone eat at least five helpings a day of fruits and vegetables. Such advice is prudent because it will result in an increased intake of dietary fiber as well as vitamins such as A and C. The former is important because dietary fiber is strongly linked to a reduction of colorectal cancer risk, while the latter are important in reducing risk for cancers of the stomach, esophagus, and lung. Intake of vitamins in the diet is apparently superior to intake in vitamin supplements, which may indicate that there are as-yet-unknown components of fruits and vegetables that provide protection from cancer.

Nevertheless, intake of selenium and other vitamins or minerals in supplement form has been associated with reduction in risk of some cancers. Recent research indicates that vitamin pills can reduce colon cancer risk, especially if they supply more than 5,000 International Units (IUs; the units shown on vitamin pill bottles) of vitamin A, more than 60 mg of vitamin C, and more than 30 IUs of vitamin E.[93] While intake of these vitamins certainly will not guarantee immunity from colon cancer, it may reduce risk sufficiently that many will want to consider this strategy. However, vitamin supplements should never be used to compensate for an inadequate diet. Instead, take your best shot at a balanced diet, being sure to have a high intake of fresh fruits and vegetables, then use multivitamin pills to make up for any inadvertent or temporary inadequacies of vitamin intake.

More specific recommendations are possible about daily intake of dietary fiber.[94] The average American consumes about 23 grams of fiber per day from all sources. If this intake could be increased by 70%, to 39 grams of fiber per day, there could be as many as 50,000 fewer cases of colorectal cancer each year in the United States. The increase in dietary fiber should come from an increase in consumption of fruits, vegetables, and grains, and not from an increase in consumption of fiber supplements. This is because it is possible that dietary fiber is not as important in cancer prevention as is some as-yet-undetermined constituent of fruits and vegetables.

NOTES TO CHAPTER 7

1. K.A. Steinmetz, and J.D. Potter, "Vegetables, fruit, and cancer. I. Epidemiology," *Cancer Causes Control* 2 (1991): 325–357.
2. G.B. Block, B. Patterson, A. Subar, "Fruit, vegetables, and cancer prevention: a review of the epidemiological evidence," *Nutr. Cancer* 18 (1992): 1–29.
3. *Ibid.*
4. Steinmetz, "Vegetables, fruit, and cancer. I.," 325–357.
5. *Ibid.*
6. P.K. Mills, W.L. Beeson, R.L. Phillips, G.E. Fraser, "Cohort study of diet, lifestyle, and prostate cancer in Adventist men," *Cancer* 64 (1989): 598–604.
7. R.G. Ziegler, C.J. Jones, L.A. Brinton, S.A. Norman, K. Mallin, et al., "Diet and the risk of *in situ* cervical cancer among white women in the United States," *Cancer Causes Control* 2 (1991): 17–29.
8. M.C.R. Alavanja, C.C. Brown, C. Swanson, R.C. Brownson, "Saturated fat intake and lung cancer risk among nonsmoking women in Missouri," *J. Natl. Cancer Instit.* 85 (1993): 1906–1916.
9. B. Levin, "Nutrition and colorectal cancer," *Cancer* 70 (1992): 1723–1726.
10. R.S. Sandler, C.M. Lyles, L.A. Peipins, C.A. McAuliffe, J.T. Woosley, L.L. Kupper, "Diet and risk of colorectal adenomas: macronutrients, cholesterol, and fiber," *J. Natl. Cancer Instit.* 85 (1993): 884–891.
11. *Ibid.*
12. *Ibid.*
13. K.A. Steinmetz, J.D. Potter, "Vegetables, fruits, and cancer. II. Mechanisms," *Cancer Causes Control* 2 (1991): 427–442.
14. W. Willett, M.J. Stampfer, G.A. Colditz, B.A. Rosner, F.E.

Speizer, "Relation of meat, fat, and fiber intake to the risk of colon cancer in a prospective study among women," *N. Engl. J. Med.* 323 (1990): 1664–1672.

15. *Ibid.*
16. E. Giovannucci, E.B. Rimm, M.J. Stampfer, G.A. Colditz, A. Ascherio, W.C. Willett, "Intake of fat, meat, and fiber in relation to risk of colon cancer in men." *Cancer Res.* 54 (1994): 2390–2397.
17. G.R. Howe, E. Benito, R. Castelleto, J. Cornee, J. Esteve, et al., "Dietary intake of fiber and decreased risk of cancers of the colon and rectum: evidence from the combined analysis of 13 case-control studies," *J. Natl. Cancer Instit.* 84 (1992): 1887–1896.
18. *Ibid.*
19. J.T. Dwyer, L.M. Ausman, "Fiber: unanswered questions," *J. Natl. Cancer Instit.* 84 (1992): 1851–1853.
20. E. Giovannucci, M.J. Stampfer, G. Colditz, E.B. Rimm, W.C. Willett, "Relationship of diet to risk of colorectal adenoma in men," *J. Natl. Cancer Instit.* 84 (1992): 91–98.
21. Sandler, "Diet and risk of colorectal adenomas," 884–891.
22. Alavanja, "Saturated fat intake and lung cancer risk among non-smoking women in Missouri," 1906–1916.
23. *Ibid.*
24. Dwyer, "Fiber: unanswered questions," 1851–1853.
25. *Ibid.*
26. Steinmetz, "Vegetables, fruits, and cancer. II," 427–442.
27. *Ibid.*
28. *Ibid.*
29. *Ibid.*
30. N.J. Wald, S.G. Thompson, J.W. Densem, J. Boreham, A. Bailey, "Serum beta-carotene and subsequent risk of cancer: results from the BUPA Study," *Br. J. Cancer* 57 (1988): 428–433.
31. *Ibid.*
32. H.B. Stahelin, K.F. Gey, M. Eichholzer, E. Ludin, "Beta-carotene and cancer prevention: the Basel Study," *Am. J. Clin. Nutr.* 53 (1991): 265S–269S.
33. *Ibid.*
34. A. Shibata, A. Paganini-Hill, R.K. Ross, M.C. Yu, B.E. Henderson, "Dietary beta-carotene, cigarette smoking, and lung cancer in men," *Cancer Causes Cont.* 3 (1992): 207–214.
35. *Ibid.*
36. G.W. Comstock, K.J. Helzlsouer, T.L. Bush, "Prediagnostic serum levels of carotenoids and vitamin E as related to subsequent cancer in Washington County, Maryland," *Am. J. Clin. Nutr.* 53 (1991) 260S–264S.

37. *Ibid.*
38. R.G. Ziegler, "Vegetables, fruits, and carotenoids and the risk of cancer," *Am. J. Clin. Nutr.* 53 (1991): 251S–259S.
39. S.T. Mayne, D.T. Janerich, P. Greenwald, S. Chorost, C. Tucci, et al., "Dietary beta-carotene and lung cancer risk in U. S. nonsmokers," *J. Natl. Cancer Instit.* 86 (1994): 33–38.
40. *Ibid.*
41. C. Mettlin, S. Selenskas, N. Natarajan, R. Huben, "Beta-carotene and animal fats and their relationship to prostate cancer risk: a case-control study," *Cancer* 64 (1989): 605–612.
42. *Ibid.*
43. A.W. Hsing, J.K. McLaughlin, L.M. Schuman, E. Bjelke, G. Gridley, et al., "Diet, tobacco use, and fatal prostate cancer: results from the Lutheran Brotherhood Cohort Study," *Cancer Res.* 50 (1990): 6836–6840.
44. S.T. Mayne, S. Graham, T. Zheng, "Dietary retinol: prevention or promotion of carcinogenesis in humans?," *Cancer Causes Control* 2 (1991): 443–450.
45. H.B. Simon, *Staying well: your complete guide to disease prevention* (New York: Houghton Mifflin Co., 1992), p. 98.
46. P.A. van den Brandt, R.A. Goldbohm, P. van't Veer, P. Bode, E. Dorant, et al. "A prospective cohort study on selenium status and risk of lung cancer," *Cancer Res.* 53 (1993): 4860–4865.
47. *Ibid.*
48. R.W. Kneller, W-D. Guo, A.W. Hsing, J-S. Chen, W.J. Blot, et al., "Risk factors for stomach cancer in sixty-five Chinese counties," *Cancer Epidemiol. Biomarkers Prev.* 1 (1992): 113–118.
49. *Ibid.*
50. K.J. Helzlsouer, G.W. Comstock, J.S. Morris, "Selenium, lycopene, alpha-tocopherol, beta-carotene, retinol, and subsequent bladder cancer," *Cancer Res.* 49 (1989): 6144–6148.
51. *Ibid.*
52. Mayne, "Dietary retinol," 443–450.
53. *Ibid.*
54. D.J. Hunter, J.E. Manson, G.A. Colditz, M.J. Stampfer, B. Rosner, et al., "A prospective study of the intake of vitamins C, E, and A on the risk of breast cancer," *New Engl. J. Med.* 329 (1993): 234–240.
55. *Ibid.*
56. Ziegler, "Vegetables, fruits, and carotenoids and the risk of cancer," 251S–259S.
57. Mayne, "Dietary retinol," 443–450.
58. Ziegler, "Vegetables, fruits, and carotenoids and the risk of cancer," 251S–259S.

59. G.R. Bunin, R.R. Kuijten, J.D. Buckley, L.B. Rorke, A.T. Meadows, "Relation between maternal diet and subsequent primitive neuroectodermal brain tumors in young children," *N. Engl. J. Med.* 329 (1993): 536–541.

60. *Ibid.*

61. J. VanEenwyk, F.G. Davis, N. Colman, "Folate, Vitamin C, and cervical intraepithelial neoplasia," *Cancer Epidemiol. Biomarkers Prev.* 1 (1992): 119–124.

62. *Ibid.*

63. E. Giovannucci, M.J. Stampfer, G.A. Colditz, E.B. Rimm, D. Trichopoulos, et al., "Folate, methionine, and alcohol intake and risk of colorectal adenoma," *J. Natl. Cancer Instit.* 85 (1993): 875–884.

64. *Ibid.*

65. G. Block, "Vitamin C and cancer prevention: the epidemiological evidence," *Am. J. Clin. Nutr.* 53 (1991): 270S–282S.

66. *Ibid.*

67. G.R. Howe, T. Hirohata, T.G. Hislop, J.M. Iscovich, J-M. Yuan, et al., "Dietary factors and risk of breast cancer: combined analysis of 12 case-control studies," *J. Natl. Cancer Instit.* 82 (1990): 561–569.

68. *Ibid.*

69. Hunter, "A prospective study of the intake of vitamins C, E, and A on the risk of breast cancer," 234–240.

70. *Ibid.*

71. *Ibid.*

72. VanEenwyk, "Folate, Vitamin C, and cervical intraepithelial neoplasia," 119–124.

73. *Ibid.*

74. Bunin, "Relation between maternal diet and subsequent primitive neuroectodinal brain tumors," 536–541.

75. Simon, *Staying well*, 161.

76. P. Knekt, A. Aromaa, J. Maatela, R.-V. Aaran, T. Nikkari, et al., "Vitamin E and cancer prevention," *Am. J. Clin. Nutr.* 53 (1991): 283S–286S.

77. Ibid.

78. R.M. Bostick, J.D. Potter, D.R. McKenzie, T.A. Sellers, L.H. Kushi, et al., "Reduced risk of colon cancer with high intake of Vitamin E: the Iowa Women's Health Study," *Cancer Res.* 53 (1993): 4230–4237.

79. *Ibid.*

80. *Ibid.*

81. *Ibid.*

82. M.P. Longnecker, J.-M. Martin-Moreno, P. Knekt, A.M.Y. Nomura, S.E. Schober, et al., "Serum alpha-tocopherol concentration in relation to subsequent colorectal cancer: pooled data from five cohorts," *J. Natl. Cancer Instit.* 84 (1992): 430–435.
83. *Ibid.*
84. Comstock, "Prediagnostic serum levels of carotenoids," 260S–264S.
85. *Ibid.*
86. M.S. Menkes, G.W. Comstock, J.P. Vuilleumier, K.J. Helsing, A.A. Rider, R. Brookmeyer, "Serum beta-carotene, Vitamins A and E, selenium, and the risk of lung cancer," *N. Engl. J. Med.* 315 (1986): 1250–1254.
87. S.J. London, E.A. Stein, I.C. Henderson, M.J. Stampfer, W.C. Wood, et al., "Carotenoids, retinol, and vitamin E and risk of proliferative benign breast disease and breast cancer," *Cancer Causes Cont.* 3 (1992): 503–512.
88. *Ibid.*
89. L. Le Marchand, L.R. Wilkens, J.H. Hankin, N.J. Haley, "Dietary patterns of female nonsmokers with and without exposure to environmental tobacco smoke," *Cancer Causes Control* 2 (1991): 11–16.
90. *Ibid.*
91. Shibata, "Dietary beta-carotene, cigarette smoking, and lung cancer in men," 207–214.
92. *Ibid.*
93. Bostick, "Reduced risk of color cancer with high intake of Vitamin E," 4230–4237.
94. Giovannucci, "Intake of fat, meat, and fiber in relation to risk of colon cancer in men" 2390–2397.
95. Steinmetz, "Vegetables, fruits, and cancer. II," 427–442.
96. B.N. Ames, "Dietary carcinogenogens and anticarcinogens: oxygen radicals and degenerative diseases," *Science* 211 (1983): 1256–1264.

8

····································

RADIATION AND CANCER

Radiation is probably the most widely recognized and intensively studied of all causes of cancer. The last days of World War II, and the Cold War that followed, made everyone very aware of the damaging potential of radiation. Yet the level of understanding of radiation by most people is strikingly poor. Radiation is harmful because it can interact with the atoms of any material that is irradiated. If the radiation is energetic enough, it will cause electrons to be ejected from irradiated atoms, in a process called ionization. The ejected electrons can then interact with other atoms to produce highly reactive chemicals called free radicals. If radiation is even more highly energetic, it can interact directly with the atomic nucleus, so that the nucleus of the atom itself is broken down into ionized particles. If human tissue is exposed to radiation, the major damage to the cells is usually caused indirectly, by ionized particles, rather than directly by the radiation itself.

WHAT IS THE ACTUAL CANCER RISK
FROM RADIATION?

The clearest data available on the relationship between radiation exposure and cancer induction in humans have come from a thorough follow-up of Japanese survivors of the atomic bomb blasts.[1] About 227,000 men, women, and children who lived in either Hiroshima or Nagasaki at the time of the attack, and who survived the atomic blast, were enrolled in a study to determine the effects of high-dose radiation. These people have been followed ever since, and data on cancer mortality were analyzed in 1982, so in some cases there is 37 years of follow-up data. These data have been used to calculate the increased risk of dying from various cancers for persons exposed to 1 Gray of radiation, as compared to unexposed persons. A Gray is a unit used to describe the amount of energy absorbed per unit volume of tissue. For comparison, the total exposure to radiation occurring during radiotherapy is typically in the range of 30 to 60 Gray,

152

with radiation often fractionated into many small exposures of 1.5 to 2.5 Gray each. But there is a major difference between radiation exposure during radiotherapy and the radiation exposure received by atomic bomb survivors, in that radiotherapy involves exposure of a very small portion of the body to radioactivity, while atomic bomb survivors usually received whole-body exposures.

The most striking effect of whole-body irradiation is an increased mortality from leukemia. The relative risk of dying from leukemia was increased nearly four-fold among bomb survivors exposed to 1 Gray radiation.[2] Leukemia incidence reached a peak only five to seven years after radiation exposure, which is an extremely short time for cancer induction. At its peak incidence, the relative risk of leukemia was nearly 10-fold higher than in an unexposed group of Japanese, but the annual incidence rate of leukemia has been dropping progressively since the early 1950s. At present, the annual relative risk of leukemia among atomic bomb survivors is still elevated two-fold with respect to a normal population. Thus, for unknown reasons, cells that form blood are more prone to malignancy after radiation exposure than are other cells in the body. In fact, 56% of all leukemia deaths among persons exposed to at least 0.01 Gray can be attributed to radioactivity.

Between 1945 and 1982, relative mortality from all other cancers combined was elevated about 30% in bomb survivors with respect to an unirradiated group of people.[3] Radiation was responsible for excess mortality from cancers of the esophagus, stomach, liver, lung, breast, colon, ovary, bladder, and kidney, as well as from multiple myeloma. The greatest increases in risk (after leukemia) were seen for the bladder, where the relative risk of cancer was 1.8-fold higher than normal, the breast (1.7-fold higher risk), and the ovary (1.5-fold higher risk). Women suffered a greater risk of these cancers than did men: for all cancers except leukemia, the relative risk of cancer from radiation was increased 11% in men and 25% in women.[4] However, radiation was unrelated to cancers of the brain, gall bladder, pancreas, rectum, uterus, prostate, kidney, and liver, nor was it responsible for lymphoma.[5]

Nearly 23% of all cancers of the bladder could be directly attributed to the single radiation exposure that most atomic bomb survivors experienced.[6] A very strong relationship exists between the total radiation dose and the relative risk of bladder cancer. The relative risk of bladder cancer has increased slightly with time, indicating that this is a slow-growing tumor and that malignancy may not develop for many years after radiation exposure.

About 22% of all breast cancers among atomic bomb survivors could be directly attributed to the radiation exposure.[7] Breast cancer incidence increased strikingly among Japanese women exposed to radiation, particularly if radiation exposure occurred at less than 30 years of age. For women exposed to whole-body radiation at a young age, breast cancer mortality increased by 70% with respect to unirradiated Japanese women. The risk of radiation-induced breast cancer increased with decreasing age at exposure, and even children less than 10 years old at radiation exposure suffered a higher risk of breast cancer.[8] All of these estimates of increased mortality from radiation exposure are subject to a certain amount of error. Estimates are based on a 37-year follow-up of the atomic bomb survivors; if certain cancers induced by radiation take longer than 37 years to develop, then incidence of these cancers would be underestimated.

The accepted criterion for determining whether a particular agent causes cancer is determining if a dose-response relationship exists between exposure to that agent and cancer incidence. For example, if radiation causes cancer, one would expect persons exposed to high levels of radiation to have a higher incidence of cancer than persons exposed to low levels of radiation. This dose-response relationship has been clearly shown for leukemia in the Japanese bomb survivors, for all cancers combined (excluding leukemia), and for cancers of the breast. However, these dose-response calculations are open to question; clearly, the response is known, since a thorough follow-up of Japanese survivors has revealed response in great detail. But the initial dose level cannot be known in detail, because there was no way to measure radiation exposure at the time. Therefore, any dose calculations were done after the fact and have relied on complex theoretical models of expected yield of radiation from detonation of the bombs and on approximations of the average radiation exposure for persons near those detonations. These calculations are complicated by the fact that the bomb dropped on Hiroshima was unlike anything ever used since, whereas the bomb dropped on Nagasaki was more like modern atomic weapons. In addition, dose calculations must take into account meteorological and topographical features unique to the two cities. If any of these assumptions or calculations is incorrect, then all of the dose-response calculations derived from the Japanese atomic bomb survivors could be incorrect.

Recently, evidence has come to light suggesting that calculations of the past radiation exposure for Japanese atomic bomb survivors may be somewhat in error. A substantial number of measurements of residual radioactivity at or near the center of the Hiroshima bomb blast have found higher-than-predicted levels of radioactivity.[9] This suggests that the earlier calculations may have underestimated neutron exposures for people at a distance greater than one kilometer from the hypocenter. This distance is, of course, more relevant for survivors, since persons at less than one kilometer from the bomb blast were likely to be killed immediately. The latest calculations suggest that exposure to low-energy neutron radiation may have been two- to 10-fold higher than previously predicted.[10] At present, no easy way is available to resolve this discrepancy, so an effort has been made to determine the radiation dose-response elsewhere—to confirm or refute the Japanese data.

Independent characterization of the relationship between radiation and risk has been made by examining the cancer mortality of groups of people exposed to various sources of radiation. For example, patients exposed to radiation during treatment for tuberculosis have been monitored over time to determine their cancer risk.[11] In the past, treatment for tuberculosis involved injecting air into the thorax, in the space around the lungs, to collapse one lung and force lung tissue away from the chest wall. This was typically done while the lungs were imaged with fluoroscopy, a medical imaging technique that involves exposure to X-rays. This procedure was often repeated two to three times a month over several years, so that the cumulative radiation exposure could be quite high. However, in this case, radiation exposure differed from the exposure to atomic bomb survivors, since patients undergoing fluoroscopy received many small doses, while the atomic bomb survivors received one massive dose. In any case, a total of 6,285 tuberculosis patients from Massachusetts, all of whom were treated with lung collapse and fluoroscopy between 1925 and 1954, were studied in 1986. These patients had been examined by X-ray fluoroscopy an average of 77 times each, and their cancer incidence was measured an average of 25 years after treatment. The average radiation exposure for these patients was calculated to be 0.75 Gray (Gy) for the breast, 0.84 Gy for the lung, 0.80 Gy for the esophagus, and 0.09 Gy for the bone marrow. Overall, these patients were no more likely to die of all cancers combined than any group of unexposed persons. However, when cancer mortality at specific sites was studied, a different picture emerged.

Female patients who received fluoroscopy were 1.4-fold more likely to develop breast cancer, with the greatest risk occurring at a point 20 to 29 years after radiation exposure.[12] Young women were at greater risk than older women, and a clear dose-response relationship was shown between radiation exposure and breast cancer. The excess relative risk of breast cancer in this study was 57% per Gray of exposure, which compares well with the estimate of breast cancer risk among atomic bomb survivors, for whom excess risk was 63% per Gray. Thus the breast is apparently one of the organs most sensitive to the carcinogenic effect of radiation. Male patients who received fluoroscopy were 4.2-fold more likely to develop bone cancer and 2.2-fold more likely to develop cancer of the oral cavity.

Male and female patients combined were 2.1-fold more likely to develop cancer of the esophagus, with the greatest risk occurring during the first 10 years.[13] If risk was calculated for the 10 years after exposure to radiation, these patients were 7.5-fold more likely than normal to develop esophageal cancer, but risk returned to near-normal levels by 20 years after treatment. Risk of leukemia or lung cancer was not significantly increased by exposure of these patients to X-ray fluoroscopy. Despite a rather high radiation dose to the lungs, ranging up to 8 Gy in some patients, there was no evidence of a dose-response relationship between radiation exposure and lung cancer risk. This is in contrast to past studies, which showed an increase in risk of lung cancer following radiation to the thorax. These results suggest that exposure to fractionated radiation, or radiation that is given in multiple small doses, is not as harmful as single exposures, even when the total radiation dose is the same.[14] This is good news for cancer patients, because cancer patients who receive radiation therapy usually receive fractionated radiation.

Another approach to investigating the relationship between radiation exposure and cancer risk has been to study cancer mortality among groups of people exposed to radiation because of their occupation. For example, a large study determined the causes of mortality in a group of 8,318 men who worked at Oak Ridge National Laboratory, Tennessee, between 1943 and 1972.[15] These men were followed through 1984, at which time a total of 1,524 men had died of various causes. Relatively low overall mortality was found in this group of men, compared to that of the general population in the United States. This is not a surprise since men at Oak Ridge tended to be better educated and more affluent than average, and education and affluence both reduce cancer risk in the population at large. However, the mortality from leukemia specifically was 1.6-fold higher than expected. Among workers who had been monitored for potential internal contamination with radioactivity, the leukemia risk was 2.2-fold higher than normal. After controlling for the effects of age and other variables, radiation was found to be responsible for a substantial elevation in cancer risk. The elevation in cancer risk only became apparent 20 or more years after radiation exposure, as an earlier study of the same group of men in 1977 failed to find any relationship between radiation and cancer risk.[16]

A rather frightening aspect of this analysis is that the dose-response estimates reported for Oak Ridge are about an order of magnitude higher than those reported for the atomic bomb survivors.[17] This discrepancy suggests that there may be racial differences in radiation response, a possibility that could call into question the general utility of the dose-response estimates derived from Japanese survivors. However, neither the dose-response estimates calculated for Oak Ridge nor those of the

Japanese atomic bomb survivors should be accepted at face value. Calculating radiation dose-response retrospectively is extremely difficult, because it amounts to reconstructing the entire radiation exposure history for scores of individuals. Such reconstruction is based on the average radioactivity present, the average duration and degree of contact with that radiation, and the resulting average exposure. Needless to say, these calculations are fraught with potential sources of error. What is most important is that all studies agree that radiation is a potent carcinogen and most studies agree as to which tissues are most at risk of radiation damage. Ultimately the only way to resolve any discrepancies between the various studies is to repeat the analysis with other groups of people in order to converge on the correct answer.

Another recent study investigated the relationship between radiation and cancer risk by studying mortality of workers in the British atomic weapons industry.[18] A total of 95,217 workers, 92% of whom were male, were followed from their date of employment until 1988. The follow-up period for these workers was rather short (less than 15 years on average) compared to the follow-up period for atomic bomb survivors. Furthermore, the average worker was only 44 years old at the close of the study, so their rate of mortality from cancer should be low compared to a group of older persons. Nevertheless, this study enrolled a large number of people, and data on their radiation exposure were far more detailed and precise than the radiation exposure data available for most other studies (including the atomic bomb survivors). Of the original workers in the study, 91% were alive at the end of the study, while another 7% had died of various causes by 1988. Overall, mortality of these workers was 15% lower than expected for such a large group, and mortality from cancer specifically was 14% lower than expected. Mortality from all cancers including leukemia was either lower than normal or no different from normal, except for mortality from thyroid cancer, which was three-fold higher than normal. Even among workers first exposed to radiation 30 years in the past, the mortality rate was less than expected. The unexpectedly low mortality rate is probably attributable to the fact that professional workers generally have a lower mortality rate than non-professional workers, presumably as a result of better health habits, better health care access, or both. When the dose-response was calculated for radiation-exposed workers, only leukemia was found to increase with increasing radiation exposure. However, cancers described as "ill-defined or secondary neoplasms" also increased with radiation dose. This is worrisome because it implies that radiation may be associated with particularly aggressive cancers whose origin is hard to determine. The risk estimates for all cancers, and for leukemia specifically, are strikingly similar to the risk estimates derived from study of the atomic bomb survivors, implying that the earlier risk estimates are reasonably accurate. This is very reassuring, since modern radiation safety standards are usually based on the atomic bomb survivor data.[19]

The warming of relations between the West and Eastern Bloc countries may provide a windfall of data on cancer risk from low-level radiation.[20] An area of what was once East Germany, between Dresden and Plauen in the Ore Mountains, was a major site of uranium mining and processing for the Soviet nuclear weapons program. This area suffered terrible pollution, as more than 500 million tons of chemical and low-level radioactive waste was spread over an area of only 1,200 square kilometers. Meticulous medical records were kept for over 450,000 uranium miners and workers in a "yellow cake" factory (where uranium ore was processed). These records, recently brought to light by a courageous young German technician, may help answer questions about the risk of cancer from low-level chronic radiation exposures. These records could also settle questions about gender or racial differences in cancer susceptibility after radiation exposure and to what extent radiation exposure interacts with exposures to various toxic chemicals.

Records kept by the German uranium mining companies indicate that nearly 21,000 miners have already died from lung disease induced by radiation or toxic dust.[21] About 15,000 of these people died from silicosis, a deterioration of the lungs brought on by chronic exposure to inhaled dust. Another 6,000 have died from a form of lung cancer associated with radiation exposure. It is projected that new lung cancer cases will continue to be diagnosed for years to come, and that eventually as many as 15,000 more lung cancer cases may be diagnosed. A complete analysis of this data has not been completed, but the German government has funded research to examine the data. Files have been found for many of the 450,000 workers, and most of the files include results from medical exams, lung X-rays, and hospital stays. There are even autopsy reports and preserved samples of lung tissue from those who died of lung cancer. It will be nearly a decade before this mountain of data is fully analyzed, but researchers may then be able to accurately calculate risk for chronic low-level radiation exposures.

At present, the dose-response relationship between radiation exposure and cancer induction is known only for people exposed to high levels of radiation. Although several studies have determined the cancer risk associated with exposure of small tissue volumes to radiation, or with exposure of tissue to repeated small doses of radiation, the risk associated with low levels of radiation is generally very poorly understood. For example, a thorough study of thyroid cancer risk after childhood X-ray exposure has shown a dose-response relationship for this organ. If cancer incidence is plotted against the cumulative radiation dose to the thyroid, a clear dose-response relationship is seen. However, these data are for radiation exposures of between 1 and 7 Gray, and little or no data are available for exposures of less than 0.1 Gray. When the dose-response data are plotted, radiation exposures above 1 Gray form a line, which implies that cancer risk increases linearly with exposure and that there is no threshold of exposure below which radiation is harmless. However, it is also possible that there is a threshold effect, so that little or no risk is incurred from very low levels of exposure. We simply do not have enough high-quality data at low levels of exposure to settle the question of whether or not such a threshold exists. This is a nagging issue, not only in radiation exposure, but in other types of carcinogen exposure as well.

COMMON SOURCES OF RADIATION EXPOSURE

For most people, there are relatively few ways in which exposure to radiation can occur. Natural sources of radiation make up about 87% of the average person's radiation exposure; the most abundant source of natural exposure is radon gas leaching from the soil.[22] Radon alone accounts for 47% of the total exposure to radiation. The remaining sources of natural exposure to radiation include exposure to: gamma rays (14% of total), consumption or inhalation of radioactive particles (12%), cosmic rays from space (10%), and thoron in soil (4%).

Artificial or man-made sources of radiation exposure account for only 13% of the average total radiation exposure.[23] These sources include exposure to diagnostic medical radiation (12% of total), exposure to radioactive fallout (0.4%), occupational exposure to radiation (0.2%), or miscellaneous exposures (0.4%).[24] For most people, exposure to medical radiation sources is by far the most important source of exposure to artificial radiation. Recently, concerns have been raised that irradiation of food (to prevent spoilage) may result in radiation exposure for people who consume the sterilized food. However, all indications suggest that food irradiation does not induce any significant level of radioactivity in food and that irradiated food is not a significant risk factor for any cancers.[25]

RADON EXPOSURE

Radon is an odorless, tasteless, colorless gas that is not actually absorbed by the body.[26] However, radon gas can decay into "radon daughters," which are solid particles that emit radioactivity as they undergo further decay, and these particles can be deposited in the lungs. If an abundance of radon gas is confined to a space such as a mine or basement, then radon daughter particles can accumulate to relatively high concentrations. If these particles are inhaled and deposited in the lungs, they can expose the lung surface to a fairly high local radiation dose.

To investigate the relationship between exposure to radon and subsequent mortality from lung cancer, a large retrospective study was undertaken.[27] Participants in this study were former miners from the Radium Hill uranium mine, which operated in South Australia from 1952 until 1961. A total of 2,574 workers, all of whom had been exposed to radon gas in the mineshaft, were identified from mine records. The extent of exposure to radon was estimated from historical records of radon gas concentrations in the mine and from individual job histories. Exposures of these miners were generally low by comparison with other mines of the same period, since workers tended to work an average of only seven months. Only about two-thirds of the total group of miners could be located again in 1987, so the follow-up was long but not very complete. However, among those miners traced until the end of 1987, lung cancer mortality was increased 194-fold compared to the Australian national population during the same period. This high level of mortality may be somewhat misleading, because the incidence of smoking among miners was much higher than among the rest of the Australian population. Nevertheless, when miners were compared with surface workers at the same mine, lung cancer mortality was still markedly higher among miners exposed to radon for more than 40 months. Although smoking and other variables were largely comparable between miners and surface workers, miners had an incidence of lung cancer that was 5.2-fold higher. These results suggest strongly that radon exposure can be a potent lung carcinogen and support current moves toward more stringent radiation control in the workplace. Nevertheless, it is not clear from this study to what extent tobacco and radon interact, and whether significant risk attaches to the lower levels of radon found in most homes.[28]

The first clear indication that radon gas interacts with smoking to increase cancer risk came from a study of uranium miners exposed to high levels of radon.[29] A total of 383 cases of lung cancer in uranium miners were studied, and 93% of the case individuals were smokers. Among miners exposed to very high levels of radon, there was a 22% excess of lung cancer among smokers, while non-smokers had a lung cancer incidence 69% lower than expected. Lung cancers developed in smoking miners at lower levels of radon exposure than in non-smoking miners. This clearly indicates an interactive effect between the two carcinogens, but it also shows that cigarette smoking plays the dominant role in causing lung cancer.[30]

Under certain circumstances, radon gas alone is a potent lung carcinogen, even without an interaction with cigarette smoke.[31] A study of lung cancer mortality among non-smoking uranium miners found that lung cancer rates were much higher in men exposed to radon than among other non-smokers. A sample of 516 men, all of whom had never smoked, was selected from a total of 4,138 men who had mined uranium on the Colorado Plateau. These non-smokers were followed from 1950 through 1984, and their mortality was compared to that of control men. Overall, lung cancer mortality rate was 12.7-fold higher than expected for non-smokers, and a crude dose-response relationship was found. This confirms that exposure to radon daughters is a potent carcinogen even in the absence of smoking. But miners exposed to low levels of radon gas experienced no increase in lung cancer mortality, even though these men cumulatively experienced radon levels more than 4,000-fold higher than the typical homeowner's cumulative exposure to radon.[32]

Some uranium miners are believed to have been exposed transiently to radon levels 10,000-fold higher than the radon levels in a typical home.[33] Because of the discrepancy between dose levels experienced by miners and dose levels experienced by almost everyone else, the Environmental Protection Agency has little solid evidence to prove that exposure to typical domestic levels of radon poses a significant lung cancer risk. Moreover, the radon level varies enormously from place to place in homes in the United States, and there is even variation from house to house within an area. Houses that are weather-sealed to minimize heating and cooling costs tend to have higher levels of radon gas, especially if the house is built in an area of granitic rock formations containing trace uranium (e.g., Maine and Pennsylvania).[34]

Very recently a study in Sweden explored the link between lung cancer and chronic exposure to the levels of radon typical of a home.[35] This study compared 1,360 men and women diagnosed with lung cancer and 2,847 healthy men and women. Cases and controls were chosen from 109 different towns across Sweden, and towns were selected so that about half had a high natural abundance of radon, while half had a low natural abundance of radon. Each person in the study answered a questionaire that probed smoking habits, occupation, and personal and family medical history. In addition, questions were asked about potential residential exposures to radon; each individual was required to list his or her residential addresses since 1947, and questions were asked about the type of house, the building materials used, the heating system, the amount of time spent at home, and so on. Then researchers actually went to the listed addresses and measured radon levels in 8,992 residences. In each of the residences, sophisticated radon monitors were placed in the bedroom and in the living room, for at least three months during the heating season. The monitors were able to accurately measure and record residential radon levels, so that cumulative radon exposures since 1947 could be estimated for both cases and controls. The researchers were able to make measurements in about 73% of all the residences listed, so a good basis for comparison between cases and controls was established.

The risk of lung cancer was found to increase with increasing radon exposure, even though the cumulative radon levels experienced by subjects were much lower than for miners.[36] Persons experiencing an approximately average level of radon exposure were no more likely to get lung cancer than those at the lowest level of exposure, but persons at the highest level of exposure were nearly twice as likely to develop lung cancer. There was also a very powerful interaction between smoking and radon exposure, such that a smoker experiencing an average level of radon was about six-fold more likely to develop lung cancer than a non-smoker. Since risk increased with both radon exposure and numbers of cigarettes smoked, some of the smokers were at a much higher risk of lung cancer. For example, an individual in the upper quartile (25%) of radon exposure who also smoked more than 10 cigarettes per day was at an 11.8-fold higher risk of cancer. By comparison, a former smoker experiencing the same radon exposure was at a 3.2-fold higher risk of lung cancer, while non-smokers did not have an elevated lung cancer risk at all.

Radon levels varied over an extremely broad range in Swedish homes.[37] The average level of radon measured in 8,992 Swedish residences was 2.9 picoCuries of radiation per liter of air, yet the highest level recorded was 63-fold higher. About 2% of the subjects chronically experienced an average radon exposure more than 138-fold higher than average, and these people had a dramatically elevated risk of lung cancer. For non-smokers experiencing a mean residential radon exposure greater than 10.8 picoCuries of radiation per liter of air, lung cancer risk was 1.2-fold higher than normal. But for light smokers (< 10 cigarettes per day) at the same level of radon exposure, lung cancer risk increased to 25.1-fold higher than normal, while heavy smokers experienced a 32.5-fold higher risk. These data suggest that radon exposure can be an important cause of lung cancer, especially among smokers.

Nevertheless, these results must be kept in perspective. Radon has clearly been shown to be the second leading cause of lung cancer after smoking,[38] yet this is not very compelling, since tobacco is by far the most important cause of lung cancer. About 90% of all lung cancers are caused by tobacco smoke, so arguing about the second leading cause of lung cancer is almost gratuitous. Smokers should be far more worried about their smoking habit than about their radon exposure, and most non-smokers probably don't need to worry. Checking levels of radon in your home may be wise, especially in certain parts of the country, to make sure that your home is not one of the few in which radon levels are extremely high. Beyond that, the best advice is to stop smoking. Tobacco smoke is a potent carcinogen in itself, but there are also naturally occurring radioactive particles in tobacco that are inhaled by the smoker, and these may be carcinogenic by the same mechanism as radon gas itself. A smoker inhales about 77% more radioactivity in a year than does a non-smoker, so a substantial amount of radioactivity is inhaled in tobacco smoke.[39]

MEDICAL RADIATION EXPOSURES

In the United States, about 80% of all exposure to man-made sources of ionizing radiation comes from medical X-rays.[40] The relationship between cancer and the low doses of radiation used for diagnostic purposes is controversial, but evidence exists that diagnostic irradiation of the trunk can be associated with an increased risk of at least one form of leukemia (chronic myelogenous leukemia or CML). This is very worrisome, because the use of diagnostic radiation is increasing steadily in the United States. In fact, several scientists believe that up to 16% of all leukemias in the United States are caused by diagnostic radiation,[41] although this figure is not widely accepted.

A very clear example of human cancer caused by diagnostic radiation is seen in the case of Thoratrast and liver cancer.[42] Thoratrast is a chemical, used during the 1930s and 1940s in North America, Europe, and Japan, that was injected into patients about to undergo X-ray exams. Thoratrast improved image contrast, so that it was easier to see certain structures in an X-ray image, but Thoratrast is also radioactive. It accumulates in the liver, spleen, and bone marrow, where it remains for decades, all the while emitting radioactivity. A study, initiated in Denmark in 1949, followed more than 1,000 patients who received an injection of Thoratrast prior to imaging of the brain. The cumulative risk for all cancers reached 86% at 50 years, meaning that 86% of all individuals who received Thoratrast developed cancer within 50 years. The relative risk of liver cancer was elevated 126-fold with respect to normal, while the risk of leukemia was elevated 10-fold. Thoratrast injection also caused a 14-fold increase in cancer of the gall bladder, a 12-fold increase in risk of metastatic cancer, a nine-fold increase in cancer affecting the lining of the abdominal cavity, and a five-fold increase in multiple myeloma. This is a very clear indication that even low-level radiation can be a significant risk factor for a range of different cancers, given a long enough time of radiation exposure.[43]

However, the Thoratrast example does not prove that exposure to the low levels of radiation typically used in modern diagnostic imaging procedures is a risk factor for cancer. To determine the risk associated with modern diagnostic imaging, a study compared the radiation exposure of a group of leukemic patients to that of a control group of healthy persons.[44] A total of 136 case patients with CML were compared to a control group of similar age and background. During the time period from three to 20 years prior to diagnosis of CML, more cases than controls had an X-ray examination of the trunk, and cases were much more likely to have had multiple X-ray exams. In fact, persons who had five or more radiographic examinations were 12-fold more likely to develop CML than normal. The risk of developing CML increased with the total radiation exposure, so that a person receiving at least 2 rads of radiation had more than double the risk of developing CML. Radiation caused the most significant increase in CML six to 10 years after exposure, and there was a trend of increasing risk with increasing radiation dose.[45]

However some contradictory evidence exists that suggests that risk of leukemia and lymphoma is not strongly linked to X-ray exposure.[46] A total of 565 patients diagnosed with leukemia (all types), 318 patients diagnosed with lymphoma, and 208 patients with multiple myeloma (another immune system cancer), were compared to 1,390 healthy controls. Patients and controls together had undergone a total of more than 25,000 X-ray procedures, or an average of more than 10 exams each. Comparison of patients and controls showed that patients were more likely to have undergone an X-ray exam in the recent past, probably to diagnose conditions related to their cancer. If these recent exams were excluded, patients were only slightly more likely to have had X-ray exams in the past. Earlier X-ray exposure raised the relative risk of leukemia by 17%, but here there was no evidence of a dose-response relationship between X-ray exposure and leukemia. This suggests that diagnostic X-ray procedures are at least not a major risk factor for leukemia or lymphoma.[47]

Another recent study purports to show that dental X-ray examinations are a risk factor for cancers of the brain.[48] Researchers interviewed 168 men between the ages of 25 and 69 years, all of whom had previously been diagnosed with a brain glioma, and these cases were compared to 177 matched healthy men who served as controls. Men who had undergone full-mouth X-rays after the age of 25 were found to be at a somewhat greater risk of glioma, and risk seemed to increase with dose. Men who were examined by X-ray at intervals longer than five years did not have an increased risk of glioma, but men who were examined once a year were at a three-fold higher glioma risk. This elevation in risk was actually not significant in a statistical sense, given the small sample size, but the trend toward increasing risk with increasing radiation exposure was significant.[49] However, these results must be taken with a grain of salt: clearly, a man with a brain tumor is likely to be searching for causes of his misfortune and may be more likely to remember an event such as a dental X-ray examination. A relatively small number of men were studied, and a statistically weak relationship was found between radiation exposure and brain tumor risk. Therefore, even though these results are consistent with the biases and expectations of many, they are simply not very convincing.

These contradictory results emphasize how difficult it is to calculate an accurate dose-response curve when the doses are all in the past and the responses are all in the present. This problem is common to virtually every study of radiation carcinogenesis, and it is likely to be a particularly acute problem when small numbers of subjects are studied. Both this and the previous study had small sample sizes, and both studies were done retrospectively (rather than prospectively). For these reasons, neither of the last two studies is definitive. However, although we do not know whether diagnostic X-rays are a cause of cancer, we know very well that therapeutic X-ray exposure can be a significant cause of cancer.

Patients who received therapeutic radiation to the spine for treatment of ankylosing spondylitis, a type of arthritis that affects the spine, are much more likely to develop leukemia.[50] A total of 14,106 patients who received radiation treatment for ankylosing spondylitis between 1935 and 1954 were followed until 1983. There was a three-fold increase in the risk of leukemia, and the appearance of excess leukemias began in as little as two years after radiation exposure. Relative risk of leukemia peaked between 2.5 and 4.9 years after radiation exposure, which is an astonishingly short time. The risk of leukemia was elevated 12.5-fold over normal between 2.5 and 4.9 years after exposure, but risk declined sharply after that. However, leukemia risk was still elevated two-fold with respect to normal even 25 years after radiation exposure. Of the four major types of leukemia, risk was greatest for acute myeloid leukemia (AML), but risk was also elevated for acute lymphatic leukemia (ALL) and chronic myeloid leukemia (CML). Risk of chronic lymphatic leukemia (CLL) was not elevated by radiation exposure, a finding that is consistent with data from Japanese survivors of the atomic bomb.

Patients irradiated for ankylosing spondylitis also suffered an increase in risk of non-leukemia cancers.[51] Mortality from all cancers except leukemia increased 28% with respect to normal. However, closer inspection of the data shows that cancer risk increased up to 71% in the time period 10 to

12.4 years after radiation exposure. This suggests that radiation causes cancer after a relatively short lag period, and that if cancer incidence is examined 20 to 30 years after exposure, many people will already have died from radiation-induced cancer. Risk was highest for cancers of the spinal cord (relative risk (RR) increased 4.7-fold) and bone (RR up 3.0-fold) within the irradiated area. The risk of cancer of the esophagus was elevated more than two-fold even 25 years after radiation exposure, which implies that this cancer progresses very slowly. Between five and 25 years after exposure, the risk of cancers of the lung, breast, spinal cord, and immune system increased, which implies that these cancers also tend to progress slowly.[52]

A large international study examined the incidence of second cancers in women who received radiation therapy as treatment for cervical cancer.[53] A total of 182,040 women from eight countries were followed, and their cancer risk was compared to that of women in the general population of the various countries. Overall, there was a 9% increase in the incidence of cancer, with more than half of this increased incidence directly attributed to radiation. Risk of cancer was higher in organs close to the cervix, since radiation does not have an effect on tissues distant from the site of irradiation. The relative risk of cancer was elevated about 10% in organs close to the cervix, with the greatest risk affecting the bladder, rectum, uterus, ovary, small intestine, and bone. There was also a 30% increase in the incidence of leukemia, although this represents a smaller increase in risk than would be predicted on the basis of current radiation risk estimates. Interestingly, women who received radiation treatment for cervical cancer had a risk of breast cancer 30% lower than normal. This probably was caused by radiation damage to the ovaries, causing them to secrete less estrogen. Since estrogen is a major cause of breast cancer, radiation-induced underproduction of estrogen has a protective effect for the breast.[54]

A more recent study examined the risk of cancer in the contralateral breast after radiation therapy for breast cancer.[55] Breast cancer affects approximately one in nine women, and women with one breast cancer have a three-fold increase in risk of a second primary breast cancer. It is possible that radiation therapy for the first cancer actually increases the risk of a second breast cancer, because of accidental exposure of the opposite breast to radiation. Scientists studied the medical records of 41,109 women who developed breast cancer between 1935 and 1982 in Connecticut, and identified 655 women in whom a second breast cancer developed. The radiation exposure of these women was compared to that of 1,189 women from the same group who did not develop a second breast cancer. The dose of radiation to the opposite breast was estimated from records kept by the radiotherapist at the time of treatment. Women who developed a second breast cancer were found to have received on average 13% more radiation to the opposite breast than women who did not develop a second cancer. Women who were later diagnosed with a second breast cancer were exposed to more than 3 Gray of radiation, a substantial exposure. The relative risk of a second breast cancer was highest 10 to 14 years after radiation treatment, and risk was greatest for women who were young at the time of irradiation. Among women who survived at least 10 years after their first cancer, radiation treatment was responsible for a 33% increase in breast cancer risk. Radiation is thus responsible for a relatively small increment in risk, since breast cancer patients have a high risk of second breast cancers even in the absence of treatment. Less than 3% of all second breast cancers studied could be directly attributed to radiation treatment, and radiation treatment after the age of 45 entails little if any risk of radiation-induced breast cancer.[56]

However, radiation has also been used in treatment of benign breast disease, and here radiation can cause problems.[57] Since the rate of breast cancer among women with benign breast disease is not significantly higher than among women without benign disease, the effects of radiation are more clearly seen. Radiation was used in Sweden to treat benign breast conditions such as mastitis, a breast inflammation or infection common at childbirth (or later for women who breast-feed). A total of 1,216 women who received radiation therapy between 1925 and 1954 were compared to 1,874 women with benign breast disease who were not treated with radiation. The average radiation dose level for women in the treated group was 5.8 Gray, meaning that a substantial radiation dose was used for a relatively minor problem. The follow-up period for these women was up to 60 years after first exposure. Treated women were found to be 3.6-fold more likely to get breast cancer than women who did not receive radiation treatment. Risk increased with radiation dose, was higher for younger women, and remained elevated even 40 to 60 years after radiation exposure. Total radiation dose, age at first exposure, and time since first exposure were all major factors in determining breast cancer risk.[58]

An earlier study that also examined the risk of breast cancer after radiation therapy for mastitis found virtually identical results.[59] A total of 601 women who had been treated for mastitis with radiation during the 1940s and 1950s were followed for an average of 29 years. The relative risk for breast cancer was elevated 3.2-fold for the irradiated breast. Total radiation dose was the only important variable, as the number of separate doses, the number of days between treatments, or the dose per treatment had no effect on breast cancer risk. This is potentially an important finding, since modern therapeutic radiation is usually done in many separate small fractions in an effort to reduce radiation damage to normal tissue. This study of breast cancer risk following radiation treatment for mastitis may mean that radiation dose fractionation is ineffective in reducing radiation damage to the breast.[60] The study also confirms the importance of using low doses of radiation in mammographic examinations of the breast.

These various studies show clearly that therapeutic radiation can be a significant risk factor for cancer, and that diagnostic radiation may also be a risk factor, at least for leukemia. There has even been a suggestion that the cancer risk from radiation can be passed from one generation to the next. Results of a small study suggest that the offspring of women who underwent diagnostic radiation during pregnancy may suffer a higher incidence of childhood leukemia.[61] A total of 128 children with acute lymphoblastic leukemia (ALL) were studied, and these children were compared to 301 other children. In this small sampling, it was found that the relative risk of ALL was elevated 1.8-fold among children whose mothers had undergone an X-ray examination during pregnancy. There was also an effect of maternal smoking on risk of ALL, as the children of smoking mothers had a 2.2-fold higher risk of ALL. When smoking and maternal X-rays were combined, the relative risk of childhood ALL increased to 3.6 higher than normal.[62] However, these are very strong claims based on a very small sample size. Little or no information is given as to how women were irradiated, so determining the radiation dose to the fetus or the uterus is impossible. This is an important point, because it is very difficult to imagine why maternal irradiation should have an effect on the risk of ALL in offspring, unless the fetus was directly exposed to radiation. Even more difficult to imagine is a responsible radiologist irradiating a fetus, especially in the recent era of medical malpractice suits. Therefore, these results should be regarded more as a cautionary flag than as a real indication of risk.

Radiation-induced leukemia is a significant clinical problem for the cancer patient, since about 70% of all cancer patients receive radiotherapy at some point during their treatment. Therefore, treatment of a cancer can itself be carcinogenic, and can conceivably induce a second malignancy. While the risk of cancer induction from radiation therapy alone is thought to be low, combinations of radiation and chemotherapy have been linked to an increased incidence of AML and solid tumors in the radiation field. Several studies have shown that Hodgkin's lymphoma patients treated with radiation and chemotherapy together have a 5–10% increase in the risk of developing AML within 10 years of treatment.[63] Yet the advantages of radiation treatment for cancer generally far outweigh the disadvantages; if radiation is administered with care and caution, it remains one of the most effective therapies for cancer.

It should also be noted that, although radiation is a potent carcinogen for breast tissue, the radiation exposure typical of a mammographic examination is probably not a significant risk factor for breast cancer. Although an increased incidence of breast cancer was evident among Japanese atom bomb survivors, these women typically received large doses of radiation (0.10 to > 5.00 Gray) to the breast. High-quality mammograms can be obtained with a very low radiation dose (less than 0.01 Gray), so the level of breast cancer risk is correspondingly lower. Since mammography can definitely help in the diagnosis of breast cancer, and there is only an as-yet-unproven potential to induce breast cancer, the benefits appear to greatly exceed the risks.

OCCUPATIONAL EXPOSURE TO RADIATION

Occupational exposure to radiation is, on average, a minor source of exposure, as only about 0.2% of the average person's total exposure occurs at work. However, this figure incorporates data from many people who have no on-the-job radiation exposure whatsoever. For persons in certain occupations, actual occupational exposure to radiation is much higher than 0.2% of their total exposure. In fact, some of the earliest studies of radiation effects involved people who were exposed to very high levels of radiation while hand-painting luminescent dials on watch faces. Modern occupations that can entail significant radiation exposure include working at a nuclear defense plant, atomic waste disposal facility, or atomic energy generating station, uranium mining, and certain medical specialities such as radiology, radiation oncology, or medical research. We have already discussed several studies of cancer risk due to occupational exposure to radiation; some of these studies enrolled so many subjects that they were able to address general issues such as the dose-response relationship in radiation exposure. However, several other studies were designed to study cancer risks specific to a particular occupation.

For example, one study investigated cancer mortality among British doctors who entered the field of radiology at a time when less was known about radiation safety.[64] Due to carelessness or ignorance, many of these men were exposed to multiple doses of stray X-rays, particularly to their arms and hands. Men who joined the British Institute of Radiology or the Royal College of Radiologists between 1897 and 1954 were studied, and the sources of their mortality were analyzed. Men who entered these societies early are of particular interest because the first issuance of safety guidelines for the use of radioactivity did not occur until 1921. Radiologists prior to 1921 practiced at a time when safety precautions were often not taken, and when chronic exposure to moderately high levels of radiation was rather routine. Among radiologists practicing before 1921, the cancer mortality was 75% higher than that of other medical doctors. In particular, the risk of skin cancer was 7.8-fold higher, the risk of leukemia was 6.2-fold higher, the risk of pancreatic cancer was 3.2-fold higher, and the risk of lung cancer was 2.2-fold higher than the cancer risk of other similar men. Radiation did not cause an increased risk of cancer of the digestive tract (oral cavity, esophagus, stomach, liver, small intestine, or rectum), bone, or bone marrow, which suggests that most of the exposures involved radiation that was only weakly penetrating. For radiologists after 1921, the cancer risk was not significantly higher than that of other physicians. However, there was evidence suggesting that cancer risk increased among men who practiced radiology for a long time. Unfortunately, it was not possible to make accurate estimates of how much radioactivity these men were exposed to, since the cumulative whole-body radiation dose could have been anywhere between 1 and 5 Grays of radiation. Interestingly, the non-cancer mortality rate of radiologists was one of the lowest of all men in England and Wales. This may mean that physicians have a lower rate of premature death overall, or it may simply mean that fewer radiologists survived cancer long enough to die of other causes. Nevertheless, these findings do not support the idea that radiation causes a syndrome of rapid aging.[65]

EXPOSURE FROM LIVING NEAR A NUCLEAR POWER PLANT

The first suggestion that living near a nuclear power plant could constitute a risk factor for cancer came from a television news program about childhood leukemia in West Cumbria, England.[66] This program, first aired in 1983, claimed that there was an excess of leukemia near the Sellafield nuclear plant (also called Windscale) and that this excess might be caused by accidental release of radioactive materials from the power plant. To investigate this possibility, a study was undertaken in which 52 children with leukemia and 22 children with non-Hodgkin's lymphoma (NHL), all from West Cumbria, were compared to 1,001 children from the same area. It was found that the relative risk of leukemia and NHL was higher in children born near Sellafield. Children living within four kilometers of Sellafield had more than a five-fold higher risk of leukemia and NHL than children living farther than five kilometers from the nuclear plant. However, children whose fathers were employed at Sellafield at the time of conception were at a 2.4-fold higher risk of leukemia or NHL, and children of fathers who were accidently irradiated (5 mGy or more) were at a 6.4-fold higher risk of these cancers. This implies that the geographical association of cancer with Sellafield might really be explained on the basis of parental employment at Sellafield, since employees are more likely to live near the plant. The children's risk of leukemia increased directly with the fathers' dose of radiation during the six months prior to conception, and fathers who received more than 0.5 mGy of radiation had nearly a five-fold higher risk of having children with leukemia or NHL. These relationships could not be explained on the basis of X-ray exposure, maternal age or medical history, diet, or playing near the power plant. Therefore, physical proximity to the power plant is apparently not the problem. Rather, the high incidence of leukemia and NHL near Sellafield is attributable to the fathers' employment history. It has been proposed that exposure of the male reproductive organs to radiation somehow causes an increased incidence of leukemia in offspring, but there is also the possibility that leukemia was caused by inadvertant contamination of the home. These results are extremely controversial because no one can explain why exposure of one generation to radiation should be leukemogenic for the next generation. Furthermore, these results contradict an earlier study of 7,387 Japanese men, irradiated during the atomic bomb blasts, for whom no next generation increase of leukemia incidence was found.[67]

In light of the suggestion that living near a nuclear power plant could be a risk factor for cancer, a large study was also undertaken of persons living near nuclear power plants in the United States.[68] The mortality of persons living in 107 "case counties" with power plants was compared to the mortality of persons living in 292 "control counties" distant from power plants but in the same geographic areas as the case counties. A total of 900,000 cancer deaths between 1950 and 1984 in case counties were compared to 1.8 million cancer deaths in the same period in control counties. Deaths due to leukemia or other cancers were not more frequent in the case counties than in the control counties. If case counties were compared to control counties before a power plant started up, and then again after the power plant started up, there was also no significant difference. These findings suggest that simply living near a nuclear power plant is not a risk factor for cancer, even for childhood leukemia.[69] However, this study did not specifically address risk from a parent working at a power plant.

Another recent study confirms that no major cancer risk is incurred by living near a nuclear power plant.[70] The incidence of childhood cancers was studied in 20 areas near nuclear power plants in West Gernany, and these areas were compared to matched control areas. A computer record of childhood cancer in West Germany showed that 1,610 cases of leukemia were diagnosed in children less than 15 years old between 1980 and 1990. When the incidence of leukemia near power plants was compared to leukemia incidence far from power plants, no major difference was found. However, if the incidence of acute leukemia at less than five years of age was examined, or when lymphomas in particular were studied, there was a very slight excess of cases near nuclear power plants. It was also found that the incidence of cancer was higher in areas where nuclear power plants were planned but not yet built.[71] This implies that areas where nuclear power plants are sited are somehow inherently different from areas with no power plants. It may well be that industrialization itself is associated with childhood cancer, and that power plants are simply more likely to be built in industrialized areas where they are needed. Therefore, childhood cancer may not be due to the power plants, but rather to the economic conditions that made it worthwhile to build a power plant in a certain area. In any case, nuclear power plants were not found to be associated with any major increase in childhood cancer.

EXPOSURE FROM NUCLEAR FALLOUT

Surprisingly little effort has been devoted to studying the long-term health effects of fallout from nuclear weapons testing. When nuclear weapons are tested, substantial quantities of radioactive iodine can be produced, since iodine is a breakdown product of uranium and plutonium.[72] Radioactive iodine is relatively stable, so it can contaminate foods and enter the foodchain. Most of the iodine in the human body accumulates in the thyroid gland, so radioactive iodine can expose the thyroid gland specifically to relatively high doses of radiation. A recent study examined a group of 2,473 schoolchildren who had lived in communities near the Nevada Test Site between 1951 and 1958, and who were thus potentially exposed to fallout from nuclear tests. These children were sought out as adults in 1985 and 1986, so there was a period of follow-up that lasted between 27 and 35 years. Information was obtained by telephone interview from these subjects about their consumption of milk and vegetables during the fallout period. This information was combined with information from the Department of Energy on radioactive fallout rates to calculate an estimate of radiation exposure for each subject. This calculation was necessarily very crude, because it relied on recollections of diet 30 years in the past and because the figures provided by the Department of Energy would be an average, thus not specific to the fallout exposure of individuals. Radiation doses calculated in this way ranged between 0 and 4.6 Gray, so this spans a range of radioactivity comparable to that of many other studies. Children who lived in southwestern Utah, closest to the bomb test site, experienced an average exposure of 0.17 Gray—a fairly low level radiation exposure. Nevertheless, radioactive fallout was found to be associated with an increased incidence of thyroid cancer. For 169 individuals who had been exposed to more than 0.4 Gray of radiation, the risk of thyroid cancer was elevated 3.4-fold with respect to unexposed persons.[73] However, this study is weakened by the small number of affected individuals in the study and by the retrospective nature of the radiation dose calculations.

While this study does not provide definitive data on the cancer risk associated with radioactive fallout, neither does it provide a compelling reason to replicate the study with more subjects. We are therefore caught in a gray area; given the decline in funding for cancer research that we are now experiencing, this study is probably not high on the list of those that must be replicated. It is actually somewhat reassuring that fallout is associated with an increased incidence of only one cancer, given the cavalier manner in which personal risk was disregarded in the Cold War era.

EXPOSURE TO HIGH-VOLTAGE ELECTRICITY AS A RISK FACTOR

Over the past decade public awareness of cancer risks that may be associated with high-voltage electrical lines has greatly increased. These electrical lines create extremely low-frequency electric or magnetic fields (EMFs) which have been linked with several forms of cancer, particularly cancers affecting children.[74] For example, an early study reported an inordinately high incidence of high-voltage electrical lines near the homes of children who died of cancer. Since building materials effectively shield home occupants from electrical fields, it was suspected that magnetic fields around the electrical lines might be the culprit. However, home wiring and household applicances can create electrical fields, so it is presently unclear whether electric or magnetic fields are of greater importance. Nevertheless, several very recent studies have found evidence, albeit equivocal, suggesting that EMFs might be a risk factor for cancer.

One large study was undertaken in Finland, to investigate the risk of cancer in children living near overhead power lines.[75] A total of 68,300 boys and 66,500 girls were identified, all of whom were less than 19 years old in 1989, and all of whom lived within 500 meters of overhead power lines (110–400 kiloVolts). These children were identified by linking computerized data on power lines to a national register of buildings, which contains information on almost every building in Finland. Buildings located within 500 meters of a power line were identified, then all children who lived in those buildings between 1970 and 1989 were identified from census data. Because so many children were identified, the cohort included nearly a million person-years of risk factor exposure, or about 4% of the person-years lived by all Finnish children less than 19 years old during the study period. In other words, this study is so large that one would expect it to have great sensitivity to even very small increases in risk and to be able to accurately determine the magnitude of any risk factor identified.

The minimum level of power line voltage examined in this study was calculated to expose children to magnetic field densities of at least 0.01 microTeslas (μT), although only 5% of the children in the study experienced magnetic fields greater than 0.2 μT.[76] In the entire cohort of 134,800 children, only 140 cases of childhood cancer were identified, whereas statistically, 145 cases were expected. Among children exposed to less than 0.2 μT, there was no increase in risk of any cancer, including leukemia, lymphoma, or cancers of the brain and nervous system. For children exposed to more than 0.2 μT, there was still no significant increase in risk of leukemia and lymphoma, although there was an increase in risk of brain tumors among boys only (not girls). These results may have been confounded though, because three tumors were found in the same boy, and this boy suffered from neurofibromatosis, a hereditary condition that predisposes to the development of nervous system tumors. Therefore, one must conclude that EMFs from high-voltage power lines do not constitute a major public health problem.[77] Some caution must be exercised though, because this study included very few children who experienced magnetic field densities higher than 0.2 μT; it is still possible that exposure to extremely high magnetic fields is harmful.

Another very recent study conducted in Denmark seems to suggest that extremely high voltage levels in overhead power lines may indeed be a risk factor for cancer.[78] This study examined 1,707 case children under the age of 15, all of whom had been diagnosed with leukemia, lymphoma, or cancer of the nervous system, and compared these children with 4,788 healthy control children. EMF exposure of all cases and controls was determined by measuring the distance between their dwelling and the nearest high voltage line and by determining the average current carried by the power line in question. Children exposed to less than 0.4 μT of magnetic field density did not have a significantly higher risk of any cancer, consistent with the results of the study described above. However, children exposed to a magnetic field density greater than 0.4 μT had a 5.6-fold higher risk of childhood cancer, and specifically a higher risk of leukemia, lymphoma, and brain tumor. Furthermore, cases were far more likely than controls to have been exposed to magnetic field densities greater than 0.8 μT; in fact, none of the controls experienced an average exposure greater than 0.8 μT, while about 20% of cases experienced an average exposure of 1.6 μT. Nevertheless, this high level of exposure to EMF is exceedingly rare in the population at large, as only three out of 4,698 children in the control group were exposed to greater than 0.4 μT. A survey of Danish dwellings found that the average level of EMF is about 0.06 μT, or only about 15% of the EMF level associated with risk of childhood cancer. Therefore, while the risk of childhood cancer from extremely high levels of magnetic field density appears to be real, the proportion of childhood cancers caused by EMF is still probably very small.[79]

A connection has also been made between EMFs and brain cancer in adults. One study compared 226 German brain tumor patients with 418 control individuals from the same part of Germany.[80] Women employed as electrical workers were found to be five-fold more likely to have brain tumors than women working in other fields. This study was very problematic though, because men employed as electrical workers were no more likely than anyone else to have brain tumors. The number of women employed as electrical workers is quite small, so there is a possibility that this association between employment and brain cancer arose purely by chance. Furthermore, there is a very real problem associated with studying widely publicized cancer risk factors, in that memory bias is more likely to be a problem. If people are already aware that EMFs are implicated in brain cancer (as many electrical workers were in 1990), they are far more likely to remember relevant EMF exposures if they already have cancer than if they are still healthy. To add to the confusion, it is very difficult to objectively measure past exposure to EMFs, particularly in a profession such as electrical work, where transient exposure to very high EMF levels is possible.[81] Finally, in any study comparing cases with controls, the type of controls chosen is critical. In a study of cases, many of whom are employed as electrical workers, the best comparison might be to other electrical workers who did not get brain cancer. To compare ill electrical workers with healthy people in a broad spectrum of other professions does not seem valid, since electrical workers may be exposed to a whole range of carcinogens. But if cases and controls are both electrical workers, this comparison would be insensitive to EMFs as a cause of cancer, since both groups experience EMFs. Therefore, the choice of control subjects can have a major impact on the findings, and it is all too easy to choose an inappropriate control group.

Another recent study examined the risk of brain tumors among men in Los Angeles County.[82] A group of 272 men between the ages of 25 and 69, all of whom had been diagnosed with a brain tumor, were compared to a similar group of 272 healthy men from the same neighborhoods. It was found that a type of brain tumor called an astrocytoma is 1.8-fold more likely to affect men in occupations that involve exposure to high-level EMFs. A crude dose-response relationship was found, such that men who were exposed to high-level EMFs for less than five years had a risk level that was 1.4-fold higher than normal, while men who worked in these jobs more than five years had a risk level that was 1.8-fold higher than normal.[83] This study had many of the same flaws as the previous one: a minor risk factor for a rare cancer, identified in a small group of cases, simply cannot make a convincing case.

Exposure to EMF has also been implicated in the causation of breast cancer.[84] The rationale for this is basically that breast cancer risk is higher in industrialized countries, so something about industrialization may affect incidence of breast cancer. There has been a great deal of speculation that either EMFs or the background level of "light at night" (LAN) could be causative, perhaps operating through an influence on synthesis of the hormone melatonin. Frankly, there is something appealing about this argument; breast cancer incidence is strikingly higher in countries with high levels of EMF and LAN, and there is no other known reason for this association. However, one must be wary of ideas and theories unsupported by real data.

Most studies of cancer risk associated with EMFs have been highly controversial, and some of them have been badly flawed.[85] A real problem is that biologists can think of no reason whatsoever why EMFs should have a carcinogenic effect on cells, hence they are very reluctant to accept inconclusive data in the absence of firm theory. This may seem as though biologists are putting the cart of theory before the horse of data, but science today is done in an environment of diminishing resources. If either the theory or the data were strong, then EMFs would be a compelling research project. But with weak theory, weak data, and limited money for health research, scientists prefer to spend what money they have on projects that have a better chance of finding something useful. This is especially true since a government-sponsored panel of scientists (the Oak Ridge Associated Universities Panel on Health Effects of Low-Frequency Electric and Magnetic Fields) concluded in 1993 that, since there are "decreasing resources available for basic health and science research, we believe. . . . there are currently more serious health needs that should be given higher priority".[86]

INTERACTIONS BETWEEN RADIATION AND OTHER FACTORS

Radiation is thought to interact with relatively few other factors, because the mechanism by which radiation damages cells is quite different from the mechanisms by which most other carcinogens damage cells. However, recent evidence has come to light that an unusual hereditary condition can make certain people more sensitive to radiation damage.

Individuals with a condition called ataxia-telangiectasia (AT) are at an elevated risk of cancer.[87] This condition is transmitted by inherited genes such that, if a child inherits two copies of the gene from the parents, the child will get AT, whereas if the child inherits only one copy of the gene, the child is a disease carrier but does not develop symptoms. Persons with AT are at a higher risk for a range of cancers, including cancers of the breast, colon, rectum, lung, and prostate. However, persons who merely carry one gene for AT are also at higher risk for many of the same cancers, including breast cancer. A group of 1,599 persons who carry one AT gene was followed for more than six years, and the incidence of breast cancer among women in this group was 5.1-fold higher than in women who do not carry the gene.

To determine breast cancer risk factors for AT carriers, the sub-group of female carriers who developed breast cancer was closely studied.[88] Among 854 female AT carriers identified beforehand, only 19 women developed breast cancer, so the results of this study are weakened by the small number of affected women. Nevertheless, a comparison between AT carriers with breast cancer and AT carriers who did not develop breast cancer was instructive. Women with breast cancer were 5.8-fold more likely to have been exposed to radiation than women who did not develop breast cancer. This difference in exposure cannot really be translated into an estimate of the risk from radiation exposure, since this study was designed to identify risk factors, not quantify them. However, it is thought that between 9% and 18% of all breast cancer patients may be AT gene carriers. What this implies is that women who are AT carriers should stringently avoid radiation exposures such as chest X-rays or fluoroscopic examinations. There is probably no good reason to avoid mammographic exams, because the benefits of this test seem to outweigh the risks. Since AT gene carriers are at a higher risk of breast cancer anyway, early diagnosis of these cancers is a compelling consideration.[89] Unfortunately, no genetic tests are yet available to identify AT gene carriers who do not express the disease. However, an AT carrier must be a close blood relative of a patient diagnosed with AT and will probably be a member of a family that has been heavily affected by cancer.

TABLE 8-1
WEIGHTED RISK CALCULATIONS FOR RADIATION RISK FACTORS

RISK FACTOR	RELATED CANCER	RELATIVE RISK	RELATIVE FREQUENCY	WEIGHTED RISK
High radon (mines) x tobacco	Lung	194	5	970c
Thoratrast infusion	Liver	126	2	252b
High radon (home) x tobacco	Lung	32.5	5	163b
High radon (mines)	Lung	12.7	5	64b
Average radon (home) x tobacco	Lung	11.6	5	58b
Radiation x AT gene carrier	Breast	5.8	5	29b
Thoratrast infusion	Leukemia	10	2	20b
Mastitis therapy	Breast	3.4	5	17b
Thoratrast infusion	Gall bladder	14	1	14b
Whole-body irradiation	Leukemia	4.9 (1 Gy)	2	10a
Whole-body irradiation	Breast	2.0 (1 Gy)	5	10a
High radon (home)	Lung	1.8	5	9a
Spinal irradiation	Spinal cord	4.7	2	9b
Whole-body irradiation	Lung	1.5 (1 Gy)	5	8a
Whole-body irradiation	Bladder	2.1 (1 Gy)	4	8a
Whole-body irradiation	Colon	1.6 (1 Gy)	5	8a
Moderate radon (home)	Lung	1.3	5	7a
Repeated fluoroscopy	Breast	1.4	5	7a

RISK FACTOR	RELATED CANCER	RELATIVE RISK	RELATIVE FREQUENCY	WEIGHTED RISK
Whole-body irradiation	All cancers	1.4 (1 Gy)	5	7a
Breast radiation therapy	Breast	1.3	5	7b
Average radon (home)	Lung	1.1	5	6a
Exposure to EMF	Childhood cancer	5.6 (> 0.4 μT)	1	6a
Whole-body irradiation	Myeloma	2.9 (1 Gy)	2	6a
Spinal irradiation	Leukemia	3.2	2	6b
Whole-body irradiation	Ovary	1.8 (1 Gy)	2	4a
Repeated fluoroscopy	Bone	4.2	1	4b
Repeated fluoroscopy	Esophagus	2.1	2	4b
Maternal X-ray exam	Childhood leukemia	1.8	2	4c
High EMF levels	Brain	1.8	2	4c
Whole-body irradiation	Esophagus	1.4 (1 Gy)	2	3a
High-dose radioactive fallout	Thyroid	3.4	1	3b
Atomic weapons lab work	Leukemia	1.6	2	3b
Spinal irradiation	Bone	3.0	1	3b
High EMF levels	Leukemia	1.4	2	3c
Multiple X-rays	Leukemia	1.4	2	3c
Whole-body irradiation	Stomach	1.2 (1 Gy)	2	2a
Pelvic radiation therapy	Pelvic	1.1	2	2b
Living near nuclear plant	Leukemia	1.1	2	2c

Tabulated estimates of risk from whole-body exposure are based exclusively on the most recent estimates of radiation dosimetry.[93]

The only other significant interaction between radiation and another cancer risk factor is that between radon exposure and smoking. Given that both of these risk factors specifically affect cells lining the airways of the lungs, it should not be surprising that there is a strong synergy between radon and tobacco.

SUMMARY

If there is an excess cancer risk from the sundry sources of environmental radiation that we are routinely exposed to, that risk remains undetected by current methods.[90] But cosmic rays and gamma rays are so ubiquitous in the environment that it is impossible to find a control group not exposed to them. Similarly, we are all exposed to some level of radiation in the food we eat and the air we breathe. It has not been practical to assess the level of risk due to these environmental exposures because everyone suffers the same exposures.

On average, radon gas exposure seems to have relatively little effect on cancer risk except for lung cancer risk in smokers. Even for smokers, radon is a far less important risk factor than is smoking itself. Therefore, to minimize the risk from radon gas, the most effective measure is simply to quit smoking. Houses that are sited near mining areas, especially where uranium is mined, or with foundations sunk in granitic soil, should be tested for radon levels in the basement. If radon levels in the basement are high, then further testing is warranted in the rest of the house. Measures should also be taken to seal the basement from gas leaks and to vent gas from the soil beneath the basement. But if basement radon levels are low, then levels throughout the house will probably also be low.

Occupational exposure to radiation accounts for only 0.2% of the average person's exposure to radiation, so for most people this is not a concern. Clearly, someone who is routinely exposed to radiation on the job should do whatever possible to minimize this exposure, but for most people, there is not much scope for improvement here. Similarly, routine emissions from modern nuclear power plants and from weapons testing seem to add little to the overall cancer risk. Massive emissions of radiation, such as occurred at Chernobyl, are clearly a global health hazard, and every possible measure should be taken to ensure that this does not happen again. Many reactors in Eastern Europe are similar to the one at Chernobyl, and even the Chernobyl reactor is back on line, so diplomatic efforts are required to mitigate this potential source of risk. Even a vastly lower level of radiation release, such as occurred at Three Mile Island, is a potential health hazard, so careful regulation of the domestic nuclear industry is also necessary.

Since the effects of radiation on the body are cumulative, limiting radiation exposure whenever possible is sensible. But many types of radiation exposure are unavoidable, so the issue becomes, how can radiation exposure be limited? One practical way of limiting radiation exposure is to minimize diagnostic medical imaging. Diagnostic imaging that involves radiation exposure is already becoming less common, as computed tomographic (CT) scanning is gradually being replaced by magnetic resonance imaging (MRI).

It should also be possible to reduce radiation exposure in CT exams by reducing both the number of exams and the radiation dose delivered during each exam.[91] New guidelines for radiological exams have been issued in England, and these guidelines should result in a substantial reduction in the total number of radiological exams. Chest X-rays are suggested only for patients about to undergo cardiac or pulmonary surgery, or for patients with suspected cancer or tuberculosis. Chest X-rays should not be part of a routine physical at any age, and they should not be used for occupational screening. This latter is an important point, because in 1983, approximately 140,000 employment-related chest X-rays were done in England.

Mammographic exams are still recommended, especially for women over the age of 50, because the radiation exposure involved in a mammographic examination is quite low and the benefits almost certainly outweigh the risks. However, a skull film should not be routinely taken after head injury, but should be reserved only for cases in which skull fracture is suspected.[92] Any suspected injury or abnormality of the brain itself should be evaluated by MRI whenever possible, because MRI is far superior to CT for showing soft tissue pathology. Basically, radiologists should be prepared to justify each request for an examination involving radiation exposure, since there is a certain amount of risk involved in every exposure to ionizing radiation.

NOTES TO CHAPTER 8

1. D.L. Preston, H. Kato, K.J. Kopecky, S. Fujita, "Studies of the mortality of A-bomb survivors. 8. Cancer mortality, 1950–1982," *Radiat. Res.* 111 (1987): 151–178.
2. *Ibid.*
3. *Ibid.*
4. *Ibid.*
5. Y. Shimizu, H. Kato, W.J. Schull, "Studies of the mortality of A-bomb survivors. 9. Mortality, 1950–1985: Part 2. Cancer mortality based on recently revised doses (DS86)," *Radiat. Res.* 121 (1990): 120–141.

6. Preston, "Studies of the mortality of A-bomb survivors. 8.," 151–178.
7. *Ibid.*
8. M. Tokunaga, C.E. Land, T. Yamamoto, M. Asano, S. Tokuoka, et al., "Incidence of female breast cancer among Atomic Bomb survivors, Hiroshima and Nagasaki, 1950–1980," *Radiat. Res.* 112 (1987): 243–272.
9. T. Straume, S.D. Egbert, W.A. Woolson, R.C. Finkel, P.W. Kubik, et al., "Neutron discrepancies in the DS86 Hiroshima dosimetry system," *Health Phys.* 63 (1992): 421–426.
10. *Ibid.*
11. F.G. Davis, J.D. Boice, Z. Hrubec, R.R. Monson, "Cancer mortality in a radiation-exposed cohort of Massachusetts tuberculosis patients," *Cancer Res.* 49 (1989): 6130–6136.
12. *Ibid.*
13. *Ibid.*
14. *Ibid.*
15. S. Wing, C.M. Shy, J.L. Wood, S. Wolf, D.L. Cragle, El Frome, "Mortality among workers at Oak Ridge National Laboratory: evidence of radiation effects in follow-up through 1984," *J. Amer. Med. Assoc.* 265 (1991): 1397–1402.
16. *Ibid.*
17. *Ibid.*
18. G.M. Kendall, C.R. Muirhead, B.H. MacGibbon, J.A. O'Hagan, A.J. Conquest, et al., "Mortality and occupational exposure to radiation: first analysis of the National Registry for Radiation Workers," *Brit. Med. J.* 304 (1992): 220–225.
19. *Ibid.*
20. P. Kahn, "A grisly archive of key cancer data," *Science* 259 (1993): 448–451.
21. *Ibid.*
22. F. Godlee, "Environmental radiation: a cause for concern?" *Brit. Med. J.* 304 (1992): 299–304.
23. *Ibid.*
24. *Ibid.*
25. A. Olszyna-Marzys, "Radioactivity and food preservation," *Nutr. Rev.* 50 (1992): 162–165.
26. E.J. Hall, *Radiobiology for the radiologist.* 2nd ed. (Philadelphia: J. B. Lippincott Co., 1988), 535.
27. A. Woodward, D. Roder, A.J. McMichael, P. Crouch, A. Mylvaganam, "Radon daughter exposures at the Radium Hill uranium mine and lung cancer rates among former workers, 1952–1987," *Cancer Causes Control* 2 (1991): 213–220.

28. *Ibid.*
29. G. Saccomanno, G.C. Huth, O. Auerbach, M. Kuschner, "Relationship of radioactive radon daughters and cigarette smoking in the genesis of lung cancer in uranium miners," *Cancer*, 62 (1988): 1402–1408.
30. *Ibid.*
31. R.J. Roscoe, K. Steenland, W.E. Halperin, J.J. Beaumont, R.J. Waxweiler. "Lung cancer mortality among nonsmoking uranium miners exposed to radon daughters," *J. Am. Med. Assoc.* 262 (1989): 629–633.
32. *Ibid.*
33. P.H. Abelson, "Mineral dusts and radon in uranium mines," *Science* 254 (1991): 777.
34. J.S. Neuberger, "Residential radon exposure and lung cancer: An overview of published studies," *Cancer Detect. Prev.* 15 (1991): 435–443.
35. G. Pershagen, G. Akerblom, O. Axelson, B. Clavensjo, L. Damber, et al., "Residential radon exposure and lung cancer in Sweden," *New Engl. J. Med.* 330 (1994): 159–164.
36. *Ibid.*
37. *Ibid.*
38. C. Bowie, S.H.U. Bowie, "Radon and health," *Lancet* 337 (1991): 409–413.
39. *Ibid.*
40. B.E. Henderson, R.K. Ross, M.C. Pike, "Toward the primary prevention of cancer," *Science* 254 (1991): 1131–1138.
41. *Ibid.*
42. M. Andersson, H.H. Storm, "Cancer incidence among Danish Thoratrast-exposed patients," *J. Natl. Cancer Instit.* 84 (1992): 1318–1325.
43. *Ibid.*
44. S. Preston-Martin, D.C. Thomas, M.C. Yu, B.E. Henderson, "Diagnostic radiography as a risk factor for chronic myeloid and monocytic leukaemia (CML)," *Br. J. Cancer* 59 (1989): 639–644.
45. *Ibid.*
46. J.D. Boice, M.M. Morin, A.G. Glass, G.D. Friedman, M. Stovall, et al., "Diagnostic X-ray procedures and risk of leukemia, lymphoma, and multiple myeloma," *J. Amer. Med. Assoc.* 265 (1991): 1290–1294.
47. *Ibid.*
48. S. Preston-Martin, W. Mack, B.E. Henderson, "Risk factors for gliomas and meningiomas in males in Los Angeles County," *Cancer Res.* 49 (1989): 6137–6143.

49. *Ibid.*
50. S.C. Darby, R. Doll, S.K. Gill, P.G. Smith, "Long term mortality after a single treatment course with X-rays in patients treated for ankylosing spondylitis," *Br. J. Cancer* 55 (1987): 179–190.
51. *Ibid.*
52. *Ibid.*
53. J.D. Boice, N.E. Day, A. Andersen, L.A. Brinton, R. Brown, et al., "Second cancers following radiation treatment for cervical cancer. An international collaboration among cancer registries," *J. Natl. Cancer Instit.* 74 (1985): 955–975.
54. *Ibid.*
55. J.D. Boice, E.B. Harvey, M. Blettner, M. Stovall, J.T. Flannery, "Cancer in the contralateral breast after radiotherapy for breast cancer," *N. Engl. J. Med.* 326 (1992): 781–785.
56. *Ibid.*
57. A. Mattson, B-I. Ruden, P. Hall, N. Wilking, L.E. Rutqvist, "Radiation-induced breast cancer: long-term follow-up of radiation therapy for benign breast disease," *J. Natl. Cancer Instit.* 85 (1993): 1679–1685.
58. *Ibid.*
59. R.E. Shore, N. Hildreth, E. Woodard, P. Dvoretsky, L. Hempelmann, B. Pasternack, "Breast cancer among women given X-ray therapy for acute post-partum mastitis," *J. Natl. Cancer Instit.* 77 (1986): 689–696.
60. *Ibid.*
61. M. Stjernfeldt, K. Berglund, J. Lindsten, J. Ludvigsson, "Maternal smoking and irradiation during pregnancy as risk factors for child leukemia," *Cancer Detect. Prevent.* 16 (1992): 129–135.
62. *Ibid.*
63. V.T. DeVita, J.E. Ultmann, "Hodgkin's disease and the lymphocytic leukemias" in *Harrison's principles of internal medicine*, E. Braunwald, et al., editors. (New York: McGraw-Hill Book Co., 1987), 1553–1567.
64. P.G. Smith, R. Doll, "Mortality from cancer and all causes among British radiologists," *Br. J. Radiol.* 54 (1981): 187–194.
65. *Ibid.*
66. M.J. Gardner, M.P. Snee, A.J. Hall, C.A. Powell, S. Downes, J.D. Terrell, "Results of case-control study of leukaemia and lymphoma among young people near Sellafield nuclear plant in West Cumbria," *Brit. Med. J.* 300 (1990): 423–429.
67. *Ibid.*
68. S. Jablon, Z. Hrubec, J.D. Boice, "Cancer in populations living near

nuclear facilities: a survey of mortality nationwide and incidence in two states," *J. Amer. Med. Assoc.* 265 (1991): 1403–1408.
69. *Ibid.*
70. J. Michaelis, B. Keller, G. Haaf, P. Kaatsch, "Incidence of childhood malignancies in the vicinity of West German nuclear power plants," *Cancer Causes Control* 3 (1992): 255–263.
71. *Ibid.*
72. R.A. Kerber, J.E. Till, S.L. Simon, J.L. Lyon, D.C. Thomas, et al., "A cohort study of thyroid disease in relation to fallout from nuclear weapons testing," *J. Amer. Med. Assoc.* 270 (1993): 2076–2082.
74. C. Poole, D. Trichopoulos, "Extremely low-frequency electric and magnetic fields and cancer," *Cancer Causes Control* 2 (1991): 267–276.
75. P.K. Verkasalo, E. Pukkala, M.Y. Hongisto, J.E. Valjus, P.J. Jarvinen, et al., "Risk of cancer in Finnish children living close to power lines," *Brit. Med. J.* 307 (1993): 895–899.
76. *Ibid.*
77. *Ibid.*
78. J.H. Olsen, A. Nielsen, G. Schulgen, "Residence near high voltage facilities and risk of cancer in children," *Brit. Med. J.* 307 (1993): 891–895.
79. *Ibid.*
80. B. Schlehofer, S. Kunze, W. Sachsenheimer, M. Blettner, D. Niehoff, J. Wahrendorf, "Occupational risk factors for brain tumors: results from a population-based case-control study in Germany," *Cancer Causes Control* 1 (1990): 209–215.
81. *Ibid.*
82. Preston-Markin, "Risk factors for gliomas and meningiomas in males in Los Angeles County," 6137–6143.
83. *Ibid.*
84. R.G. Stevens, S. Davis, D.B. Thomas, L.E. Anderson, B.W. Wilson, "Electric power, pineal function, and the risk of breast cancer," *FASEB J* 6 (1992): 853–860.
85. Poole, "Extremely low-frequency electric and magnetic fields and cancer," 267–276.
86. J.G. Davis, W.R. Bennett, J.V. Brady, R.L. Brent, L. Gordis, et al., "EMF and cancer," *Science* 260 (1993): 13–14.
87. M. Swift, D. Morrell, R.B. Massey, C.L. Chase, "Incidence of cancer in 161 families affected by ataxia-telangiectasia," *N. Engl. J. Med.* 325 (1991): 1831–1836.
88. *Ibid.*
89. *Ibid.*

90. Godlee, "Environmental radiation," 299–304.
91. *Ibid.*
92. *Ibid.*
93. Shimizu, "Studies of the mortality of A-bomb survivors. 9.," 120–141.

9

....

HORMONES, WOUND-
HEALING, AND CANCER

CHRONIC STIMULATION OF CELL GROWTH
AND CANCER

Cells grow to form new tissue, not by getting larger, but by splitting in two, so that two new daughter cells are formed, each the same size as the original mother cell. Therefore, when we talk of cell growth, we are really talking about cell division. If cells are growing rapidly, this simply means that the rate of cell division is rapid. An increased rate of cell division is induced by many different circumstances, including normal growth and maturational processes, stimulation of cell growth by hormones, or wound-healing after injury. In addition, chronic stimulation of cell growth can be caused by drugs, infectious agents, chemicals, or chronic irritation.[1]

A chronically stimulated rate of cell growth can result in the accumulation of genetic errors and can lead to the development of cancer. For example, rapid tissue growth during maturation is associated with childhood cancer; hormone stimulation is associated with cancers of sex-specific tissues such as the breast or prostate gland; and wound healing is related to many different cancers.[2] In this chapter we will focus primarily on hormones and trauma as a cause of cancer, since many of the childhood cancers were covered in the chapter on familial factors in cancer causation.

About 32% of all newly diagnosed cancers in the United States are related to hormone exposure. The very idea that hormones can cause cancer may surprise some people, but the hormone-related cancers include cancers of the breast, prostate, endometrium, and ovary. Together, these cancers took a toll of nearly 100,000 lives in 1992. In addition, hormones may play a role in cancers of the testis, thyroid, and bone.[3] By comparison, trauma is a fairly minor cause of cancer, but the mechanism of cancer causation by hormones and by wound healing after trauma is very similar.

ESTROGEN AS A RISK FACTOR FOR VAGINAL CANCER

One of the clearest indications that hormones can cause cancer has come from the study of a relatively rare cancer. Vaginal cancer, specifically clear cell adenocarcinoma of the vagina, can be induced by diethylstilbestrol (DES), a synthetic estrogen which was used in the 1940s and 50s to maintain a problem pregnancy.[4] Women who took DES were exposed to moderately high doses of the drug for many months, while their child was in the uterus. Female children were thus exposed *in utero* to high concentrations of a synthetic hormone to which their own tissues could respond. An unusual clustering of vaginal cancer cases was first described in 1971, affecting women whose mothers took DES. In some instances, vaginal cancer developed in girls as young as seven years, and vaginal cancer incidence was high in DES-exposed girls only 14 years of age.

Very clear evidence now exists that DES exposure *in utero* increases the risk of vaginal cancer in young girls. Among a group of 170 patients with clear-cell adenocarcinoma of the vagina, 65% had been exposed to DES *in utero*.[5] In a group of 110 girls exposed prenatally to DES, 56% had abnormal vaginal mucosa and 35% had a condition that is a likely precursor to cancer. Among a matched group of 82 girls who were not exposed to DES, only about 1% had abnormal vaginal mucosa and none had the precursor condition to cancer. The odds of developing cancer from DES exposure could not be calculated from this study though, because none of the DES-exposed girls in the study had cancer.

Another study was undertaken to determine what risk factors were important for vaginal cancer in DES-exposed women.[6] Risk factors were investigated in 156 patients with clear cell adenocarcinoma who had been exposed to DES, and in another 1,848 DES-exposed women of similar age who did not develop vaginal cancer. The patterns of DES exposure, the use of other hormones by the mother, the mother's age and pregnancy history, and the daughter's birth and medical history were all compared. The relative risk of vaginal cancer was higher for women whose mothers began taking DES early in their pregnancy.[7] This implies that the longer the period of exposure to DES, the greater the potential risk of vaginal cancer.

ESTROGEN AS A RISK FACTOR FOR BREAST CANCER

Mothers who took DES are themselves apparently at a higher risk of breast cancer.[8] Shortly after the association between DES and vaginal cancer was first noticed, a National Registry was established, with medical information about mothers who had been exposed to DES during pregnancy. Women in this registry were recently evaluated to determine whether they suffered a higher than normal incidence of breast cancer. A total of 3,029 women who had taken DES between 1940 and 1960 were compared to an equal number of women who had not been so exposed. Women who had taken DES were found to be 35% (1.35-fold) more likely to get breast cancer than normal, and risk was still elevated more than 30 years following DES exposure. Breast cancer incidence among DES-exposed women was similar to that of unexposed women for more than 20 years after first exposure. Only after about 22 years did the incidence of cancer among DES-exposed women began to climb sharply, suggesting that DES is a relatively weak carcinogen for the breast. Nevertheless, the results of this study are important because so few other breast carcinogens are known.[9] With the exception of family history and radiation exposure, DES exposure is one of the strongest breast carcinogens identified thus far.

The fact that a synthetic estrogen can induce a high incidence of both vaginal and breast cancer demonstrates convincingly that synthetic hormones are a risk factor for cancer. Yet this does not prove that natural hormones are also a risk factor for cancer. However, good evidence is now available that natural hormones can play a causative role in some of the most common cancers. For example, estrogen stimulates the growth of breast cells, and strong evidence exists that natural estrogen is a major risk factor for breast cancer—the most frequently diagnosed cancer in the United States.

The greatest single risk factor for breast cancer is being female, since women are more than 100 times more likely to get breast cancer than men. Estrogen is clearly implicated, since men with altered estrogen metabolism, testicular damage, or testicular atrophy (from mumps) are at greater risk than most men of developing breast cancer. Women who suffer ovarian dysgenesis, a congenital failure of the ovaries to develop normally, and have lower estrogen levels as a result, generally do not develop breast cancer. Experimental studies with animals have also shown an association between levels of active estrogen (estradiol) in the blood and breast cancer risk. Despite the simplicity of this idea, no conclusive evidence has yet been found for a direct association between hormone levels in the bloodstream and human breast cancer risk.

While direct evidence may be lacking for an association between blood estrogen levels and breast cancer risk, circumstantial evidence is abundant. For example, there is a striking difference in breast cancer incidence between Japan and the United States, and the average serum level of estrogen in Japanese and American women is also strikingly different.[10] One study measured serum estrogen in 91 post-menopausal women in Japan and in 38 post-menopausal white women in the United States. The

Japanese women were chosen from a rural agricultural area, in order to sample women who represent as closely as possible the traditional Japanese lifestyle. Estrogen levels were about 42% higher in American women than in Japanese women. However, American women also tended to be larger and more obese than Japanese women, and obesity is a known risk factor for breast cancer in post-menopausal women. When the difference in serum estrogen was adjusted for body weight, American women still had estrogen levels that were 35% higher than Japanese women. These results could explain in part why Japanese and American breast cancer rates differ in young women and begin to diverge even further after menopause.[11]

To identify other factors that can affect breast cancer incidence, a group of 20,341 Seventh-Day Adventist women in California was monitored.[12] This is a particularly good group of women to study, as Seventh-Day Adventists are often vegetarians and almost always avoid smoking and drinking. Each woman in the study completed a detailed lifestyle questionnaire in 1976, and each was followed for six years. During the study period, which involved a total of about 115,000 person-years of follow up, 215 confirmed cases of breast cancer were detected. The average age of women at diagnosis was 66 years, indicating that most of the women diagnosed were well past the menopause. Several known risk factors for breast cancer were found to have an effect on this group of women. For example, a higher breast cancer risk was associated with older maternal age at birth of the first child, or a family history of breast cancer, or obesity. In addition, age at menopause was found to be a significant risk factor, as women who experienced menopause at 50 years of age or later were 1.4-fold more likely to develop breast cancer than women who experienced earlier menopause. Since the total exposure to estrogen is determined in part by the age at menopause, these results are consistent with the idea that estrogen is a potent risk factor for breast cancer.[13]

Generally, any factor that decreases the cumulative exposure to estrogen tends to decrease the overall risk of breast cancer. The age at first menstruation (menarche) is an important breast cancer risk factor because women who have an early menarche tend to have a higher cumulative exposure to estrogen.[14] Women whose menarche occurred when they were younger than 14 years old have a breast cancer risk 1.3-fold higher than women whose menarche occurred at 16 years or older. Strenuous physical exercise in adolescence tends to result in amenorrhea, (the absence of a menstrual cycle) and women who exercise to this point are thought to be at a lower risk of breast cancer later in life.[15] Pregnancy is also protective from breast cancer, because the ovulatory cycle ceases during pregnancy, and because women who have borne children tend to have lower levels of estrogen in the bloodstream than women who have not borne children.

Women who have no children, or women who delay having children until they are older than 30 years old, are at a 1.9-fold higher risk of breast cancer than women who have their first child by 20 years of age.[16] Similarly, lactation and nursing have a protective effect from breast cancer, probably because the return to a normal ovulatory cycle is often delayed in nursing mothers.[17] All of these separate associations are consistent with the idea that estrogen levels in the bloodstream are a major risk factor for breast cancer, yet no one has ever proven this to be true.

The absence of a direct association between estrogen levels in the bloodstream and the risk of breast cancer could occur for several reasons. The nature and extent of response of a tissue (or a tumor) to a hormone is not only determined by the amount of hormone present, but also by the responsiveness of that tissue to hormone. Simply measuring blood hormone levels would thus reveal only half the picture. Furthermore, the actions of estrogen are opposed by several other hormones that vary over the course of the menstrual cycle, and estrogen itself is present to a variable degree depending upon the menstrual cycle. Nevertheless, if the cumulative amount of estrogen exposure is a major risk factor for breast cancer, then estrogen replacement therapy (ERT) after menopause should lead to an increased breast cancer incidence.

Several recent studies have shown that estrogen replacement therapy does cause an increased risk of breast cancer. The prospective study of Seventh-Day Adventist women explored the link between breast cancer and use of exogenous estrogen, either as ERT or as oral contraceptives (OCs).[18] After taking into account various potentially confounding variables, current use of ERT was associated with a 1.7-fold increase in breast cancer risk. A 1.5-fold higher risk of breast cancer was associated with use of ERT even in the absence of a history of maternal breast cancer. If a woman had other risk factors, then use of ERT further increased breast cancer risk: women with prior benign breast disease who used ERT experienced a 2.8-fold higher risk than normal, and women who experienced menopause at 44 years of age or later experienced a 1.6-fold higher risk than normal. No significant increase in breast cancer risk was associated with use of OCs in this population, although women who used both OCs and ERT incurred a 1.4-fold increase in breast cancer risk. However, this study was weakened because there was not a convincing increase in breast cancer risk with increasing duration of ERT use, so a dose-response relationship could not be determined.[19]

Another large prospective study also examined the risk of breast cancer after ERT. A total of 23,244 Swedish women, all 35 years of age or older, who had filled estrogen prescriptions in the Uppsala region of Sweden were studied.[20] During the follow-up period of nearly six years, breast cancer was diagnosed in 253 women. Compared with other women in the same part of Sweden, the women who had taken estrogen had an overall risk of breast cancer that was 10% higher than normal. Risk was found to increase with the duration of estrogen treatment, so that risk reached a level 1.7-fold higher than normal after nine years of ERT. Since estrogen can be administered in several forms, an effort was also made to examine the relative risk for each of the major forms of ERT. Estradiol, which was used in 56% of the ERT treatments in these women, was associated with a high risk of breast cancer, since risk reached 1.8-fold higher than normal after only six years. On the other hand, no increase in breast cancer risk was found for the 22% of women who used conjugated estrogens, or for the 22% of women who used other forms of estrogen such as estriol. The highest risk of breast cancer in any subgroup of women was seen in the 10% of women who took estrogen plus progestin in combination for extended periods. For women who used only this combination for more than six years, the relative risk of breast cancer was elevated 4.4-fold, with respect to untreated women. Therefore, long-term ERT use by perimenopausal women is associated with an increased risk of breast cancer, especially if estrogen is combined with progestin.[21]

A more recent and much larger study has confirmed the major findings of these earlier studies.[22] The effect of ERT on breast cancer risk was assessed prospectively as a part of the Nurses' Health Study, which followed 121,700 women between the ages of 30 and 55 years. At the beginning of the study, nurses were given a questionnaire that surveyed known and suspected causes of cancer and cardiovascular disease. Specifically, women were asked about family history of breast cancer, menopausal status, and post-menopausal use of hormones, as well as diet and other risk factors. These women were re-surveyed every two years for a total of eight years to update information on cancer risk factors and to ascertain whether major medical events had occurred. There were 722 cases of breast cancer diagnosed during a total of 367,187 person-years of follow-up. When hormone use of the cases as compared to that of other women in the group, it was found that past use of ERT was found not to be a risk factor for breast cancer. However, current use of ERT increased the risk of breast cancer 1.4-fold with respect to women who did not use hormone supplementation. Risk from using ERT tended to increase with age, as women aged 39 to 44 had a breast cancer risk 1.1-fold higher than normal while using ERT, while women aged 60 to 64 had a breast cancer risk 2.1-fold higher than normal while using ERT. However, a long duration of ERT use seemed to have no affect on breast cancer risk when compared to short duration use. Therefore, current use of ERT is responsible for a rather modest increase in breast cancer risk, while ERT may also be responsible for a large decrease in the risk of cardiovascular disease and hip fractures. On balance, the benefits of long-term ERT use may outweigh the risks, since breast cancer risk may drop rapidly after discontinuation of ERT.[23]

Another recent study combined the results of 16 different studies to quantify the effect of ERT on breast cancer risk.[24] The dose-response relationships in separate studies were combined mathematically, using a technique called meta-analysis, to derive an estimate for risk of breast cancer given the duration of estrogen use. This approach should be more accurate because it combines so much data, but problems always arise in combining data from different studies. In any case, the proportional increase in risk of breast cancer was calculated for each year of estrogen use. For post-menopausal women, breast cancer risk did not increase until after at least five years of ERT use. After 15 years of ERT, breast cancer risk was increased about 1.3-fold with respect to women who did not use ERT. The higher breast cancer risk associated with ERT in some earlier studies was found to be due largely to the inclusion of premenopausal women in the study, or to the higher risk for women who use estradiol with progestin. Also found was an interaction between ERT and a family history of breast cancer. Among women with a family history of breast cancer, those who had ever used ERT had a 2.3-fold higher risk of breast cancer than those who had not.[25]

These studies of breast cancer risk from ERT are very convincing when taken together: many of them were prospective, so that risk factors were carefully defined before cancers were diagnosed; most were careful to match women in the study with a reasonable control group of women; and the three studies together characterized breast cancer risk in a total of 165,285 women. Whether to take ERT during the menopause is a question of personal choice that should be discussed on an individual basis with a physician. Short-term use of ERT, for no more than about five years after completing the menopause, has many things to recommend it: menopausal symptoms such as "hot flashes" are ameliorated, and there is a substantial protective effect from cardiovascular disease, osteoporosis, and bone fractures, but there is also a marginally higher risk of breast cancer. For many women, the increased risk of breast cancer will be enough to convince them not to use ERT. However, no single answer is right for all women, and this question calls for an informed personal choice.

ORAL CONTRACEPTIVES AS A RISK FACTOR FOR BREAST CANCER

If estrogen is a risk factor for breast cancer, then it is logical to expect that oral contraceptives (OCs) could also result in a significant breast cancer risk, since OCs contain some form of estrogen. In order to test this idea, the association between breast cancer risk and OC use was examined in 401 breast cancer patients and in 519 women who entered a New York City hospital for other reasons.[26] No evidence was found linking breast cancer risk and the duration of OC use, either in women who had children or in women who were childless. In fact, use of OCs actually seemed to confer protection from breast cancer for women under 50 years of age. Women who had used OCs for less than five years were 10% less likely to develop breast cancer than non-users, and women who had used OCs for more than five years were 60% less likely to develop breast cancer than nonusers. No interactive effects were identified between OC use and other breast cancer risk factors such as family history, having no children or having them late in life, or abstaining from breastfeeding.[27] However, these results do not conclusively prove that OCs are protective from breast cancer, since the group of women studied was fairly small and because the study was retrospective. A retrospective study relies on memory, many years after the fact, to reconstruct risk factor exposure, so this opens the door for memory bias and similar problems.

The study that claimed that OCs are not a risk factor for breast cancer is directly contradicted by the results of another larger prospective study.[28] As a part of the Nurses' Health Study, a group of 118,273 women between 30 and 55 years old was entered into a prospective study of breast cancer risk factors. These women answered questionnaires about various risk factors including OC use. For each woman, the duration of OC use, the duration of use prior to the first pregnancy, and the duration of use prior to reaching 25 years of age was calculated. Women were followed for 10 years, so a total of 1,137,415 person-years of follow-up were involved in this study. This is a massive follow-up effort, which should have great power to accurately determine the effect of even relatively small risk factors. During the 10-year follow-up period, a total of 1,799 new cases of breast cancer were diagnosed. Women who had used OCs at any point in the past were found to have a risk of breast cancer 7% higher than women who had never used them. For women who were currently using OCs, the breast cancer risk was increased by 53%, or 1.5-fold, over never-users. This discrepancy between the risk of current OC use versus past OC use suggests that estrogen can act to promote the growth of an existing tumor, but that it is not a very effective carcinogen by itself.

The highest category of risk was found for current OC users between 40 and 44 years of age, for whom relative risk was increased 2.7-fold.[29] It is unknown why the age group from 40 to 44 appears to be most vulnerable to breast cancer induced by OCs, although this is the age group in which breast cancer incidence tends to increase sharply anyway. In addition, current use of OCs seemed to increase the risk of a late stage tumor that was either large or metastatic. Finally, breast cancers diagnosed in women who were past users of OCs were more likely to test positive for estrogen receptor expression than cancers diagnosed in women who never used OCs.

The only potential flaw that could be identified in the Nurses' Health Study is that nurses are not a random sample of the population and may not represent the general population very well. Many women have gone into nursing because of an early family experience of catastrophic illness, which may mean that nurses are not a good surrogate for the rest of the female population. But this is minor quibbling; the Nurses' Health Study was a very large, well-designed, well-executed study that was able to provide clearcut answers to an important question. A prospective study is almost always better than a retrospective study, and a large study is almost always better than a small one, so on balance, the findings of the Nurses' Health Study should be given precedence.

ESTROGEN AS A RISK FACTOR FOR OVARIAN CANCER

Just as estrogen has been identified as a risk factor for breast cancer, it has also been associated with cancers of the ovary. The relationship is quite complicated, since the effects of estrogen interact with the effects of other hormones in a complex interplay that is repeated every menstrual cycle. Estrogens are actually secreted by the ovary, although a small percentage of total estrogens are made by fat cells, which can convert other hormones into estrogen. The only alternative source of estrogen before menopause is oral contraceptives (OCs), while the only alternative source of estrogen after menopause is estrogen replacement therapy (ERT).

Ovarian cancer usually develops from cells that form a covering over the ovary, and these cells are induced to grow during the process of ovulation. This is essentially similar to what happens during wound healing, since the cells induced to grow are those cells that "heal" the small lesion formed during ovulation. Factors that prevent ovulation (e.g., pregnancy) protect against ovarian cancer, and the degree of protection conferred is related to the length of time that ovulation is blocked. An elevated risk of ovarian cancer is found in women who ovulate for more than 40 years, who have never given birth, or who first gave birth after age 30. Because estrogen can be synthesized by fat cells, obesity is also a risk factor for ovarian cancer, as is consumption of a diet high in calories.

Because OCs actually prevent ovulation and thus prevent the growth of some cells in the ovary, there is good reason to expect that they would be protective against ovarian cancer. To test this idea, 150 ovarian cancer patients under the age of 50 were individually matched with healthy control women, to compare the pattern of fertility and OC use in the two groups.[30] All of the women were interviewed by telephone about their reproductive and menstrual history, their use of hormones, and their family history of cancer. It was found that the risk of ovarian cancer decreased with increasing numbers of live births, with increasing numbers of incomplete pregnancies, and with the use of OCs. These three factors could be amalgamated into a single index, called "protected time," by considering them all as periods of non-ovulation. The total time of exposure to estrogen could be calculated by determining the time interval between the menarche and the diagnosis of ovarian cancer (or the cessation of menses), and subtracting the "protected time." The total time of exposure to estrogen was strongly related to risk of ovarian cancer. Several other factors found to be associated with ovarian cancer risk were obesity, cervical polyps, and gall bladder disease. There was an indication that family history was also important, since seven patients, but no controls, could recall a family history of ovarian cancer.[31]

Another more recent study focused on risk factors for ovarian cancer in both black and white women.[32] This comparison is of particular interest because white women have a higher incidence of ovarian cancer than do black women. Data were combined from seven different studies to form a large meta-analysis of cases and controls. The case patients were 110 black women diagnosed with ovarian cancer between 1971 and 1986, while the controls were 365 healthy black women. In addition, the exposure to identified risk factors was examined in 246 healthy black women and 4,378 healthy white women. In comparing black cases to black controls, women who had four or more children were found to have an ovarian cancer risk 47% lower than women who had borne fewer children. In addition, breast feeding for six months or longer reduced ovarian cancer risk by 15%, and use of OCs reduced ovarian cancer risk by 38%. All of these results are consistent with the idea that a period of non-ovulation is protective from ovarian cancer.[33]

When black controls were compared to white controls, it was found that black women generally had more "protected time," during which they avoided exposure to estrogen. For example, 48% of black women reported bearing four or more children, while only 27% of white women had four or more children. Similarly, 62% of black women nursed their children for six months or more, while only 53% of white women nursed as long. However, 59% of white women took OCs, while only 51% of black women did.[33] If these racial differences in "protected time" are also present in black and white women who develop ovarian cancer, this would be consistent with the idea that estrogen causes ovarian cancer.

A recent review of the literature concluded that women who have used OCs for at least five years have a risk of ovarian cancer that is reduced 40% relative to that of nonusers.[35] But the situation is more complex than it first appears; modern OCs are combinations of estrogen and progesterone, taken in daily doses for 21 days, followed by seven days with no treatment. The ovary is exposed to "unopposed" estrogen only on those days when no contraceptives are taken, at a time when blood levels of estrogen are naturally low because of the menstrual cycle. Prior to the introduction of modern combination OCs, contraceptives were made of estrogen that alternated with progesterone in sequence. Sequential OCs have been linked with an increased risk of ovarian and endometrial cancer, since they function, in principle, much like ERT. Thus the protective effect of OCs is limited exclusively to modern combination OCs.

ESTROGEN AS A RISK FACTOR FOR UTERINE CANCER

Combination OCs are also protective from cancer of the uterine endometrium, that portion of the uterus where a fertilized egg would implant. A study of cancer trends in England and Wales has shown that, over the last 20 years, the proportion of women who use OCs has increased fairly dramatically.[36] During the same time period, every other known risk factor for endometrial cancer has also increased. Therefore, the incidence of endometrial cancer should have increased unless OCs have a protective effect. Over the last 20 years in England and Wales, mortality from endometrial cancer has declined by 41%, suggesting that OCs have had a major effect on endometrial cancer mortality.

Another recent study has directly examined combination OCs as a risk factor for endometrial cancer. This study compared 405 women with endometrial cancer to 297 healthy women of similar age, race, and geographic area.[37] Each of these women were interviewed about various possible risk factor exposures. It was found that use of combination OCs was associated with a 60% reduction in risk of endometrial cancer. Long-term OC use, defined as more than 10 years, was associated with an 80% reduction in risk of endometrial cancer. Women who had used combination OCs but had discontinued this use more than 20 years in the past still enjoyed a 30% reduction in endometrial cancer risk compared to women who had never used OCs. These results persisted even when corrected for other risk factors such as age, menopausal status, obesity, number of children borne, smoking history, or history of infertility. The magnitude of the protective effect was diminished in women who had never given birth or in women who had used estrogen replacement therapy (ERT) for more than three years. Perhaps the most surprising aspect of this study is that the protective effect of OCs can persist for more than 20 years.

These results are confirmed by another recent study that examined endometrial cancer risk and OC use by women in Switzerland.[38] A case group of 122 women aged 75 or less with endometrial cancer was compared to a control group of 309 women who were in a hospital for reasons unrelated to OC use. It was found that cases were about half as likely to have used OCs as controls, showing that the risk of endometrial cancer is reduced by OCs. For women who had used OCs for two to five years, endometrial cancer risk was reduced by 50%, while for women who had used OCs more than five years, risk was reduced 70%. Again, the protection conferred by OC use seemed to last more than 20 years, as women who had used OCs 20 years in the past had a risk of endometrial cancer that was still 20% lower than normal.

All told, many separate small studies concur that OC use tends to reduce endometrial cancer risk by about half.[39] However, all of these studies are case-control studies, in which cases who already have cancer are matched with healthy controls, and reasons are sought for why one group is healthy and the other is not. These studies are necessarily retrospective, with the inherent problems of memory bias, and all were rather small. This means that, while OCs are probably indeed protective from endometrial cancer, the degree of protection is somewhat open to question.

Interestingly, a recent study has found that an alternate method of birth control is also protective from endometrial cancer.[40] In this study, the use of intrauterine devices (IUDs) was compared between a case group of 437 women with endometrial cancer and a control group of 3,200 women from the same geographic areas. Use of IUDs was found to reduce the rate of endometrial cancer by about half. Generally, the longer IUDs were used, the stronger the protective effect, but a real dose-response relationship could not be identified with certainty. The protective effect of IUDs was achieved without regard to how old a woman was when she either started or stopped using them. It was proposed that IUDs exert their protective effect in much the same way as OCs—by blocking the monthly sequence of changes that the cells of the uterine wall go through as part of the menstrual cycle.

The relationship between estrogen replacement therapy (ERT) and endometrial cancer risk has been explored to a very limited extent. We have already noted a study that reported that the protective effect of OCs from endometrial cancer could be partly blocked by use of ERT for three years or more.[41] Beyond that, there is little to go on. We know that prevention of ovulation by pregnancy reduces endometrial cancer risk, so it is reasonable to assume that exposure to estrogen in ERT will increase endometrial cancer risk. What is needed is a retrospective case-control study that can quickly determine the degree of risk conferred by use of ERT.

OC'S AS A RISK FACTOR FOR LIVER CANCER

There is some evidence that use of OCs can increase the risk of cancers affecting the liver.[42] A study examined the risk factors of all women aged 18 to 39 years who died of liver cancer in Los Angeles County during the period from 1975 to 1980. This was a total of only 11 evaluable cases, because this is an unusual cancer in women, and quite rare in young women. Because there were so few cases to study, any conclusions about risk factors for this cancer are necessarily weak. Perhaps the 11 individuals might accidently share a trait that is not a risk factor, but that is blamed as a risk factor anyway, whereas an accidental trait common to 100 or 1,000 case individuals is harder to imagine.

Nevertheless, 11 female patients with a type of liver cancer called hepatocellular carcinoma were matched with 22 control women selected from the same neighborhoods.[43] Ten of the 11 women with liver cancer had taken OCs, and the remaining case woman had taken nine months of hormone injections, immediately prior to her diagnosis, to control menstrual bleeding. By comparison, only 59% of the control women had taken OCs at any point in the past. The average duration of OC use in the 11 liver cancer cases was 65 months, while the average duration of OC use in controls was only 27 months. None of the cases differed in any marked way from controls except for this difference in OC use. Unfortunately, the relative risk associated with OC use cannot be calculated from this type of study, but we can be sure that the absolute risk is small because the cancer is so rare.

TESTOSTERONE AS A RISK FACTOR FOR CANCER

Evidence is clear that the male hormone testosterone is a risk factor for prostate cancer.[44] Castrated males apparently never get prostate cancer, and castration has a palliative effect on men who have already been diagnosed with prostate cancer. Men with cirrhosis rarely ever get prostate cancer, because alcohol depresses the levels of circulating testosterone. Finally, men with prostate cancer tend to have higher levels of circulating testosterone than do healthy controls of the same age.

Black men in the United States have the highest prostate cancer rate in the world, a rate nearly double that of whites in the United States.[45] The increased rate of prostate cancer in blacks is already apparent at age 45, the age at which the earliest prostate cancers occur. This suggests that whatever factors are responsible for the difference in prostate cancer rate are present early in life. The level of testosterone in the bloodstream was measured in a group of 50 black and 50 white college students in Los Angeles. The average level of testosterone in blacks was 15% higher than in whites, after adjustment for differences in age, weight, alcohol use, cigarette smoking, and use of prescription drugs. This degree of difference in circulating testosterone could account for about a two-fold difference in prostate cancer rate.[46]

Furthermore, pregnant black women have higher levels of testosterone than do pregnant white women, so black male children are exposed to higher levels of testosterone in the uterus.[47] Early developmental exposure to an active hormone that has an effect on fetal tissue is, in essence, similar to the exposure of female fetuses to DES, which we have already seen has a strong effect on later incidence of cancer. In black male children, the *in utero* exposure to testosterone could be responsible for the higher incidence of prostate cancer or testicular cancer among adult black men.

Recently, several reports have suggested that vasectomy can have a strong effect on the risk of prostate cancer. One study examined prostate cancer risk retrospectively in the spouses of women in the Nurses' Health Study.[48] These men were initially identified because their wives had reported, as part of the earlier study, that vasectomy was the major form of contraception that they used. A total of 14,607 men who had vasectomies were compared to an equal number of age-matched men who did not have vasectomies. All men were followed for more than 12 years, during which time 96 men with vasectomies developed prostate cancer. It was found that men with a vasectomy had a prostate cancer risk that was 1.6-fold higher than normal. The relative risk of prostate cancer increased with time since the vasectomy, so that men who had vasectomies for 20 or more years were at a risk 1.9-fold higher than men with no vasectomy. This elevation in risk persisted even when odds were adjusted for smoking, alcohol consumption, educational level, body mass, and geographical area of residence. Risk appeared to be greater for men who had their vasectomy at or after the age of 40. Strangely, vasectomized men were also found to have a lower risk of cardiovascular disease or colorectal cancer.

Why vasectomy should alter the risk of prostate cancer is unknown, although vasectomy is known to alter the function of the prostate gland. For some reason, the volume of secretion from the prostate gland declines after vasectomy. It has been proposed that, following vasectomy, the prostate is no longer directly exposed to male hormones moving from the testicles through the prostate during ejaculation. This change also occurs during normal aging, and aging is known to sharply increase the incidence of prostate cancer. Thus a vasectomy may mimic the conditions that are present in the prostate during normal aging.[49]

Another smaller, prospective study also showed that vasectomy increases the risk of prostate cancer.[50] A total of 10,055 male health professionals who had a vasectomy were compared prospectively to 37,800 similar men who had not had a vasectomy. All of these men were between 40 and 75 years of age in 1986, and they were followed for a total of four years. During the follow-up period, a total of 300 men were diagnosed with prostate cancer. It was found that vasectomy was associated with a 1.7-fold higher risk of prostate cancer. Among men who had vasectomies for more than 22 years, the risk of prostate cancer was 1.9-fold higher than among men without vasectomies. The consistency of the results between the two studies, and the increased risk with time since vasectomy, suggests that vasectomy causes prostate cancer by an unknown mechanism.[51]

WOUND-HEALING AND CANCER

The role of wound-healing in cancer is much less clear-cut and much less important than the role of hormones. Nevertheless, wound-healing and hormones both seem to induce cancer by a similar mechanism. Both act as a stimulus for rapid cell growth, and both cause changes in gene regulation within the cell. In the case of wound-healing, a mature differentiated cell responds to injury by first turning into an undifferentiated cell, and then re-differentiating into a range of different cell types, in order to replace all the cells lost or damaged during wounding. This involves many changes in the way that genes are regulated, because different genes are required for each of the different cell types. Similarly, in the case of hormones, a relatively undifferentiated cell responds to hormone stimulation by differentiating into a range of specialized cell types. This also calls for changes in gene regulation, and it can actually be shown that genes are "turned on" in response to hormone exposure.

The classic example of wound-healing as a risk factor for cancer is the relationship between head injury and brain tumor, a relationship which was first described more than 60 years ago. Recent evidence has been obtained to show that this relationship is real, and that head injury can increase the risk of a specific brain tumor called a meningioma.[52] A group of 70 men, all aged between 25 and 69 and all diagnosed with meningioma in Los Angeles County, were compared to an equal number of matched healthy control men. Men who had a serious head injury 20 or more years in the past were 2.3-fold more likely to get a meningioma than normal men. "Serious head injury" was defined as any condition that led to loss of conciousness, dizziness, or a medical examination. In fact, nearly one-third of all the meningioma patients had had a serious head injury in the past. There was a clear dose-response relationship between head injury and meningioma: men with only one serious head injury 20 years in the past were at a 1.3-fold higher risk of meningioma than normal, but men with three or more serious head injuries were at a 6.2-fold higher risk of meningioma.[53]

Probably the best known example of wound-healing and cancer is the widely known, and widely misunderstood, case of asbestos exposure and lung cancer. Since the turn of the century, asbestos has been recognized as a public health hazard and asbestosis, a lung scarring disease, was a leading cause of death for men in some industries. But occupational safety regulations have been in effect for many years, and asbestosis incidence has been declining in the United States for nearly 40 years. The relationship between asbestos and lung cancer risk is well known because of efforts by the Environmental Protection Agency (EPA) to regulate public exposure to asbestos fibers shed from building insulation. But this relationship is also widely misunderstood; for example, it is not widely appreciated that the strongest link between asbestos and cancer involves, not lung cancer, but a rare form of cancer called mesothelioma. Mesothelioma affects the membranes, or pleura, lining the cavities of the thorax and abdomen. About 80% of all mesotheliomas occur in men exposed to asbestos in the workplace, or occasionally in family members who either live near asbestos mines or are exposed to asbestos fibers brought home on clothing. By contrast, only a tiny fraction of lung cancers are linked to asbestos.

The average period between first exposure to asbestos and a diagnosis of mesothelioma is 35 to 40 years, with most deaths occurring in patients well over 60 years of age. This long period of latency makes it very difficult to determine with surety the risk associated with asbestos fiber exposure, since so many people with fiber exposure die of other causes. Nevertheless, a group of 17,800 male asbestos insulation workers in the United States and Canada was followed from 1967 until 1986.[54] During this period, 356 of the men died of malignant mesothelioma. Because mesothelioma is ordinarily so rare, this number of deaths indicates that asbestos causes a very large increase in relative risk of this cancer. But, given that these men were exposed to asbestos fiber concentrations vastly higher than normal, asbestos still does not seem to be the potent carcinogen that the EPA has implied. Furthermore, more than half of these asbestos insulation workers were known to be heavy smokers, while the smoking habits of another third of the workers could not be determined. This is important because there may well be an interactive effect between asbestos and smoking in the causation of mesothelioma, as there is known to be in the causation of lung cancer.

Asbestos fiber exposure has also been linked to an increased risk of lung cancer. However, as noted earlier, most people exposed to high levels of asbestos fibers are also smokers, and separating the two causes is often difficult. For example, in the above study of 17,800 asbestos insulation workers, the incidence of lung cancer was actually lower than expected among non-smoking workers exposed to asbestos fibers. In fact, lung tumors are rare among asbestos workers who do not smoke, and it has not been absolutely proven that asbestos acting alone can cause lung cancer in non-smokers. Exposure to asbestos fibers has been estimated to increase the relative risk of lung cancer by no more than a factor of three.[55] Four major industries were likely to involve exposure to asbestos fibers in the past: the greatest risk was associated with the textile industry and with mining of tremolite, while lesser risk was associated with exposure to asbestos in cement and other mixed products, and low levels of risk were associated with mining of chrysotile and manufacture of friction products. In the cases of textile manufacture or tremolite mining, the relative risk of lung cancer is elevated two- to three-fold, even for workers routinely exposed to 200 asbestos fibers per cubic centimeter of air. At the same level of exposure, workers exposed to asbestos fibers in cement and other mixed products suffered a relative risk less than two-fold higher than normal. Workers exposed to asbestos fibers during chrysotile mining had a relative risk scarcely higher than that of people who were not exposed to asbestos fibers at all.

Part of the problem with asbestos is that the situation is quite complex, and these complexities were not understood or appreciated at the time laws were being passed. The word asbestos can be applied to six chemically and physically distinct types of minerals (chrysotile and the amphiboles, including crocidolite, amosite, anthophyllite, tremolite, and actinolite), which are often mined from deposits containing other potentially harmful minerals.[56] Chrysotile accounts for 95% of the world's production of asbestos, but the amphiboles are believed to cause most of the health problems. However, current regulatory policy does not distinguish between chrysotile and the amphiboles. Asbestos is a strong, durable, flexible material that resists acid and heat, so it has been incorporated into many different materials. Unfortunately, as these materials age, they can shed tiny fragments of asbestos in the form of air-borne fibers that can then be inhaled. Asbestos fibers can be shed from aging insulation in schools or public buildings, but the estimated risk of death associated with asbestos in

TABLE 9-1
WEIGHTED RISK CALCULATIONS FOR HORMONAL RISK FACTORS

RISK FACTOR	RELATED CANCER	RELATIVE RISK	RELATIVE FREQUENCY	RISK WEIGHT
DES (*in utero* exposure)	Vaginal	~100	1	~100c
OC use at 40–44 years of age	Breast	2.7	5	14b
ERT x benign breast disease	Breast	2.8	5	14c
Age at first birth > 30 yrs	Breast	1.9	5	10a
Nulliparous (no children)	Breast	1.9	5	10a
ERT at ≥ 55 years	Breast	1.8	5	9b
Menopause after age 55	Breast	1.5	5	8a
Age 25–29 yrs at first birth	Breast	1.6	5	8a
Vasectomy (>22 years)	Prostate	1.9	4	8a
High levels of testosterone	Prostate	2.0	4	8c
Current OC use	Breast	1.4	5	7a
Age at first birth 20–24 yrs	Breast	1.3	5	7a

RISK FACTOR	RELATED CANCER	RELATIVE RISK	RELATIVE FREQUENCY	RISK WEIGHT
Menopause after age 50	Breast	1.4	5	7a
Vasectomy	Prostate	1.7	4	7a
Menarche at < 15 years old	Breast	1.3	5	7a
Diethylstilbestrol	Breast	1.4	5	7a
Current ERT use all ages	Breast	1.4	5	7b
Prior OCs x current ERT	Breast	1.4	5	7b
ERT use for > 3 years	Breast	1.4	5	7b
ERT at < 50 years old	Breast	1.2	5	6a
Past OC use	Breast	1.1	5	6a
ERT at 50–54 years old	Breast	1.1	5	6b
Non-use of OCs	Endometrium	2.1	3	6c
Non-use of IUDs	Endometrium	2.0	3	6c
Serious childhood head injury	Brain	2.3	2	5c
Bearing <4 children	Ovary	1.9	2	4c
Non-use of OCs	Ovary	1.6	2	3c
Breast fed < 6 months	Ovary	1.2	2	2c

The abbreviations include post-menopausal estrogen replacement therapy (ERT), oral contraceptive (OC), and diethylstilbestrol (DES).

schools is 10-fold less than the estimated risk of dying in a flood. By the EPA's own (possibly optimistic) figures, a total ban on asbestos would save the lives of 202 people over the next 13 years, at a cost ranging from $76 million to $106 million *per life*.[57] Thus, the risk of cancer from asbestos fibers appears to be quite small, even by the EPA's own estimate.

Other cases in which wound-healing (or stimulated cell growth) has been strongly linked to an increased risk of a specific cancer include:[58]

1. Skin rash from sun exposure (solar keratosis) and squamous cell skin cancer.
2. Chronic ulcerative colitis, a debilitating inflammatory condition of the colon, and colorectal cancer.
3. Gall stones and gall bladder cancer (80% of gall bladder cancer patients had stones).
   Other potential links between stimulated cell growth and cancer include:
4. Consumption of hard or highly fibrous foods and stomach cancer.
5. Exposure to excessively loud noise and acoustic nerve tumors.
6. Kidney stones and cancer of the ureter of the kidney.

Unfortunately, relatively little is known about any of these relationships in terms of levels of cancer risk. In fact, the link between cancer and these conditions of chronically stimulated cell growth is largely hypothetical (or anecdotal), and much research is needed.

SUMMARY

The most important hormone-related cancers are breast, ovary, uterine endometrium, and prostate. But there may also be a hormonal role in cancers of the testis, thyroid, and bone (e.g., osteosarcoma). As clear as our knowledge of some of these relationships is, it is not always clear how that knowledge should be used. It is neither practical nor desirable to recommend that most people undergo an ovariectomy or orchiectomy merely because surgery would decrease their relative risk of a particular cancer. Prevention of these cancers will probably depend more upon gently modifying the effect of the hormone than upon eliminating the source of the hormone.

For example, the risk of breast cancer could be substantially reduced by delaying the onset of the normal menstrual cycle and by minimizing the therapeutic use of estrogens in post-menopausal women. Delaying the menarche, or start of the normal menstrual cycle, by a few years might be achieved through a vigorous exercise program.[59] Hormonal contraceptives might also be designed to specifically decrease breast cancer risk. This possibility will be explored more fully in the discussion of chemical prevention of cancer (Chapter 15), but it has been calculated that five years use of a specially formulated contraceptive could reduce the incidence of breast cancer by nearly 40%.[60] The downside of this equation is that use of such hormonal contraceptive is essentially equivalent to a chemical hysterectomy, and the effects of the ovaries must be completely blocked. Additional (low-level) hormones could be added to the hormonal contraceptives, so that women would not lose their secondary sexual characteristics, but this is a fairly radical proposal nonetheless.

Analysis of the incidence rate of endometrial cancer as a function of age suggests that lifelong effects could be realized from even short-duration use of OCs.[61] Five years of combination-type OC use could reduce a woman's lifetime risk of endometrial cancer by some 60%. In contrast, five years of ERT use is likely to increase a woman's subsequent lifetime risk by at least 90%, since in ERT the estrogen is not usually opposed by progesterone.[62] These arguments are complicated, but the general point is simple: gentle modification or modulation of hormonal exposure is likely to play a substantial role in the prevention of hormonal cancers. Until we can determine the most effective and least disruptive ways to modulate hormone exposures, hormonal cancers are likely to remain a major cause of human mortality.

NOTES TO CHAPTER 9

1. S. Preston-Martin, M.C. Pike, R.K. Ross, P.A. Jones, B.E. Henderson, "Increased cell division as a cause of human cancer," *Cancer Res.* 50 (1990): 7415–7421.
2. *Ibid.*
3. B.E. Henderson, R.K. Ross, M.C. Pike, J.T. Casagrande, "Endogenous hormones as a major factor in human cancer," *Cancer Res.* 42 (1982): 3232–3239.
4. A.L. Herbst, S. Anderson, M.M. Hubby, W.M. Haenszel, R.H. Kaufman, K.L. Noller, "Risk factors for the development of diethylstilbestrol-associated clear cell adenocarcinoma: a case-control study," *Am. J. Obstet. Gynecol.* 154 (1986): 814–822.
5. A.L. Herbst, D.C. Poskanzer, S.J. Robboy, L. Friedlander, R.E. Scully, "Prenatal exposure to stilbestrol: A prospective comparison of exposed female offspring with unexposed controls," *New Engl. J. Med.* 292 (1975): 334–339.

6. Herbst, "Risk factors for the development of diethylstilbestrol-associated clear cell adenocarcinoina," 814–822.
7. Ibid.
8. T. Colton, E.R. Greenberg, K. Noller, L. Resseguie, C. Van Bennekom, et al., "Breast cancer in mothers prescribed diethylstilbestrol in pregnancy: Further follow-up," *J. Amer. Med. Assoc.* 269 (1993): 2096–2100.
9. Ibid.
10. H. Shimizu, R.K. Ross, L. Bernstein, M.C. Pike, B.E. Henderson, "Serum oestrogen levels in postmenopausal women: comparison of American whites and Japanese in Japan," *Br. J. Cancer* 62 (1990): 451–453.
11. Ibid.
12. P.K. Mills, W.L. Beeson, R.L. Phillips, G.E. Fraser, "Dietary habits and breast cancer incidence among Seventh-day Adventists," *Cancer* 64 (1989): 582–590.
13. Ibid.
14. J.R. Harris, M.E. Lippman, U. Veronesi, W. Willett, "Breast cancer (Part 1)," *N. Engl. J. Med.* 327 (1992): 319–328.
15. L. Bernstein, R.K. Ross, R.A. Lobo, R. Hanisch, M.D. Krailo, B.E. Henderson, "The effects of moderate physical activity on menstrual cycle patterns in adolescence: implications for breast cancer prevention," *Br. J. Cancer* 55 (1987): 681–685.
16. Harris, "Breast cancer," 319–328.
17. B.E. Henderson, R. Ross, L. Bernstein, "Estrogens as a cause of human cancer," *Cancer Res.* 48 (1988): 246–253.
18. P.K. Mills, W.L. Beeson, R.L. Phillips, G.E. Fraser, "Prospective study of exogenous hormone use and breast cancer in Seventh-day Adventists," *Cancer* 64 (1989): 591–597.
19. Ibid.
20. L. Bergkvist, H-O. Adami, I. Persson, R. Hoover, C. Schairer, "The risk of breast cancer after estrogen and estrogen-progestin replacement," *N. Engl. J. Med.* 321 (1989): 293–297.
21. Ibid.
22. G.A. Colditz, M.J. Stampfer, W.C. Willett, C.H. Hennekens, B. Rosner, F.E. Speizer, "Prospective study of estrogen replacement therapy and risk of breast cancer in postmenopausal women," *J. Amer. Med. Assoc.* 264 (1990): 2648–2653.
23. Ibid.
24. K.K. Steinberg, S.B. Thacker, S.J. Smith, D.F. Stroup, M.M. Zack, et al., "A meta-analysis of the effect of estrogen replacement therapy on the risk of breast cancer," *J. Amer. Med. Assoc.* 265 (1991): 1985–1990.

25. *Ibid.*
26. R.E. Harris, E.A. Zang, E.L. Wynder, "Oral contraceptives and breast cancer risk: a case-control study," *Int. J. Epidemiol.* 19 (1990: 240–246.
27. *Ibid.*
28. I. Romieu, W.C. Willett, G.A. Colditz, M.J. Stampfer, B. Rosner, et al., "Prospective study of oral contraceptive use and risk of breast cancer in women," *J. Natl. Cancer Instit.* 81 (1989): 1313–1321.
29. *Ibid.*
30. J. Casagrande, E.W. Louie, M.C. Pike, S. Roy, R.K. Ross, B.E. Henderson, "Incessant ovulation and ovarian cancer," *Lancet* ii (1979): 170–173.
31. *Ibid.*
32. E.M. John, A.S. Whittemore, R. Harris, J. Itnyre, and the Collaborative Ovarian Cancer Group, "Characteristics relating to ovarian cancer risk: collaborative analysis of seven US case-control studies. Epithelial ovarian cancer in black women," *J. Natl. Cancer Instit.* 85 (1993): 142–47.
33. *Ibid.*
34. *Ibid.*
35. B.E. Henderson, R.K. Ross, M.C. Pike, "Toward the primary prevention of cancer," *Science* 254 (1991): 1131–1138.
36. L. Villard, M. Murphy, "Endometrial cancer trends in England and Wales: a possible protective effect of oral contraception," *Int. J. Epidemiol.* 19 (1990): 255–258.
37. J.L. Stanford, L.A. Brinton, M.L. Berman, R. Mortel, L.B. Twiggs, et al., "Oral contraceptives and endometrial cancer: do other risk factors modify the association?," *Int. J. Cancer* 54 (1993): 243–248.
38. F. Levi, C. La Vecchia, C. Gulie, E. Negri, V. Monnier, et al., "Oral contraceptives and the risk of endometrial cancer," *Cancer Causes Control* 2 (1991): 99–103.
39. Henderson, "Estrogens as a cause of human cause," 246–253.
40. X. Castellsague, W.D. Thompson, R. Dubrow, "Intra-uterine contraception and the risk of endometrial cancer," *Br. J. Cancer* 54 (1993): 911–916.
41. Stanford, "Oral contraceptives and endometrial cancer," 243–248.
42. B.E. Henderson, S. Preston-Martin, H.A. Edmondson, R.L. Peters, M.C. Pike, "Hepatocellular carcinoma and oral contraceptives," *Br. J. Cancer* 48 (1983): 437–440.
43. *Ibid.*
44. Henderson, "Toward the primary prevention of cancer," 1131–1138.
45. R.K. Ross, L. Bernstein, H. Judd, R. Hanisch, M. Pike, B.

Henderson, "Serum testosterone levels in healthy young black and white men," *J. Natl. Cancer Instit.* 76 (1986): 45–48.

46. *Ibid.*

47. B.E. Henderson, L. Bernstein, R.K. Ross, R.H. Depue, H.L. Judd, "The early *in utero* oestrogen and testosterone environment of blacks and whites: potential effects on male offspring," *Br. J. Cancer* 57 (1988): 216–218.

48. E. Giovannucci, T.D. Tosteson, F.E. Speizer, A. Ascherio, M.P. Vessey, G.A. Colditz, "A retrospective cohort study of vasectomy and prostate cancer in US men," *J. Amer. Med. Assoc.* 269 (1993): 878–882 .

49. *Ibid.*

50. E. Giovannucci, A. Ascherio, E.B. Rimm, G.A. Colditz, M.J. Stampfer, W.C. Willett, "A prospective cohort study of vasectomy and prostate cancer risk in US men," *J. Amer. Med. Assoc.* 269 (1993): 873–877

51. *Ibid.*

52. S. Preston-Martin, W. Mack, B.E. Henderson, " Risk factors for gliomas and meningiomas in males in Los Angeles County," *Cancer Res.* 49 (1989): 6137–6143.

53. *Ibid.*

54. J. Ribak, R. Lilis, Y. Suzuki, L. Penner, I.J. Selikoff, "Malignant mesothelioma in a cohort of asbestos insulation workers: clinical presentation, diagnosis, and causes of death," *Brit. J. Ind. Med.* 45 (1988): 182–187.

55. B.T. Mossman, J.B. Gee, "Asbestos-related diseases," *New Engl. J. Med.* 320 (1989): 1721–1730.

56. *Ibid.*

57. Editorial: "Common sense in the environment," *Nature* 353 (1991: 779–780.

58. Preston-Martin, "Increased cell division as a cause of human cancer," 7415–7421.

59. T.J.A. Key, M.C. Pike, "The dose-effect relationship between unopposed oestrogens and endometrial mitotic rate: Its central role in explaining and predicting endometrial cancer risk," *Br. J. Cancer* 57 (1988): 205–212.

60. *Ibid.*

61. *Ibid.*

62. *Ibid.*

10

·······························

VIRUSES, MICROBES, AND CANCER

Three decades ago viruses were widely suspected to be the "missing link" in cancer causation—the element that would eventually be proven to be responsible for most human cancers. Because of this widespread conviction, an enormous amount of time and money was spent studying principles of virology and trying to isolate viruses from various human cancers. To a certain extent, these efforts were a disappointment; viruses are now known to be causative of only three or four major human cancers. However, these efforts were not wasted. Were it not for the early attention paid to viruses, it is quite likely that acquired immune deficiency syndrome (AIDS) would not have been recognized as a viral disease, and many more people could have died of AIDS.

This illustrates a critically important point: just as it was impossible to predict that cancer research would eventually help us to understand AIDS, predicting which branch of science will contribute the next major breakthrough in the war against cancer is impossible. While a major advance against cancer could certainly come from a cancer researcher who has focused on some aspect of cancer for his of her entire career, a major advance against cancer could also come from a botanist, or a developmental biologist, or an invertebrate zoologist.

Viruses are now thought to be responsible for about 15% of all human cancers,[1] while microbes and bacteria may be responsible for another 5% of human cancers. This is a much lower number than was anticipated three decades ago, but still means that viruses were responsible for about 77,000 cancer deaths in 1991, a staggeringly large figure.

WHAT ARE VIRUSES AND MICROBES?

A virus is a tiny particle, much smaller than a bacterial cell, composed of a protein shell around a core of genetic material. The genetic material is

211

usually composed of RNA, although some viruses have DNA instead. Viruses are incapable of replicating themselves unless they first invade a cell and take over the protein-synthetic machinery of that cell. After a virus has taken over the metabolic machinery of a cell, it makes viral proteins and new copies of viral RNA in order to replicate itself. After the virus has replicated itself, dozens of new viral particles are released, each of which is capable of repeating the cycle, attacking new host cells and replicating itself. While this sort of attack does not usually result in the death of the host cell, the virus can still induce the host cell to make substantial quantities of viral protein and viral RNA. In fact, up to 1% of all the RNA in an infected cell may be viral in origin, and expression of viral RNA can result in significant alterations of the form and function of the infected cell.

"Microbe" is a general term, that refers to any microscopic disease-causing organism, usually a bacterial cell. Bacterial cells can invade or attach to normal human cells, but they are not as insidious as viral particles in that they do not usurp the metabolic machinery of a cell quite as effectively as does a virus. Nevertheless, bacterial infections, especially chronic bacterial infections, can cause irritation and inflammation, and certain bacterial infections are known to increase the likelihood of subsequently developing cancer.

Generally, microbes seem to cause human cancers by inducing a chronic state of inflammation, in essence similar to a chronic state of cell wounding. This stimulates the growth rate of normal human cells, which also increases the rate at which these cells can mutate. The mechanisms by which viruses cause human cancer are unclear, but a number of viral actions might be involved in carcinogenesis. Viruses could potentially induce human cancers by: direct stimulation of cell growth; induction of a host response such as inflammation, which causes an indirect stimulation of host cell growth; suppression of the immune system of the host; or insertion of viral genetic material into the host DNA so that normal genes are abnormally expressed.

VIRUS-INDUCED CANCER

The first virus to be definitely linked to human cancer was the human T-cell leukemia-lymphoma virus, called HTLV-I. This virus is closely linked to a form of leukemia-lymphoma prevalent in coastal areas of Japan, in the Caribbean, and in regions of central Africa. The virus is transmitted by breast feeding, sexual intercourse, blood transfusions, or needle sharing. The time period between viral infection and development of leukemia-lymphoma can be up to several decades, suggesting that viral exposure alone is not sufficient for development of cancer. HTLV-I antibodies are present in more than one million people in Japan, suggesting that exposure to the virus is very widespread. But only about 500 patients a year develop the associated cancer, meaning that only one in every 25 to 30 people infected with the HTLV-I virus will progress to leukemia-lymphoma.[2] It is not known to what extent infection with HTLV-I increases the relative risk of cancer, but the cancer is rare or absent in areas without the HTLV-I virus. Therefore, the virus may act as a potent risk factor for this very rare cancer.

In recent years, viruses have also been linked to a number of more common cancers. The hepatitis B virus (HBV) causes hepatitis, a chronic inflammation of the liver, and it has also been linked to liver cancer. Areas of the world with high levels of chronic HBV infection, such as China, southeast Asia, and West Africa, tend to have a very high incidence of liver cancer. In these parts of the world, liver cancer can account for up to 30% of all cancers, making it regionally the most prevalent form of cancer. For example, the incidence of liver cancer in Japan is roughly five-fold higher than in the United States, while in Mozambique liver cancer incidence is nearly 35-fold higher than in the United States. Liver cancer, properly known as hepatocellular carcinoma, usually does not occur until decades after a persistent HBV infection, suggesting that an interaction between HBV and other risk factors may be necessary to cause cancer.

The relative risk of hepatocellular carcinoma after infection with HBV was assessed in a classic study from a decade ago that still represents the state of the art.[3] This study was undertaken in Taiwan, where the incidence of hepatocellular carcinoma is quite high and where a public health insurance system made it relatively easy to determine health outcomes in a large number of people. A group of 22,707 Chinese male civil servants was enrolled in the study between 1975 and 1978, and these men were followed for an average of 3.3 years each. At the time of enrollment, each man donated a blood sample and completed a brief questionnaire about their state of health. Blood samples were used to determine if the men had been exposed to HBV, as shown by whether or not the blood carried antibodies to the virus. Because the exposure to virus could be objectively determined at the beginning of the study, this means that the study was prospective. Furthermore, since a large group of men was followed for approximately 75,000 man-years of time, the results of this study are likely to be quite definitive. During the follow-up period, a total of 41 men died of hepatocellular carcinoma and 266 men died of other causes, so nearly 15% of all deaths were due to liver cancer.[4]

About 15% of all men in the study had been exposed to HBV, as shown by the presence of antibodies to the hepatitis B surface antigen. Nearly

42% of all deaths in the HBV-positive group were due to hepatocellular carcinoma, while less than 1% of all deaths in the HBV-negative group were due to this cancer. HBV infection also seemed to cause an increased incidence of cirrhosis of the liver, as non-cancerous liver disease was responsible for 16% of all deaths in the HBV-positive men. The relative risk of hepatocellular carcinoma increased steadily with age, which suggests again that the interval from infection to induction of cancer is long. The fact that at least one HBV-negative man died of hepatocellular carcinoma proves that HBV is not the only cause of this cancer, but the association between HBV and liver cancer is exceedingly strong. All other factors being equal, the relative risk of hepatocellular carcinoma in HBV-positive men was 223-fold higher than in noninfected men.[5]

A recent study in which hepatocellular carcinoma cases were compared to healthy controls was able to confirm the findings of the earlier study. This study was done to evaluate the roles of HBV exposure, cigarette smoking, and alcohol use in causation of hepatocellular carcinoma in the United States.[6] One of the major purposes of this study was to evaluate the effect of smoking on liver cancer risk among HBV-negative persons. This was done because it had been suggested that smoking had a more powerful effect on HBV-negative persons than on HBV- positive persons. A total of 86 hepatocellular carcinoma cases were compared to 161 healthy controls in this study. Eighteen percent of the cases and none of the controls were found to have been chronically infected with HBV, confirming that HBV is a major risk factor for liver cancer. However the study did not find that cigarette smoking is a risk factor for hepatocellular carcinoma, and there was no relationship between quantity of cigarettes smoked and risk of liver cancer. Thus, HBV infection is the only major known risk factor for hepatocellular carcinoma in the United States.[7]

The data relating HBV infection to hepatocellular carcinoma are so strong that several clinical trials are now underway to test whether vaccination against HBV will protect a vulnerable population from liver cancer. These studies are primarily being conducted in Africa and Asia, where the incidence of hepatocellular carcinoma is much higher than in the United States. However, if the results show that vaccination reduces the incidence of this terrible cancer, then it may be worthwhile to implement vaccination programs in the United States as well. The vaccine presently being tested is cheap and seems to be effective, and hepatitis is a very damaging disease even in people who never progress to hepatocellular carcinoma. In the United States in 1992, a total of about 12,000 people died of hepatocellular carcinoma, so the vaccination may be a very practical way to lower the incidence of a major cancer.

The Epstein-Barr virus (EBV) has been linked to about four different kinds of human cancer. EBV antibodies are present in about 90% of the population of the United States, and in virtually 100% of the population in other parts of the world, indicating that most people have been exposed to the virus at some point in the past. In the United States, EBV exposure often occurs in adolescence, when it can cause infectious mononucleosis. The EB virus persists in the infected person throughout his or her life, and virus is regularly shed in the saliva. Antibodies to the EB virus appear months to years before the clinical onset of cancer of the nasopharynx, and the antibodies define populations at higher risk for this cancer.[8] Infection with EBV has also been strongly associated with Burkitt's lymphoma, and may cause Hodgkin's lymphoma and non-Hodgkin's lymphoma as well. Because all lymphomas are cancers of the immune system, it has long been suspected that chronic viral infection somehow causes some immune cells to become cancerous. The link between EBV infection and lymphoma is clearest in AIDS patients and in transplant patients who are immunosuppressed to prevent organ rejection. Nevertheless, exactly how viral infection results in cancer is unclear.

Active EBV has been found in tumor cells from patients with cancer of the nasopharynx, and roughly a third of all patients with Hodgkin's lymphoma have viral proteins expressed in certain of their tumor cells. EBV infection is also implicated as a cause of non-Hodgkin's lymphoma (NHL), which is a frightening possibility, because EBV exposure is epidemic and the incidence of NHL has increased more than 50% in the last 15 years.[9] One study explored the link between EBV exposure and NHL using blood samples that were collected from 104 people prior to their diagnosis of cancer.[10] This study used the resources of a serum bank that kept frozen blood serum samples from a total of 240,000 people. Serum samples from the NHL patients had been taken an average of 63 months before NHL was diagnosed, and the case samples were matched with 259 control individuals, who were similar in terms of age, sex, ethnic group, and date of blood collection. When EBV antibodies were measured in the blood samples of cases and controls, cases were found to be much more likely to be EBV-positive. Antibodies directed against EBV were associated with a roughly three-fold elevation in NHL risk. The particular pattern of antibodies suggests that EBV-exposed persons may actually suffer a type of immunosuppression. Overall, at least 10% of NHL patients have viral gene products in their tumor,[11] and one study found that 35% of patients with NHL had EBV viral DNA in their tumor cells.[12]

Therefore, the EB virus may be important in causing a subset of NHL tumors. This is difficult to understand, since most adults throughout the world have been infected with EBV. It is not clear why an epidemic virus should be associated with a relatively rare cancer, or why some infected persons progress to cancer, while most do not. Furthermore, why should incidence of this cancer be increasing now, when incidence of the virus has been high for many decades? There is a good possibility that EBV infection alone is not sufficient to cause NHL and that some other factor is needed to induce cancer formation. Changes in the prevalence of exposure to some unknown risk factor could thus be responsible for the increase in NHL.[13]

HUMAN PAPILLOMAVIRUS AS A RISK FACTOR FOR CERVICAL CANCER

One of the clearest cases of viral infection leading to cancer is the relationship between human papillomavirus (HPV) and cervical cancer. HPV is also thought to cause other genital cancers, as well as cancers of the anal region. Exposure to the virus probably occurs during sexual activity, so cervical cancer has been referred to as a venereal cancer. Together these anogenital cancers make up about 10% of the cancers occurring world-wide. Viral DNA is found in about 90% of all cervical cancer cells, with the viral DNA usually being integrated into the DNA of the tumor cells. As with the other cancer viruses, infection with HPV alone is not sufficient for development of cancer, but viral infection is one step on the road to malignancy. More than 60 different types of HPV have been described, and about a third of these are known to cause cervical cancer.

Recent evidence suggests that HPV may cause at least 76% of all cervical cancers.[14] The techniques used to detect viral gene products have become very much more sensitive in just the last few years, so it is now possible to detect viral involvement in cases where previous tests would have shown none. In one study conducted in Oregon, a group of 500 women with early stage cervical cancer were compared to an equal number of healthy control women. Each of these women underwent a Pap smear and a cervicovaginal lavage, in which a gentle stream of water was used to wash the cervix and vagina and these washings were collected. Cells that had been dislodged from the cervical and vaginal walls were screened for expression of viral gene products. In addition, each woman answered a series of questions that related to various known risk factors for cervical cancer. It was found that 81% of the case subjects were infected with HPV, while only 18% of the control women were similarly infected. When special tests were conducted to identify specific types of HPV, two HPV types in particular were found to be associated with high cervical cancer risk. Infection with HPV-16 or HPV-18 increased the relative risk of cervical cancer 51-fold, with respect to uninfected women. Infection with another series of HPV types (HPV-31, -33, -35, -39, -45, -51, or -52) increased risk about 33-fold over normal, while a third series of HPV types (HPV-6, -11, or -42) increased risk nine-fold over normal. Some women had multiple infections with HPV, which may have further increased their overall risk of cervical cancer.

Many of the case subjects showed a typical epidemiological profile of the cervical cancer patient.[15] Cases tended to have had more sexual partners, to have had intercourse at an earlier age, to be cigarette smokers, and to be of a lower socio-economic status. However, when these separate risk factors were corrected for viral exposure, it was found that viral exposure was a better predictor of cervical cancer risk than any of the other risk factors. For example, women who had 10 or more sexual partners in their lifetime were at a four-fold higher risk of cervical cancer than women who had only one sexual partner. But, if viral exposure is considered, having 10 or more sexual partners only increased the risk of cervical cancer two-fold with respect to a woman who had one partner. Evidently, having many sexual partners is a risk factor for cervical cancer, at least in part because multiple sexual partners increase the risk of exposure to a venereal virus such as HPV. This is clearly shown by the fact that women with 10 or more sexual partners who were HPV-positive were not at any greater risk of cervical cancer than women who were HPV-positive but who had only one sexual partner. The only previously known risk factor that appeared to be at least partly independent of HPV exposure was parity; women who had four or more children were at an increased risk of cervical cancer whether or not they had been exposed to HPV. Careful analysis of the data suggests that at least 76% of all cases of cervical cancer could be attributed to infection with HPV.[16]

These stunning results are largely consistent with an earlier study that prospectively followed a group of 241 women in Seattle.[17] These women were treated at a sexually transmitted disease clinic in Seattle, Washington, between 1984 and 1989. All of these women were found to be free of cervical cancer at presentation, and all were treated for the symptoms that first required the clinic visit. Each woman was then asked to complete a questionaire about risk factors for cervical cancer, to undergo a complete physical examination, and to have cervical cells collected for HPV screening. Because of their prior history of venereal disease, these women were at an increased risk of cervical cancer, so each was examined for cervical cancer every four months, for an average follow-up period of 25 months. Over the course of follow-up, a total of 28 women developed cervical cancer, and most of these women were HPV-positive. In fact, the incidence of cervical cancer was 28% among women with a positive test for HPV, and only 3% among women who were HPV-negative. The risk of cervical cancer was highest among women with HPV-16 or -18, as these women were 11-fold more likely to develop cervical cancer than women who were uninfected with HPV. About half of the women who were positive for HPV-16 or HPV-18 developed cervical cancer within 12 months of entering the study, and all of the women who developed cervical cancer did so within 24 months of their first positive HPV test. This suggests that HPV can cause cervical cancer in a strikingly short period of time. A number of other risk factors for cervical cancer were also identified in this study. The greatest risks were associated with prior exposure to chlamydia, gonorrhea, or cytomegalovirus, but none of these risks was as potent as infection with HPV.[18]

Infection with HPV also may affect cancer risk in men, as HPV-positive men appear to have a higher risk of cancer of the penis.[19] One study compared a group of 110 case men, all diagnosed with penile cancer, with 355 randomly selected healthy men who served as controls. Each man was interviewed about various known risk factors for penile cancer, including past sexual activity, history of sexually transmitted diseases, smoking history, and previous medical conditions of the penis. In addition, a small sample from each tumor was tested for evidence of HPV, using an exquisitely sensitive new technique. Nearly half of the penile tumors showed evidence of viral involvement, suggesting that the tumors may have been induced by HPV. Infection of men with the HPV virus often causes genital warts, so a comparison was also made between cases and controls, to determine whether the incidence of genital warts differed. It was found that men with genital warts were nearly six-fold more likely to have cancer of the penis. Nevertheless, this does not prove that men with genital warts will develop penile cancer, since genital warts can be caused by strains of HPV that do not induce tumors. Men who were HPV-positive were more than twice as likely to have had five or more sexual partners as men who were HPV-negative, showing that HPV infection is associated with sexual activity.[20] This is consistent with evidence showing that women with multiple sexual partners are more likely to be HPV-positive.

In fact, new evidence suggests that the cervical cancer risk of women is determined in part by the sexual history of their male partner.[21] A small study was done in India, where the risk of cervical cancer is one of the highest in the world, and where sexual promiscuity by women is quite rare. These unique features of life in India made it possible to study the role of male sexual partners in cervical cancer risk. Women with a single lifetime sexual partner were found to be at a higher risk of cervical cancer if that partner was sexually active outside the marriage. For women whose sexual partner had premarital sex with more than two other women, the risk of cervical cancer was elevated 2.4-fold, compared to women with a monogamous partner. For women whose partner had both premarital and extramarital sexual relations, the risk of cervical cancer was elevated 6.9-fold with respect to the lowest risk group. These results, while really rather preliminary, are consistent with what we know of HPV epidemiology, and they suggest that male sexual partners can play a role in the dissemination of cervical cancer.[22]

An association has also been noted between the virus that causes AIDS and several ordinarily rare cancers. AIDS is caused by the human immunodeficiency virus (HIV-1), whose primary action is suppression of the patient's immune system. However, immune suppression in AIDS patients is associated with an increased incidence of several rare cancers (B-cell lymphoma and Kaposi's sarcoma). It is probable that HIV-1 does not actually cause these tumors directly, but since HIV-1 causes suppression of the immune system, these tumors may escape immune control. In fact, recent evidence suggests that Kaposi's sarcoma, a rare malignancy of the cells that form blood vessels, is actually caused by cytomegalovirus (CMV), but that chronic CMV infection usually only occurs when the patient is immunosuppressed by HIV. However, there is also some evidence that HIV-1 can cause lymphoma directly.[23]

MICROORGANISMS AND CANCER

The only well-established example of a cancer associated with bacterial infection is that of stomach cancer and a bacterium called *Helicobacter* (or *Campylobacter*) *pylori*. Apparently once a person is infected with *H. pylori*, that infection is permanent; in healthy persons under age 30, the rate of infection is only about 10%, but in persons over 60 years of age, the prevalence rate of *H. pylori* infection approaches 60%.[24] Often this infection has no ill effects, but a certain proportion of people develop either peptic ulcer or chronic gastritis. Since chronic gastritis is known to be associated with stomach cancer, scientists realized that stomach cancer could potentially be caused by chronic bacterial infection. Chronic bacterial infection could cause stomach inflammation, with damage to the stomach lining and a condition of chronic wound-healing. As we saw before, chronic wound-healing often seems to set the stage for development of cancer.

Evidence for a connection between chronic infection with *H. pylori* and stomach cancer is, at least in part, circumstantial, but that evidence is getting stronger. One study was done in China, where infection with *H. pylori* is far more common than in Europe or North America, and where stomach cancer is the leading cause of cancer mortality.[25] However, even within China, there are striking regional differences in stomach cancer incidence: stomach cancer mortality varies 74-fold between different parts of China, and the highest mortality rate in China is more than 1,000-fold higher than in the United States. To determine the frequency of infection with *H. pylori*, scientists measured the prevalence of antibodies to *H. pylori* in blood samples taken from 1,882 men. Blood samples were collected in 1983 from men aged 35 to 64 years old in 46 rural counties scattered all over China. Depending upon region, the rate of infection with *H. pylori* varied from 28% to 96% of the population. There was a general correlation between the rate of infection with *H. pylori* and the stomach cancer mortality rate, although differences in bacterial infection rate explained only about 16% of the variation in stomach cancer mortality. What this means is that, while infection with *H. pylori* is probably an important cause of stomach cancer, other unknown causes are cumulatively more important. It was also noted that no other cancer, not even colorectal cancer, showed any association with *H. pylori* infection.[26]

More recently, a large study examined the association between *H. pylori* infection and stomach cancer in 13 countries around the world, instead of just in China.[27] A total of 3,194 subjects, composed equally of men and women, were selected to fall into one of two age groups: either subjects were 25 to 34 years old, or they were 55 to 64 years old. Each subject provided a blood sample and answered a short questionnaire about certain risk factors. All of the blood samples were screened to determine which subjects were infected with *H. pylori* as shown by the presence of antibodies to the bacterium in the blood. The proportion of subjects who were infected in each country was then correlated with the prevalence of stomach cancer in that country. There was a general trend for countries with a high incidence of bacterial infection to have high rates of stomach cancer incidence and stomach cancer mortality in both men and women.[28] However, this type of "ecological study" is limited, because correlation does not imply causality; simply showing that bacterial infection rate and cancer mortality rate are correlated does not prove that infection is the cause of cancer. Furthermore, this study did not sub-divide patients depending upon what particular type of stomach cancer they had. As we shall see, separating patients by diagnosis can make a large difference in the results.

These results have been confirmed and extended by a study that examined *H. pylori* infection and gastric cancer risk in Mexico.[29] This study firstly confirmed that bacterial infection increases the risk of stomach cancer about two-fold with respect to uninfected individuals, but it went one step further. Infection with *H. pylori* was found to increase the risk of chronic gastritis about 15-fold, compared to people who were not infected. This is important because gastritis is known to be a precursor condition to stomach cancer; therefore, this study shows that bacterial infection is strongly linked with gastritis, but that most people with gastritis do not develop stomach cancer.[30]

A recent study that examined the association between stomach cancer and H. pylori infection, also separated patients by the particular type of stomach cancer they had at diagnosis.[31] Stomach cancer can affect the gastric cardia, that portion of the stomach where the esophagus opens into the stomach, or it can affect the sac-like lower portion of the stomach, which is called the antrum. When the connection between H. pylori infection and stomach cancer is closely examined, it turns out that bacterial infection is more closely associated with development of cancer of the antrum than of the cardia. This was discovered in a study conducted in Minnesota, which compared a group of 69 patients with stomach cancer with 218 patients with cancer at other sites (colon, lung, or esophagus) and with another 252 cancer-free controls. The 69 patients with stomach cancer were further sub-divided into 32 patients with cancer at the cardia and 37 patients with cancer at the antrum. Each case and control individual gave a blood sample that was screened for antibodies to H. pylori using a highly sensitive test. It was found that 65% of the patients with stomach cancer at the antrum had been exposed to H. pylori, but only 38% of the patients with stomach cancer at the cardia had been so exposed. Similarly, 38% of the cancer-free controls had also been exposed to H. pylori. Infection with this bacterium increased the odds of developing antral cancer of the stomach nearly three-fold, compared to uninfected persons. Furthermore, infection with H. pylori was found to specifically increase the likelihood of developing a type of antral cancer that is more common in China than in the United States. Therefore these results provide fairly strongly support for the idea that H. pylori infection can lead to the development of antral stomach cancer.[32]

Recently scientists studied the relationship between H. pylori infection and stomach cancer in a group of Japanese-American men living in Hawaii.[33] A total of 5,908 men were enrolled in this study between 1967 and 1970, at which time each man donated a blood sample; each man was then followed for more than 20 years. Because men were enrolled in the study while they were still healthy, this study is prospective, and the results are more likely to be unbiased. By 1989, a total of 109 cases of stomach cancer had been diagnosed in this cohort of men. The stored serum of each patient and of an age-matched control was tested for the presence of antibody to H. pylori. It was found that 94% of the men with stomach cancer and 76% of the control subjects had a positive antibody test, indicating that this bacterium is quite common in this Japanese-American population. However, men who were infected were roughly six-fold more likely to develop stomach cancer. It was also found that as the level of antibody to *H. pylori* increased, so did the risk of stomach cancer: men with low levels of antibody were at a 4.7-fold higher risk of stomach cancer, but men with high levels of antibody were 7.6-fold more likely to develop stomach cancer. The association between infection and stomach cancer risk was strong even for men in whom the diagnosis was made 10 or more years after the blood sample was taken. Nevertheless, while infection with *H. pylori* is strongly associated with an increased risk of stomach cancer, most people with an infection will still never develop stomach cancer. Thus, other factors must increase the risk of stomach cancer, and there is a pressing need to identify these other factors.[34]

Another study, published at the same time as the preceding study, has confirmed that infection with *H. pylori* increases the risk of stomach cancer.[35] This study examined a group of 128,992 men and women in California who had donated blood samples between 1964 and 1969. These people were also followed for more than 20 years, until a total of 186 people developed stomach cancer. The 186 cases were matched by age, sex, and race to a group of 186 healthy control subjects. At the end of the 20-year study period, frozen blood samples that had been collected in the 1960s were tested for antibodies to *H. pylori*. In addition, information about cigarette use, blood group, and the history of stomach disease or surgery, which had been obtained from questionnaires filled out at enrollment, was analyzed. The average interval between blood collection and the diagnosis of stomach cancer was found to be 14.2 years. It was also found that cancer of the gastric cardia was not linked to *H. pylori* infection, but that bacterial infection increased the risk of antral stomach cancer nearly four-fold with respect to normal. Infection with *H. pylori* was a particularly strong risk factor for stomach cancer in women, for whom the risk was increased 18-fold by bacterial infection, and in blacks, for whom risk was increased nine-fold by infection. This study confirms that *H. pylori* infection is strongly associated with an increased risk of stomach cancer.[36]

REDUCING EXPOSURE TO VIRAL AND BACTERIAL CARCINOGENS

Because infection with certain viruses and bacteria can apparently cause cancer, reducing the incidence of viral and bacterial infection would be a sound strategy for reducing cancer incidence. In fact, a vaccine against the hepatitis B virus (HBV) is already available, and it would be of great public health benefit if this vaccine was routinely given. The vaccine is relatively inexpensive now, and large-scale efforts at immunization would further reduce the cost. While liver cancer is not an extremely common cancer in the United States, more than 15,000 people were diagnosed with this cancer in 1992. Since many of these cases were associated with HBV infection, widespread use of the vaccine would be a practical and effective cancer preventive method.

Similarly, it would be very worthwhile to develop a vaccine against the human papilloma virus (HPV), especially those two viral strains (HPV-16 and -18) that are most closely associated with cervical cancer. But lower priority should be given to HPV vaccination than to HBV vaccination; HPV infection is largely preventable by condom use, early stage cervical cancer is easily diagnosed by Pap smear, and cervical cancer is less frequently fatal than liver cancer. Nevertheless, major public health benefits might be achieved with a widely available vaccine against HPV.

Efforts are now being made to develop a vaccine against *H. pylori*.[37] Such a vaccine would be likely to have a more important role in reducing the incidence of ulcers and chronic gastritis than in reducing the incidence of stomach cancer, because stomach cancer is rare by comparison with the other diseases. Nevertheless, stomach cancer is still a major killer and a vaccine against *H. pylori* would be welcomed in many parts of the world.

It will probably never be possible to prevent all viral and bacterial infections, and it is not clear that total prevention of infection is a practical goal anyway. An alternative to prevention of infection might be to delay the first infection of individuals as long as possible, by rigorous personal hygiene, by strict public sanitation, or by stringent quarantine of infected individuals. But there is reason to suspect that delay of infection might not always be the most appropriate strategy to reduce cancer incidence. For example, Hodgkins disease is probably stimulated by infection with the Epstein-Barr virus (EBV), although we know there are other factors that determine which EBV-infected people will go on to develop Hodgkins disease. Factors that increase the risk of early exposure to EBV actually decrease the risk of later developing Hodgkins disease. Crowded living conditions, large family size, or relatively poor public sanitation are all associated with a *lower* incidence of Hodgkins disease. In the United States, where early childhood exposure to EBV is not the rule, Hodgkins disease incidence is relatively high in young adults. In Japan, where EBV exposure is more ubiquitous, young adults seldom develop Hodgkins disease. This suggests that viral infection must occur during a particular window of time, perhaps in early adolescence, in order to result in development of Hodgkins disease. This is not an argument in favor of early exposure to viruses, it is simply an argument that many aspects of the relationship

TABLE 10-1
WEIGHTED RISK CALCULATIONS FOR VIRAL RISK FACTORS

RISK FACTOR	RELATED CANCER	RELATIVE RISK	RELATIVE FREQUENCY	RISK WEIGHT
Hepatitis B virus (HBV)	Liver	223	2	446a
Chronic immunosuppression	Lymphoma	35	3	105c
HPV-16 or 18	Cervical	51.0	2	102a
Human papilloma virus (HPV)	Cervical	33.6	2	67a
HPV-31, 33, 35, or 39	Cervical	33.0	2	66a
HPV-45, 51, or 52	Cervical	33.0	2	66a
Hp infection (Black Americans)	Stomach	9.0	2	18a
HPV-6, 11, or 42	Cervical	8.7	2	17a
High-level *Hp* infection	Stomach	7.6	2	15a
Hp infection (Japanese Americans)	Stomach	6.0	2	12a
Low-level *Hp* infection	Stomach	4.7	2	9a
Epstein-Barr virus (EBV)	Lymphoma	2.9	3	9c
Helicobacter pylori (Hp)	Stomach	3.6	2	7a
Hp infection (White Americans)	Stomach	2.9	2	6a
Genital warts (HPV)	Penile	5.9	1	6b
Sexually active male partner	Cervical	2.4	2	5c

The relative importance of a risk factor is quantified by considering three factors: the relative risk associated with the factor; the relative frequency of the related cancer; and the statistical power of the study that linked the risk factor with the cancer.

between viral infection and cancer are poorly understood. Expending great effort to eradicate viral diseases may backfire unless we acquire a more thorough understanding of viral and bacterial risk factors in cancer.

SUMMARY

Viruses and microbes are now known to be causally related to a rather small number of cancers, none of which are among the leading killers. Yet this does not negate the importance of these agents as causes of cancer, nor does it lessen the worth of preventive efforts directed against them. Hepatitis B virus (HBV) is a potent risk factor for hepatocellular carcinoma, yet this cancer is largely preventable because a vaccine already exists for HBV. Similarly, cervical cancer should be considered a preventable cancer because simple personal hygiene measures can arrest the spread of human papilloma virus (HPV). It is quite likely that a vaccine could be developed against *Helicobacter pylori* in the near future, so that stomach cancer could become a preventable cancer. If the mortality from these three cancers could be halved, this would mean that more than 25,000 lives would be saved each year in the United States alone. Furthermore, in parts of Asia and Africa, hepatocellular carcinoma is far more common than in the West, accounting for up to 30% of all deaths from cancer. Thus, the goal of preventing these cancers becomes even more compelling.

NOTES TO CHAPTER 10

1. H. zur Hausen, "Viruses in human cancer," *Science* 254 (1991): 1167–1173.
2. *Ibid.*
3. R.P. Beasley, C.C. Lin, L.U. Hwang, C-S. Chien, "Hepatocellular carcinoma and hepatitis B virus. A prospective study of 22,707 men in Taiwan," *Lancet* ii (1981): 1129–1132.
4. *Ibid.*
5. *Ibid.*
6. H. Austin, E. Delzell, S. Grufferman, R. Levine, A.S. Morrison, et al., "A case-control study of hepatocellular carcinoma and the hepatitis B virus, cigarette smoking, and alcohol consumption," *Cancer Res.* 46 (1986): 962–966.
7. *Ibid.*
8. J.W. Sixbey, Q-Y. Yao, "Immunoglobulin A-induced shift of Epstein-Barr virus tissue tropism," *Science* 255 (1992): 1578–1580.

9. S.H. Zahm, A. Blair, "Pesticides and non-Hodgkins lymphoma," *Cancer Res.* 52 (1992): 5485s–5488s.
10. N.E. Mueller, A. Mohar, A. Evans, "Viruses other than HIV and non-Hodgkins lymphoma," *Cancer Res.* 52 (1992): 5479s–5481s.
11. S.J. Hamilton-Dutoit, G. Pallesen, "A survey of Epstein-Barr virus gene expression in sporadic non-Hodgkins lymphomas," *Am. J. Pathol.* 140 (1992): 1315–1325.
12. G. Ott, M.M. Ott, A.C. Feller, S. Seidl, H.K. Muller-Hermelink, "Prevalence of Epstein-Barr virus DNA in different T-cell lymphoma entities in a European population," *Int. J. Cancer* 51 (1992): 562–567.
13. Mueller, "Viruses other than HIV and non-Hodgkins lymphoma," 5479s–5481s.
14. M.H. Schiffman, H.M. Bauer, R.N. Hoover, A.G. Glass, D.M. Cadell, et al., "Epidemiologic evidence showing that human papillomavirus infection causes most cervical intraepithelial neoplasia," *J. Natl. Cancer Instit.* 85 (1993): 958–964.
15. *Ibid.*
16. *Ibid.*
17. L.A. Koutsky, K.K. Holmes, C.W. Critchlow, C.E. Stevens, J. Paavonen, et al., "A cohort study of the risk of cervical intraepithelial neoplasia grade 2 or 3 in relation to papillomavirus infection," *N. Engl. J. Med.* 327 (1992): 12720–1278.
18. *Ibid.*
19. C. Maden, K.J. Sherman, A.M. Beckmann, T.G. Hislop, C-Z. Teh, et al., "History of circumcision, medical conditions, and sexual activity and risk of penile cancer," *J. Natl. Cancer Instit.* 85 (1993): 19–24.
20. *Ibid.*
21. S.S. Agarwal, A. Sehgal, S. Sardana, A. Kumar, U.K. Luthra, "Role of male behavior in cervical carcinogenesis among women with one lifetime sexual partner," *Cancer* 72 (1993): 1666–1669.
22. *Ibid.*
23. B.G. Herndier, B.T. Shiramizu, N.E. Jewett, K.D. Aldape, G.R. Reyes, M.S. McGrath, "Acquired immunodeficiency syndrome-associated T-cell lymphoma: evidence for human immunodeficiency virus type 1-associated T-cell transformation," *Blood* 79 (1992): 1768–1774.
24. W.L. Peterson, "*Helicobacter pylori* and peptic ulcer disease," *N. Engl. J. Med.* 324 (1991): 1043–1048.
25. D. Forman, F. Sitas, D.G. Newell, A.R. Stacey, J. Boreham, et al., "Geographic association of *Helicobacter pylori* antibody prevalence and

gastric cancer mortality in rural China," *Int. J. Cancer* 46 (1990): 608–611.

26. *Ibid.*
27. D. Forman, P. Webb, D. Newell, M. Coleman, D. Palli, et al., "An international association between *Helicobacter pylori* infection and gastric cancer," *Lancet* 341 (1993): 1359–1362.
28. *Ibid.*
29. J. Guarner, A. Mohar, J. Parsonnet, D. Halperin, "The association of *Helicobacter pylori* with gastric cancer and preneoplastic gastric lesions in Chiapas, Mexico," *Cancer* 71 (1993): 297–301.
30. *Ibid.*
31. N.J. Talley, A.R. Zinsmeister, A. Weaver, E.P. DiMagno, H.A. Carpenter, et al., "Gastric adenocarcinoma and *Helicobacter pylori* infection," *J. Natl. Cancer Instit.* 83 (1991): 1734–1739.
32. *Ibid.*
33. A. Nomura, G.N. Stemmerman, P-H. Chyou, I. Kato, G.I. Perez-Perez, M.J. Blaser, *"Helicobacter pylori* infection and gastric carcinoma among Japanese Americans in Hawaii," *N. Engl. J. Med.* 325 (1991): 1132–1136.
34. *Ibid.*
35. J. Parsonnet, G.D. Friedman, D.P. Vandersteen, Y. Chang, J.H. Vogelman, et al., *"Helicobacter pylori* infection and the risk of gastric carcinoma," *N. Engl. J. Med.* 325 (1991): 1127–1131.
36. *Ibid.*
37. J. Alper, "Ulcers as an infectious disease," *Science* 260 (1993): 159–160.

11
....

LIFESTYLE, BEHAVIOR, AND CANCER

For the purposes of the following discussion, lifestyle and behavior are both broadly defined, so this chapter is essentially a compendium of those cancer risk factors that did not fit under the headings of previous chapters. This can lead to a certain amount of confusion since the divisions are somewhat arbitrary. Smoking, which is a risk factor for many different cancers, would seem to be a lifestyle choice, but this risk factor was already discussed in the chapter on chemical causes of cancer. This is because the mechanism by which tobacco smoke causes cancer has many features in common with the mechanism by which mustard gas causes laryngeal cancer. Clearly, exposure to mustard gas is not a lifestyle choice, and exposure to carcinogenic chemicals is common enough that such chemicals warrant a chapter of their own.

The mechanisms by which lifestyle and behavioral choices induce cancer are, in many cases, not well known. Therefore, this chapter is a compendium of loose ends, risk factors that are not easily classified and that produce cancers by unknown mechanisms. Nevertheless, the relationship between several of these risk factors and certain cancers has been clearly established, so the fact that our understanding of mechanism is poor should not imply that these risk factors are trivial. In fact, several of the lifestyle risk factors are very important from a public health standpoint, either because they are associated with a very common cancer or because they are rather powerful risk factors.

OBESITY

Obesity is known to be a risk factor for mortality from many different causes. This was shown most recently by a study that followed a group of 19,297 men prospectively from middle age onward.[1] A group of Harvard alumni, at an average age of 47 years in 1964, filled out a detailed questionnaire at enrollment in the study. These men were all free of heart disease, stroke, or cancer at enrollment, and each answered questions about height, weight, smoking habits, physical activity, and medical history. Each man was then followed until 1988, by which time 4,370 men had died of various causes and there had been a total of 425,718 person-years of follow-up. The body mass index (BMI) was calculated for each man, in order to have a summary statistic that incorporated both height and weight (BMI = weight in kilograms divided by the square of height in meters). Risk of death was then determined as a function of BMI at enrollment, by comparing the proportion of men who died in each of five BMI classes. For each of the men who died, the cause of death was also determined, to see whether obesity predisposed to any particular type of mortality.

Not surprisingly, obesity was found to cause a 2.5-fold increase in the risk of cardiovascular disease for non-smoking men in the highest quintile (20%) of BMI, as compared to non-smoking men in the lowest quintile of BMI.[2] However, cancer mortality also increased with increasing BMI—the heaviest men were at a 1.5-fold higher risk of cancer than the lightest men, even when smokers were eliminated from the comparison. Cancer risk was roughly comparable for men in the three lowest quintiles of BMI (≤ 24.5) and was only slightly elevated for men in the second highest quintile (24.5 to < 26.0), so this indicates that cancer risk is strongly elevated only for the heaviest 20% of men. However, when all causes of mortality were combined among non-smoking men, the risk of death increased steadily with increasing BMI. If men in the lowest quintile of BMI (< 22.5) are used as a point of comparison, men in the highest quintile of BMI (≥ 26.0) had a 67% higher risk of death. Men in the next highest quintile of BMI (24.5 to < 26.0) had a 27% higher risk of death than the lightest men. Much of the excess mortality among obese and slightly obese men was caused by a dramatically higher incidence of cardiovascular disease. In fact, heart attack risk was nearly 50% lower for men in the lowest quintile of BMI, when compared to the whole rest of the group. Thus obesity is a general risk factor for death, particularly death from heart disease.[3] This study is very convincing because the follow-up period was so long and because there were many deaths during the follow-up. However, the study did not address obesity as a risk factor for specific cancers, so there is a certain lack of detail that makes the study less satisfying.

Recently, data from the Harvard Alumni Health Study were used to determine whether obesity is a risk factor specifically for colon cancer.[4] A group of 17,595 alumni, all of whom had completed a detailed lifestyle questionnaire between 1962 and 1966, were followed up in 1988. During the follow-up period, a total of 302 cases of colon cancer were diagnosed.

When the colon cancer risk of those men in the highest quintile of BMI was compared with those in the lowest quintile of BMI, obesity was found to increase the relative risk of colon cancer 2.4-fold. Generally, colon cancer risk increased with increasing BMI, even when the numbers were adjusted to account for age, physical activity, and a parental history of cancer. However, obesity in early adulthood did not predict cancer risk as well as did obesity in middle age. This suggests that even individuals who were overweight as young adults could potentially benefit from a subsequent loss of weight, even if the weight loss occurred in middle age.

The connection between obesity and cancer risk has been extensively studied in the case of breast cancer, since obesity was long known as a risk factor for this cancer.[5] One study of the link between weight, height, and breast cancer risk examined 567,333 women in Norway, who were followed for an average of 12 years.[6] Because this study involved more than 6.8 million person-years of follow-up, the results are quite likely definitive. Body mass index (BMI) was calculated as in the previous studies, in order to combine the data on height and weight into a single number to indicate obesity. It was found that BMI was correlated with breast cancer risk in every age category, from 30 years old up to 69 years old. However, the relationship between obesity and breast cancer risk was somewhat counterintuitive: while obesity was a strong risk factor for breast cancer in post-menopausal women, it was actually protective for pre-menopausal women. For women aged 50 years old or older, those in the highest decile (10%) of BMI were 16% more likely to get breast cancer, and 46% more likely to die of it, than women in the lowest decile of BMI. Yet, for women under age 50, women in the highest decile of BMI were 16% less likely to get breast cancer, although they are still 16% more likely to die of it, than women in the lowest decile of BMI. The higher risk of breast cancer mortality in obese women of all ages occurs because obese women tend to be diagnosed at a later stage of disease, possibly because it is harder to discover a small tumor in an obese woman. The same study also showed that tall women of all ages are somewhat more prone to breast cancer; women aged 50 or older who are in the tallest height decile are 42% more likely to develop breast cancer.[7]

The idea that obesity causes an increased risk of breast cancer has been largely confirmed by several studies in the United States. For example, the Adventist Health Study, which followed 20,341 Seventh-Day Adventist women in California for a total of 115,000 person-years, confirmed that obesity is a potent risk factor for breast cancer.[8] During the follow-up period 215 cases of breast cancer were diagnosed, so a fairly large number of case women could be compared to age-matched control women. Because each subject filled out a dietary questionnaire prospectively at the beginning of the study, the study provides a wealth of information on various risk factors for breast cancer. It was found that obesity is the fifth most important risk factor for breast cancer, and that women in the upper third of the weight distribution had a 1.6-fold higher risk of breast cancer compared to women in the lower third of the weight distribution. This study was particularly valuable because it examined many separate risk factors for breast cancer, so it was able to put obesity into a broad framework of risk factors. Overall, the five most important risk factors for breast cancer were (in decreasing order): the number of years between menarche and first giving birth; highest educational attainment; age at first giving birth; family history of breast cancer; and obesity.[9]

A more recent study also confirms that obesity increases breast cancer risk in post-menopausal women.[10] A total of 37,105 Iowa women, all between the ages of 55 and 69 years of age, were studied to determine to what extent breast cancer risk was affected by a family history of the disease. This study was prospective, so that information on race, occupation, family medical history, height, weight, and body fat distribution was gathered at the beginning of the study. Over the four-year follow-up period, 493 new cases of breast cancer were diagnosed. Overall, women in the highest quintile of body mass index (BMI) were 1.6-fold more likely to develop breast cancer than women in the lowest quintile of BMI, but obesity was not as important as family history in determining cancer risk. Compared to women in the lowest quintile of BMI, obese women with a family history of breast cancer were 2.2-fold more prone to breast cancer, while obese women without a family history of breast cancer were only 1.5-fold more prone to breast cancer. Body weight was also a predictor of breast cancer risk and it also interacted with family history in determining breast cancer risk. A women with no family history of disease, but who was in the highest quintile of body weight, was 1.6-fold more likely to get breast cancer than a lighter woman, while a woman with a family history of disease was 2.6-fold more likely to get breast cancer. In fact, in this study, weight was a better predictor of breast cancer risk than was BMI. Tall women tend to be heavier than short women, even if they are not obese, and height itself was a determinant of breast cancer risk. Therefore, weight alone predicts breast cancer risk fairly well, since heavy women are likely to be tall or obese or both. Considering only those women without a family history of breast cancer, those who weigh more than 175 pounds are at 1.6-fold higher risk of breast cancer than those who weigh less than 140 pounds. For women between 141 and 174 pounds, breast cancer risk is elevated about 1.3-fold with respect to the lightest women.[11]

Finally, there is some indication that obesity can be a risk factor for certain other cancers besides colon and breast cancer. For example, a comparison between 160 case individuals with renal cell kidney cancer and an equal number of healthy controls found that obesity was a significant risk factor for this cancer.[12] Cases and controls were matched for age, race, sex, and neighborhood of residence, and their responses to a questionnaire about risk were compared. For both men and women, those in the heaviest quartile of BMI were at a roughly three-fold higher risk of renal cell cancer than those in the lightest quartile of BMI.

EXERCISE

If obesity is a risk factor for cancer, physical exercise seems likely to be protective from cancer, since an active person is far less likely to be obese. This indeed appears to be true, based on several somewhat preliminary studies that have been published in the last few years.

The largest and most convincing study to examine physical activity level as a risk factor for cancer is the Harvard Alumni Health Study. Colorectal cancer risk was studied as a function of physical activity in 17,148 men between the ages of 30 and 79 years.[13] These men were entered into the study in 1965, at which point their physical activity was assessed on the basis of self-reported activities, such as stair climbing, walking, and sports play. Activity was assessed again in 1977, when the subjects were given a follow-up questionnaire. The study was terminated in 1988, when 225 men had developed colon cancer and another 44 men had developed rectal cancer. When the activity level of case individuals was compared to that of the control individuals, low levels of physical activity were were found to be a risk factor for colon cancer but not for rectal cancer. However, the physical activity level estimated from either of the evaluations alone was not significant; only when physical activity was sustained over the course of the study was there a protective effect. In fact, exercise did not need to be very vigorous to be protective, since moderate exercise was comparable to vigorous exercise in terms of the protection conferred. Men who exercised at a level of energy expenditure greater than 2,500 kilocalories per week were 50% less likely to get colon cancer than men who exercised at a level less than 1,000 kilocalories per week. However, men who exercised at a level between 1,000 and 2,500 kilocalories per week were 48% less likely to get colon cancer than the most sedentary men. The fact that two activity assessments together were able to predict risk with more accuracy than one separate activity assessment may mean that consistent exercise is more important than vigorous exercise. Alternatively, it may mean that a single assessment simply cannot measure physical activity with precision.[14]

When measures of physical activity were combined with measures of obesity to determine which was a better predictor of colon cancer risk, a very interesting picture emerged:[15] physical activity was protective from colon cancer even in obese men. Overall, body mass index (BMI) was predictive of colon cancer risk, so that the heaviest fifth of alumni had a 2.5-fold higher risk of colon cancer. However, when these men were classified by activity level, it was found that BMI predicted colon cancer risk only among those who were sedentary. This implies that being overweight during middle age is a risk factor for colon cancer but that, in overweight but active men, colon cancer risk may not be increased. This could be explained in a fairly simple way, since physical activity enhances bowel motility, and regular bowel movements appear to reduce colon cancer risk.[16]

The results of this recent study are consistent with an earlier study of job activity and colon cancer risk.[17] A group of 2,950 men, all of whom had been diagnosed with colon cancer in Los Angeles County between 1972 and 1981, were examined to see whether their activity was higher or lower than normal. Each man's occupation was ranked as having a high, moderate, or sedentary level of activity, then colon cancer risk was determined separately for each activity level. Men with sedentary jobs were found to be at least 1.6-fold more likely to get colon cancer, and colon cancer risk declined with increasing job activity. This was true for black, white, and Hispanic males, although physical activity was again not associated with risk of rectal cancer.[18] Thus physical activity could play a role in reducing colon cancer incidence by increasing bowel motility, and this effect may be completely independent from the effect of exercise on body weight.

Some evidence also suggests that physical activity could potentially reduce the incidence of breast cancer, also by a mechanism completely independent from the effect of exercise on body weight. Vigorous exercise has a strong effect on the female menstrual cycle, so exercise could also have an indirect effect on hormone-dependent cancers such as breast cancer. Women who engage in very strenuous physical activity are often amenorrheic, meaning that they do not experience menstrual cycles, and logic would suggest that this could be associated with a reduced incidence of breast cancer. Yet it is unknown whether moderate levels of exercise have any effect on menstrual cycles. To answer this question, a group of 166 college women were asked to monitor their menstrual cycles for 12 months, while also recording their physical activity level.[19] It was found that moderate physical exercise increased the probability of a long menstrual cycle by about 10%, and various other stresses had a similar effect on cycle time for all women. Thus activity level to a certain extent determines menstrual cycle time, which could have a long-term effect on breast cancer risk. Since longer cycles mean fewer cumulative cycles, there will be less cumulative exposure to the high levels of estrogen that are characteristic of some phases of the menstrual cycle. Since estrogen exposure has been associated with breast cancer risk, vigorous exercise could possibly reduce breast cancer risk even in obese women, just as exercise reduced colon cancer risk even in obese men. Furthermore, the probability of a "missed period," or anovular cycle, increases with increasing exercise for all women.[20] Therefore, participation in moderate physical exercise may indirectly reduce the incidence of breast cancer, although as yet little firm evidence supports this conclusion.

ALCOHOL CONSUMPTION

Excessive alcohol consumption has been estimated to be responsible for as much as 5% of all cancer deaths in the United States.[21] Alcoholics have a 10-fold higher risk of cancer at all sites, with the greatest risk associated with cancers of the head and neck, the esophagus, the stomach, the liver, and the pancreas. In addition, some evidence exists that alcohol can increase the risk of colon cancer and breast cancer. It is not at all clear how alcohol could have an effect on such diverse tissues, especially since some of these tissues never come in direct contact with alcohol. However, researchers suspect that excessive alcohol consumption may actually suppress the immune system;[22] if this proves to be true, then it would not be surprising that alcohol could cause breast cancer.

The clearest and strongest case for alcohol increasing the risk of cancer is seen in oral and upper gastrointestinal cancers. One large study compared the alcohol and tobacco use of healthy men and women with that of men and women who had been diagnosed with cancers of the mouth, tongue, and pharynx.[23] Case individuals were identified from cancer registries for 1984, and all were from one of four major metropolitan areas in the United States: Atlanta, Los Angeles, San Francisco, or New Jersey. A total of 1,114 case patients were identified, and these men and women were then matched with 1,268 control individuals on the basis of age, sex, and race. Each of the cases and controls was then interviewed about his or her history of tobacco and alcohol intake, dietary habits, area of residence, occupation, medical history, and so on. A comparison of cases and controls showed that 94% of the male and 82% of the female case patients had been drinkers of alcoholic beverages, whereas only 83% of the male and 60% of the female controls were drinkers. Of those case individuals who drank alcohol, more than 94% also smoked tobacco.

Alcohol and tobacco were a very powerful interactive risk, as people who were both heavy smokers and heavy drinkers were nearly 38-fold more likely to get oropharyngeal cancer. An exceptionally strong interactive risk was evident among those who smoked pipes or cigars and drank alcohol.[24]

Analysis of alcohol use by cases and controls shows that, even when the effects of smoking are eliminated mathematically, risk of oropharyngeal cancer increases with increasing consumption of any kind of alcohol.[25] More than half of the male cases drank 30 or more drinks per week, compared with only 14% of the controls. Similarly, nearly 25% of the female cases drank this much, while only 2% of the female controls were heavy drinkers. Heavy drinking of any kind of alcohol led to a nine-fold higher risk of oropharyngeal cancer in both men and women, but this risk dropped off dramatically for moderate drinkers, so that drinking five to 14 drinks per week increased the risk of oropharyngeal cancer about two-fold. Cancer risk was greatest for hard liquor, with beer not far behind, and wine was a distant third in terms of risk. In fact, only when wine consumption exceeded four drinks per day was there any increase in cancer risk. Cancer risk was comparable between blacks and whites, but fewer whites were exposed to high levels of the risk factors.

The results of this analysis were strong enough that it was possible to calculate the proportion of oropharyngeal cancers that could be directly attributed to drinking alcoholic beverages and smoking tobacco;[26] overall, 74% of all oropharyngeal cancers could be attributed to an interaction between drinking and smoking. In men, nearly 80% of all oropharyngeal cancers were attributable to these risk factors, while for women 61% of the cancer was due to drinking and smoking. Unfortunately, because drinking and smoking habits are so strongly correlated with one another, determining what proportion of oropharyngeal cancers were caused by drinking alone was not possible.[27]

These early results have been largely confirmed by a more recent study of oropharyngeal cancer risk, which focused on racial differences in cancer risk.[28] Racial differences in risk of oropharyngeal cancer are potentially important because the rate of these cancers is about 65% higher in blacks, and blacks are more likely to be diagnosed at a young age or at an advanced stage of disease. This study compared 1,065 oropharyngeal cancer cases with 1,182 controls and was structured so that about 17% of both cases and controls were black. This study design enabled the researchers to specifically examine risk factors for blacks and whites. Heavy drinking (30 or more drinks per week) resulted in a 17-fold increase in oropharyngeal cancer risk for blacks, and only a nine-fold increase for whites. However, blacks tended to drink more alcohol than whites, and 37% of blacks were smokers, as compared to 28% of whites. Patterns similar to the previous study were found, as risk increased with increasing alcohol consumption, and beer and hard liquor were stronger risk factors than wine. Since it could be calculated that 83% of blacks and 73% of whites developed their cancer as a direct result of exposure to both smoking and drinking, it was concluded that there was no major difference between blacks and whites in terms of oropharyngeal cancer risk. A small number of other risk factors for oropharyngeal cancer included loss of teeth, use of dentures, and presence of mouth sores, which could account for some cancer cases, but these were very minor by comparison with smoking and drinking.[29]

Alcohol has also been implicated as a potent risk factor for cancer of the larynx, and again, strong interactions were present between alcohol consumption and smoking.[30] A study conducted in Poland, where the death rate from laryngeal cancer is one of the highest in the world, compared 249 newly diagnosed men with laryngeal cancer with 965 healthy male controls. Each man was interviewed about potential risk factor exposures, such as alcohol, tobacco, diet, occupation, and other socioeconomic factors. About 65% of cases and 23% of controls consumed alcohol at least once a week, and the main type of alcohol consumed was vodka. Non-smoking men who consumed vodka regularly for more than 30 years had a nine-fold increase in laryngeal cancer risk by comparison with non-smoking non-drinkers. Smoking and drinking were strongly interactive, so that for men who drank vodka regularly for more than 15 years and who smoked 20 or more cigarettes per day, the risk of laryngeal cancer was elevated 330-fold by comparison with non-smoking non-drinkers. This extraordinary elevation of risk implies that the risk of laryngeal cancer associated with drinking actually can multiply the risk associated with smoking among men who both drink and smoke. This multiplicative effect may have been further aggravated by poor nutrition in some cases, since men who both drank and smoked were less likely to have adequate nutrition.[31]

There is also recent evidence that excessive alcohol consumption can lead to an elevated risk of colorectal cancer.[32] A study was undertaken in 1985 to determine the effect of alcohol consumption on rectal cancer risk, using patients with colon cancer as one of the control groups. This study showed that alcohol intake had a weak effect on the risk of rectal cancer, but it also accidently identified an increased risk of colon cancer due to alcohol. This demonstrates that science can occasionally advance in unexpected directions. A group of 644 men with colorectal cancer was compared with a group of 992 healthy control men using a telephone interview that inquired about various known and suspected risk factors. Alcohol was a weak risk factor for rectal cancer specifically, since alcohol use was associated with a 1.5-fold higher risk of rectal cancer. But alcohol use was also associated with a 1.8-fold increased risk of colon cancer. Colorectal cancer risk was somewhat higher for consumption of beer specifically, although risk was only elevated for those who drank five or more alcoholic beverages per day.

These results were subsequently confirmed by a meta-analysis that mathematically combined the results of 27 different published studies into one large study of alcohol and colorectal cancer risk.[33] However, even when 27 different studies were combined, alcohol was a weak risk factor for colorectal cancer. For those who consumed two alcoholic beverages daily, the relative risk of colorectal cancer was increased by only 10%. This meta-analysis also confirmed that beer was a stronger risk factor for colorectal cancer than other alcoholic beverages. Wine increased the risk of colorectal cancer by only 11%, while hard liquor increased risk by 13%, and beer increased risk by 26%. From a statistical standpoint, only beer consumption could be confidently related to colorectal cancer risk, since neither wine nor hard liquor caused a significant increase in risk.[34] Another more recent meta-analysis of alcohol consumption as a risk factor for colorectal cancer combined the results of 52 different studies from over the past 35 years.[35] This study also confirmed that alcohol is a weak risk factor; a lifelong drinker was calculated to have a two- to three-fold higher risk of colorectal cancer.

None of these studies inspire a great deal of confidence, either because they compared small numbers of cases and controls, or because they were retrospective, or because they identified alcohol as a risk factor for colon cancer after the study had already been completed. For this reason, it is not yet clear whether alcohol really is a risk factor for colorectal cancer. However, some of this confusion was cleared up by a recent study that prospectively examined the association between alcohol intake and the risk of colorectal adenoma.[36] Colorectal adenomas, small wart-like growths found on the inner surface of the large intestine and rectum, can transform into cancerous tissue. Since colorectal adenomas are a known risk factor for colorectal cancer, showing a relationship between alcohol and adenoma strongly implies a relationship between alcohol consumption and cancer.

The relationship between alcohol and adenomas was explored prospectively, using female subjects who were already enrolled in the Nurses' Health Study and male subjects who were already enrolled in the Health Professionals Follow-up Study.[37] Each of the men and women in these two studies had been given a food frequency questionnaire, which also inquired about the consumption of alcohol. Thus it was possible to look for interactions between food and alcohol intake. A total of 25,474 men and women were enrolled in these two studies, and all the subjects received an endoscopic examination of their bowel during the course of the four-to-10-year follow-up period. The endoscopic examinations revealed 895 pre-cancerous polyps, for which subjects received appropriate treatment. When individuals with polyps were compared to individuals who were free of polyps, drinkers of more than 30 grams of alcohol daily (about two drinks) were found to have an elevated risk of colorectal adenoma. Again, beer was associated with the highest risk of adenoma, closely followed by hard liquor, with wine having the least risk. However, in this study, the risk of wine was not much less than the risk of beer or hard liquor. Subjects who drank more than 30 grams of alcohol daily were at a 1.8-fold higher risk of adenoma, compared to those who did not drink at all. However, this study found that drinking less than 30 grams of alcohol daily apparently did not significantly increase the risk of adenoma, compared to people who did not drink at all. Dietary intake of folate and methionine were both somewhat protective for people who drank heavily, which suggests that folate supplementation might be considered as a cancer preventive strategy for habitual drinkers.[38]

Alcohol has also been implicated as a risk factor for breast cancer at least in one large meta-analysis that combined the results of 16 separate studies.[39] This meta-analysis compared a total of 11,378 breast cancer patients with 210,093 healthy controls, although some of the component studies were prospective, while others were case-control studies. Evidence of a dose-response relationship was found between alcohol intake and breast cancer risk. The risk of breast cancer was increased between 1.4- and 1.7-fold over that of non-drinking subjects for those with an average intake level of two drinks daily. However, because this study combined data from many separate studies, which often differed from each other in experimental design, these results must be accepted with reservation. This is especially true since some of the largest component studies were unable to find a relationship between alcohol intake and breast cancer risk. For example, one component study that compared 1,467 cases with 10,178 controls concluded that alcohol did not increase breast cancer risk at all. However, the two largest component studies, both of which were prospective and which together included 1,428 cases and 178,015 controls, found that alcohol consumption was indeed a risk factor for breast cancer. In fact, both of these component studies found a dose-response relationship between alcohol intake and breast cancer risk, although the two studies examined very different levels of alcohol intake. One can conclude that alcohol intake probably increases breast cancer risk somewhat, although the extent of increase is not well known.[40] Nevertheless, it is probably fair to say that risk of breast cancer from a daily intake of two drinks is almost certainly less than double that of a teetotaler.

Recently, alcohol intake has been found to actually increase blood levels of estrogen, the female hormone.[41] This provides a very satisfying explanation for how alcohol intake could act to increase breast cancer risk, since estrogen is a well-known risk factor for breast cancer. This ingenious study involved 34 pre-menopausal women who were given a controlled diet for six menstrual cycles, with 30 grams of alcohol consumed daily for three of those cycles and no alcohol consumed for the other three cycles. Levels of hormone were measured in blood and in urine at various points through the menstrual cycle, and hormone levels were compared for each subject with and without alcohol in the diet. Daily intake of alcohol (equivalent to two drinks) increased blood levels of estrogen by as much as 27.5%. This means that, if estrogen is the major cause of breast cancer, then alcohol intake can increase the exposure to this risk factor dramatically. This finding is consistent with data showing that alcohol is a risk factor for breast cancer.[42]

There is also some evidence that alcohol intake can increase the risk of the most common form of liver cancer, hepatocellular carcinoma.[43] A group of 85 case patients diagnosed with hepatocellular carcinoma was matched with 159 control patients diagnosed with diseases other than cancer or liver disease. Each of the cases and controls was interviewed about his or her use of tobacco and alcohol, and each donated a blood sample that was screened for evidence of infection with the hepatitis B virus. The greatest difference found between cases and controls was that 18% of the cases showed evidence of chronic viral infection, whereas none of the controls were infected with HBV. However, alcohol use differed significantly between the cases and controls; 24% of the case patients, but only 12% of the control patients, had a high total intake of alcohol over their lifetime. When regular drinkers were compared to non-drinkers, a nearly three-fold higher risk of hepatocellular carcinoma appeared among the drinkers, and there was an increasing risk of cancer with increasing frequency of alcohol intake. When risk was calculated for specific kinds of alcoholic beverages, beer was found to be associated with the highest risk of hepatocellular carcinoma, while both wine and hard liquor were not associated with a major increase in risk. When the risk from regular consumption of alcoholic beverages was compounded by a regular smoking habit, the risk of hepatocellular carcinoma was increased more than three-fold over normal. All things considered, alcohol was a significant, but not a strong, risk factor for liver cancer.[44]

COFFEE CONSUMPTION

Stories in the press suggesting that beverages such as coffee or tea can cause cancer have generated a great deal of interest. These stories were based on a small number of scientific studies and tended to exaggerate the significance of the scientific findings. For example, a study published in 1989 purported to show a link between cancer of the renal pelvis and consumption of more than six cups of coffee per day.[45] Researchers identified a group of 187 case patients diagnosed with cancer of the ureter or renal pelvis (that portion of the kidney that collects urine as it moves from the kidney through the ureters to the bladder). These case patients were matched with 187 healthy controls, drawn from the same neighborhoods as the cases. Both cases and controls were interviewed about personal and family medical history, occupational history, and use of analgesics (pain relievers), tobacco, alcohol, and coffee. When coffee consumption of cases was compared to that of controls, it was found that slightly more cases than controls were likely to drink more than six cups of coffee per day (13% versus 8%). It was calculated that, among those people classified as heavy coffee drinkers, the risk of renal pelvis and ureter cancer was increased 1.8-fold with respect to coffee non-drinkers.[46] This was reported in the media as an 80% higher risk of cancer among heavy coffee drinkers, which is, of course, consistent with what the scientists reported. However, the scientists themselves noted that these results were not statistically significant, meaning that the association between coffee and cancer may not be real, but merely the result of working with a small number of cases and controls. Furthermore, the media did not make the point that cancer of the renal pelvis is a very rare cancer, with fewer than 2,000 cases diagnosed each year, and that an 80% higher risk of a very rare cancer may still mean that the cancer is very rare. If 2,000 new cases per year are diagnosed among 250 million people in the United States, then the odds that any one person will develop the disease in a given year are only one in 125,000. If these odds are increased by 80%, due to heavy coffee consumption, then the odds that any one person will get the disease are still only about one in 69,444. An objective appraisal of the study in question suggests that essentially no risk of developing renal pelvis cancer is associated with heavy consumption of coffee.

Another study, which showed that coffee reduces colorectal cancer risk and which involved many more cases and controls than the previous study, was never widely reported by the media.[47] A group of 1,771 case patients from Milan, Italy, all diagnosed with cancers of the mouth, pharynx, esophagus, stomach, colon, rectum, liver, or pancreas, were matched with 1,944 control patients who were diagnosed with noncancerous conditions. Each person answered a questionnaire on various risk factors for gastrointestinal cancers including diet and coffee consumption. When cases were compared to controls, it was found that coffee did not increase the risk of most gastrointestinal cancers, and that it actually reduced the risk of cancers of the colon and rectum. When drinkers of three or more cups of coffee per day were compared to those who drank one or fewer cups, coffee consumption was found to reduce colon cancer risk by 36% and rectal cancer risk by 34%. Of particular note in this study was the finding that coffee did not increase the risk of pancreatic cancer, even though an earlier study had reported that coffee increased pancreatic cancer risk. Overall, coffee was not found to be a risk factor for any cancer examined, although this study did not specifically address the relationship between coffee and renal pelvis cancer.

USE OF ASPIRIN AND ANALGESICS

The study of coffee as a risk factor for renal pelvis cancer (discussed above) also reported that aspirin is a risk factor for this cancer.[48] Again, this conclusion was based on a retrospective comparison of 187 cases with an equal number of controls, so a certain amount of skepticism is appropriate. Nevertheless, regular use of aspirin was reported to increase the risk of renal pelvis and ureter cancer 1.9-fold and prolonged use of analgesics (more than 30 consecutive days) was a potent risk factor. In fact, it was concluded that if an individual used pain relievers containing aspirin, acetaminophen, phenacetin, or any combination of these analgesics for more than 30 days, then the risk of developing renal pelvis and ureter cancer was increased more than two-fold, in comparison to nonusers. This study was consistent with two earlier studies of renal pelvis risk factors, but the rarity of these tumors and the relatively small increase in risk associated with use of analgesics suggest that these results should be accepted with great caution. This is especially true because several subsequent studies have shown that analgesics generally reduce the risk of cancer.

A great deal of interest has been expressed in aspirin as a potential cancer preventive agent because experimental research with animals has shown that anti-inflammatory drugs are often very effective at suppressing cancer growth.[49] Aspirin is a very effective anti-inflammatory agent that does not have the side effects associated with similar agents such as steroids. Because of this interest in aspirin, a large prospective study was done to determine the risk of fatal cancer as a function of aspirin use. This study, initiated in 1982 by the American Cancer Society, enrolled more than 635,031 men and women drawn from all 50 states. Each participant answered a questionnaire about diet, use of medications, smoking history, alcohol intake, physical activity, occupation, height, weight, family medical history, and other potential risk factors. The average age of participants at enrollment was 57, and these participants were followed until 1988, at which time there was a total of more than 3.7 million person-years of follow-up. During the follow-up period, 91.4% of the participants remained alive, 6.7% of the participants died of various causes, and 1.8% were lost to follow-up. When those who died were compared with those who survived, the death rate from cancers of the esophagus, stomach, colon, and rectum was found to be lower among frequent aspirin users. However, aspirin use seemed to have little or no effect on mortality from respiratory, urinary or genital cancers, and the frequency of cancers of the brain, nervous system, or immune system was also unaffected.

Frequent aspirin users (those who use aspirin 16 times per month or for more than one year) were about 40% less likely to die from gastrointestinal cancers than non-users.[50] The greatest reduction in risk for women was a 51% reduction in stomach cancer risk among frequent users, while for men the greatest reduction was a 56% reduction in risk of rectal cancer. For both men and women, frequent aspirin use led to a 37% reduction in risk of colon cancer, which is one of the most common and devastating of all cancers. The trend of decreasing risk was strongest among those who had used aspirin for 10 years or more. Among people who were frequent aspirin-users for 10 years or more, colon cancer risk declined 64%, rectal cancer risk declined by 61%, stomach cancer risk declined by 48%, and there was a 46% reduction in esophageal cancer risk. Since more than 81,000 people died from these cancers in 1992, a modest reduction in risk would be significant, and the effects of aspirin were so strong that aspirin was recommended as a cancer preventive agent.[51]

These results have been partially confirmed by several recent studies that examined aspirin as a cancer preventive agent. In one study, the incidence of cancer was determined in a large group of Swedish men and women with rheumatoid arthritis, among whom the use of aspirin and other anti-inflammatory drugs was higher than normal.[52] Site-specific incidence of cancer was determined in a group of 11,683 rheumatoid arthritis sufferers, and this was compared to the expected incidence rate for Swedish men and women. It was found that rheumatoid arthritis was associated with a reduced risk of gastrointestinal cancers: stomach cancer incidence was 37% lower; colon cancer incidence was 37% lower; and rectal cancer incidence was 28% lower. However, also found was a two-fold higher risk of lymphoma among rheumatoid arthritis sufferers,[53] which is consistent with the idea that both arthritis and lymphoma are diseases of the immune system.

Several studies have now shown that aspirin use is associated with a reduced risk of colorectal cancer. However, these findings could be explained in any of several ways: perhaps patients with early stage colorectal cancer avoid aspirin because they already feel nauseated or perhaps aspirin use decreased the manifestation of cancer symptoms, so that a diagnosis of colorectal cancer was delayed among aspirin users.[54] Thus the possibility exists that (in a small study) aspirin use could decrease the rate of diagnosis of colorectal cancer without actually being protective. To get around this problem, a recent study examined the relationship between aspirin use and the risk of colorectal polyps. If aspirin is truly protective from colorectal cancer, then it should also reduce the incidence of polyps or colorectal adenomas. A group of 793 patients, all of whom had at least one previous colorectal adenoma, were enrolled in a prospective study of the relationship between aspirin use and the incidence of additional adenomas. Patients were followed for a year, then all were examined with a colonoscope as a part of the follow-up. Both men and women who reported regular aspirin use were 48% less likely to have new adenomas at the colonoscopic exam, by comparison with patients who did not use aspirin. These findings, together with those previously discussed, provide very strong evidence that aspirin may protect against colorectal cancer.

CONTRACEPTION, CHILDBIRTH, AND CHILD REARING

The impact of hormonal contraceptives was discussed in detail in the chapter on hormonal causes of cancer and that discussion will not be repeated here, even though hormones are the most important cancer risk in all contraceptives. This section will be limited to a discussion of the link between nonhormonal contraceptives and cancer. Although relatively few cases are known in which nonhormonal contraceptives have an effect on cancer, a recent study did show that tubal ligation can reduce the incidence of ovarian cancer.[55] This is potentially an important finding because ovarian cancer is the fourth leading cause of cancer death in women, and it is a particularly insidious cancer because it is very difficult to diagnose. This study used the resources of the Nurses' Health Study to assess whether tubal ligation or hysterectomy can affect the subsequent risk of ovarian cancer. This by-now-familiar study was a prospective study that enrolled 107,868 married female registered nurses who were 30 to 55 years of age in 1976, when the study began. These nurses answered a broad range of questions at enrollment, among them questions about medical and reproductive history, diet, hormone use, contraceptive practices, and various other cancer risk factors. During the 12-year period over which the women were followed (over 859,791 person-years of follow-up), a total of 260 cases of ovarian cancer were diagnosed. Although 14% of the women in the study had a tubal ligation for contraceptive purposes, only 6% of the ovarian cancer cases affected women with tubal ligations. This implies that tubal ligation can somehow protect women from ovarian cancer. However, the comparison is not completely straightforward, since women with tubal ligations tended to have more children and were more likely to have used oral contraceptives, especially for longer durations. Thus many potential variables had to be carefully controlled in this study.

When a rigorous comparison was made between women with tubal ligations and women without, with various other confounding factors controlled, ligation was found to reduce the risk of ovarian cancer by 67%.[56] In fact, the longer the time since tubal ligation, the lower the risk of ovarian cancer appeared to be. Hysterectomy also seemed to be a weakly protective effect, since having had a simple hysterectomy reduced the risk of ovarian cancer by about 33%. Condom use or vasectomy in the male partner does not seem to affect the risk of ovarian cancer, although use of oral contraceptives prior to tubal ligation apparently could further reduce the risk of ovarian cancer. These findings strongly suggest that women who have decided not to bear more children should consider tubal ligation as a long-term contraceptive strategy because of the reduced risk of ovarian cancer.

Childbirth practices, particularly maternal age at birth of the first child, have a major effect on the incidence of breast cancer. This was shown clearly by a large prospective study of Seventh-Day Adventist women in California, which made it possible to determine the relative importance of various breast cancer risk factors.[57] A total of 20,341 women were enrolled in the study in 1976, and each woman completed a detailed questionaire about personal, medical, childbearing, and menstrual history, and about risk factors such as diet and obesity. At the end of a six-year period (about 115,000 person-years of follow-up), a total of 215 women had developed breast cancer. Because of the broad coverage of questions asked at enrollment, it was possible to put each of the risk factors into perspective and to rank their importance with respect to one another. Dietary causes of breast cancer were not very important and the consumption of high fat animal products was not consistently related to breast cancer risk. The three most significant risk factors for breast cancer identified in this study were, in order of declining importance: total number of years between menarche (first menstruation) and first childbirth; highest educational level obtained; and mother's age at birth of the first child. Therefore, two of the three most important risk factors identified for breast cancer are "lifestyle decisions" relating to contraception and childbirth.

These results have been at least partly confirmed in several recent studies. One prospective study, designed to examine the combined effect of family history and reproduction on breast cancer risk, followed 37,105 women between the ages of 55 and 69.[58] During the four-year follow-up period, a total of 493 new breast cancer cases were diagnosed. In comparing cases to controls, a powerful interaction between family history and other risk factors was found. For example, women who gave birth to their first child at age 30 were at a higher risk of breast cancer than women who had their first child when they were less than 20 years old. The risk of breast cancer was about two-fold higher for an older first-time mother with no family history of disease, whereas an older first-time mother with a family history of breast cancer had a risk nearly six-fold higher than a young mother with no family history. Thus, among women who have their first child at age 30 or older, the risk of breast cancer is affected by the family history of breast cancer, but reproductive factors are also clearly critical in determining breast cancer risk.

For reasons that remain unknown, women who bear more than two or three children have a reduced risk of breast cancer.[59] Compared to women who have no children, women with five or more children have a 17% lower risk of breast cancer if they have no family history of the disease, and a 43% lower risk of breast cancer if they do have a family history of breast cancer. But the importance of family history is overstated by this type of analysis, as nearly 88% of women in the study reported having a family history of breast cancer. Since breast cancer is such a common disease, and since "family history" was defined to include breast cancer in any close relative (mother, grandmother, aunt, sister, or daughter), it is not surprising that a great majority of women claim a family history of breast cancer. Overall, a family history of breast cancer increased breast cancer risk only 1.5-fold, whereas many other risk factors are more powerful.

Another study has concluded that age of the mother at first birth, and the parity of the mother, can have a large impact on breast cancer risk.[60] A meta-analysis approach was used to mathematically combine the results of eight different studies in the Nordic countries, where the incidence of breast cancer is quite high. The meta-analysis approach was used because several of the smaller separate studies had failed to identify age and parity as significant risk factors for breast cancer. This meta-analysis compared a total of 5,569 breast cancer cases with 136,015 healthy control women, so the larger sample of women surveyed could potentially enable researchers to identify even subtle risk factors. The meta-analysis confirmed that both age and parity are important risk factors, and that each risk factor could have an effect independent of the other. Overall, nulliparity (bearing no children) was associated with a 30% increase in risk compared to parous women, and for every two births, breast cancer risk was reduced about 16%. There was also a trend toward increasing breast cancer risk with increasing age at first birth, as women who gave birth after the age of 35 years had a 40% higher risk of breast cancer than women who gave birth before age 20. Thus, the increased risk associated with late age at first birth or low parity is rather small, which may explain why several of the smaller studies were unable to detect increases in risk.

The trend to delayed childbearing in the United States may lead to an increase in breast cancer over the coming decades.[61] How great this increase will be is a matter of some debate, since this estimate is contingent upon an accurate indication of the relative risk from delaying childbirth. One study suggested that women born between the years of 1945 and 1949 will have a 5% greater incidence of breast cancer than those women born between 1935 and 1939, since women in the latter cohort tended to have children at a younger age. However this estimate assumed that nulliparous women had roughly twice the risk of breast cancer as women who had their first children before age 20. Subsequent studies have generally shown this risk to be smaller, so that the increase in incidence of breast cancer would also be smaller. Yet even if these figures are wrong, the point is well taken that private decisions, such as when to have children, can have ramifications for public health, and that breast cancer incidence is likely to increase over the coming years.

Very recent research suggests that lactation may reduce the relative risk of breast cancer.[62] These findings were the result of a retrospective analysis of all women in Wisconsin, western Massachusetts, Maine, and New Hampshire who were diagnosed with breast cancer between 1989 and 1991 and who were less than 75 years of age. These women were identified from the Cancer Registry in their respective states, and each woman was contacted through her physician. A total of 5,878 women, or nearly 81% of those eligible, were contacted and agreed to participate in this study. Each woman answered survey questions about pregnancy, duration of lactation and breast feeding, and use of drugs to inhibit lactation. In addition, a total of 8,216 healthy women were randomly selected and interviewed as controls. When cases and controls were compared, lactation was found to be associated with a slight reduction in the risk of breast cancer among pre-menopausal women, although there was no difference in post-menopausal women. Pre-menopausal women who had lactated were at a 22% lower risk of breast cancer than women who had never lactated. Risk tends to decrease with increasing duration of lactation, as pre-menopausal women who had lactated for one to two years were at a 34% lower risk of breast cancer. Whether sufficient milk was produced to satisfy the child, or whether hormones were used to maintain milk production, seemed to have no effect on breast cancer risk. Among pre-menopausal women who first lactated at less than age 20, the risk of breast cancer was reduced 44%. However, this protective effect seemed to disappear once women had gone through menopause, which suggests that pre-menopausal breast cancer is somehow fundamentally different from post-menopausal breast cancer.

Since lactation had a strong effect on the relative risk of breast cancer, scientists were able to estimate the public health impact of lactation.[63] It was calculated that, if women who do not breast-feed or who breast-feed for less than three months were to increase the duration of breast-feeding to four to 12 months, breast cancer among parous pre-menopausal women could be reduced by 11%. If all women with children lactated for 24 months or longer, the incidence of breast cancer could be reduced by as much as 25%. The reduction in risk would be even greater among women who first lactate at an early age. This same study also confirmed that age at birth of the first child was an important risk factor for breast cancer. Women who bore children after 29 were at a 1.3-fold higher risk of breast cancer than women who bore children before age 20. In addition, breast cancer risk declined with parity as follows: two children reduced risk by 8% by comparison with women who bore one child; three children reduced risk by 20%; and four or more children reduced risk by 24%. The mechanism of all of these effects is believed to be estrogen, since young age at first birth, multiple parity, and extended lactation would all reduce the exposure to estrogen.[64]

URBAN LIVING

Analysis of the incidence of cancer in various regions in the United States has shown that incidence is highest in the industrial Northeast; in fact, the incidence of cancer is 11.8% higher in the urban Northeast than in the more rural northern parts of the United States that stretch from Minnesota and Wisconsin to Oregon and Washington.[65] This suggests that there may be something about living in an urban setting that causes cancer.

Many features of urban living could potentially cause cancer, but one of the most obvious possibilities is air pollution. Recently a strong association was identified between air pollution and the incidence of lung cancer, based on a survey of cancer mortality in six cities.[66] The six cities selected for comparison in this study ranged from highly polluted (Steubenville, Ohio; St. Louis, Missouri), to moderately polluted (Harriman, Tennessee; Watertown, Massachusetts), to fairly pristine (Topeka, Kansas; Portage, Wisconsin). A cohort of about 1,350 people was chosen in each city, and these individuals were followed prospectively for 15 years, for a total of 111,076 person-years of follow-up. Individuals averaged 49 years at enrollment and were roughly equally divided between men and women. During the follow-up period there were 1,430 deaths in the cohort; most of these deaths could be directly attributed to cigarette smoking. However, if the mortality rate was corrected for smoking prevalence, the number of deaths per 1,000 person-years differed strikingly in the different cities. The lowest adjusted death rate was found in Portage, Wisconsin, one of the most pristine cities, while the highest adjusted death rate was found in Steubenville, Ohio, the most polluted of the six cities. The death rate in Steubenville was nearly 30 higher than in Portage, while the death rate in St. Louis was 14% higher than in Portage.

Air pollution was correlated with death from lung cancer and from cardiopulmonary disease, but not with death from other causes.[67] Overall, the relative risk of mortality from all causes was 1.26-fold higher in the most polluted city, compared to the least polluted city. The relative risk of lung cancer was 1.37-fold higher in the most polluted city, even after correction for age, sex, smoking habits, occupational exposures, education, and obesity. Coincidentally, the relative risk of mortality from cardiopulmonary disease was also elevated 1.37-fold in the most polluted city. Mortality rate in the six cities correlated very closely with the average number of fine particles in the air, as well as the average number of sulfate particles in the air. There was an interactive effect between smoking and air pollution, as smokers in the most polluted cities were 11% more likely to die (from all causes) than non-smokers in the most polluted cities, and eight-fold more likely to get lung cancer than non-smokers. These risk estimates are likely to be fairly accurate because the study was large and prospective, because there were 111,076 person-years of follow-up involved in the study, and because results are drawn from six widely separated cities. This study therefore validates the recent emphasis on reduction of urban air pollution.[68]

Another recent study seems to suggest that several additional risk factors may be associated with living in an urban setting. One study, which was actually designed to determine why breast cancer incidence rates are four to seven times higher in the United States than in China or Japan, came across evidence that rural living is somehow protective from breast cancer.[69] A case-control study was done of Asian-American women, all of whom were first- or second-generation immigrants from China, Japan, or the Philippines. A total of 597 such women who were diagnosed with breast cancer were the case subjects, while a total of 966 healthy Asian-American women served as the control subjects. It was found that Asian-American women born in the West had a 60% higher risk of breast cancer than Asian-American women born in the East. However, for Asian-American women born in the East, relative risk of breast cancer was determined, in part, by whether their communities prior to immigration were rural or urban. Migrants from urban areas had a 1.3-fold higher risk of breast cancer than migrants from rural areas. Among Asian-American women who had been in the United States for less than seven years, the risk associated with urban life was even clearer. Recent migrants to the West who had lived in an urban area in the East for most of their life were at a two-fold higher risk of breast cancer than recent migrants who had previously lived in a rural area. No specific risk factors were identified in this study, so it may well be that air pollution is a contributory factor to the elevated breast cancer risk. Nevertheless, this study clearly implicates something in the urban environment as causative of breast cancer.[70]

EDUCATIONAL ATTAINMENT

Most epidemiological studies of cancer risk involve a comparison of cases and controls to determine the impact of a particular risk factor on cancer incidence. Whenever such a comparison is made, care must be taken to eliminate from consideration those variables that might cause a spurious result. For example, in the study of tubal ligation discussed above, it was found that women with tubal ligations were, on average, of higher parity and more likely to have used oral contraceptives for long periods. Since parity and oral contraceptive use could both have a strong effect on ovarian cancer risk, both of these variables had to be mathematically eliminated from consideration. In the course of doing many such analyses, epidemiologists have learned that several variables can have a strong impact on cancer risk, and these variables are carefully considered in any reputable study. For example, age has a very powerful effect on the risk of cancer, and any study that fails to consider age as a variable is likely to generate incorrect conclusions. Epidemiologists are therefore always vigilant for variables that have an impact on the conclusions, even if the effect of the variable cannot be explained.

One variable that seems to have an effect on cancer incidence is educational attainment, even though it is not at all obvious why education should affect cancer risk. Generally, educated persons seem to be less likely to get cancer, although this generalization is untrue in the case of breast cancer. Perhaps educated persons have better access to the health care system or they may be better able to make use of whatever resources are available to them. Educated persons may also be more likely to recognize the warning signs of disease and the help of a physician may be more affordable for them. Alternatively, occupational exposure to carcinogens may simply be is lower among white collar workers. In any case, the level of educational attainment seems to be an important variable in many epidemiological studies, and education generally acts to reduce cancer risk.

For example, a large prospective study of Seventh-Day Adventist men found that education reduced prostate cancer risk.[71] A group of about 14,000 men were followed for a total of more than 78,000 person-years of follow-up, during which time 180 cases of prostate cancer were identified. Analysis of these cases showed that educational attainment was more closely linked to prostate cancer risk than any other risk factor, including smoking history, alcohol intake, obesity, diet, marital status, and even a history of previous prostate problems. The risk of prostate cancer decreased with educational attainment in a dose-dependent fashion, such that the greater the education, the lesser the risk of prostate cancer. If prostate cancer risk is referenced to men with less than a high school education, then a high school graduate has a 25% lower risk of prostate cancer, a college graduate has a 36% lower risk, and a man with a post-graduate education has a 59% lower risk of prostate cancer. The reason why education should reduce prostate cancer risk is completely unknown, but the data are reasonably convincing. While it is still too soon to recommend that education be obtained to prevent cancer, this finding is very thought-provoking.

SUNLIGHT EXPOSURE

Certain wavelengths of light, particularly in the ultraviolet (UV) range, are known to cause skin cancer. However, the evidence linking UV light to skin cancer is somewhat tenuous, because non-melanoma skin cancer is not a major cancer killer and has not been the subject of much research. There is clear evidence that extreme sunlight exposure increases the risk of skin cancer, and the relationship between exposure and risk shows a dose-response effect. But the degree to which normal or low-level sunlight exposure elevates risk in an otherwise healthy person is unclear. Of the three types of UV light in sunlight, UV-B has been most closely linked to skin cancer. UV-A light is less damaging, and UV-C light, while very dangerous, is effectively absorbed by the Earth's atmosphere. UV-B light is present in the lamps used in tanning salons, so indoor tanning can potentially also be carcinogenic.

One of the best recent studies of the relationship between sun exposure and skin cancer was done in Australia, the country that is reported to have the highest rate of skin cancer in the world.[72] An interview approach was used to determine the incidence of skin cancer during a 12-month period preceding the survey in a group of 30,747 Australians over the age of 14.

This large sample of people had 1,179 cases of nonmelanoma skin cancer that were reported to have been diagnosed within the last year. Those who indicated that they had skin cancer within the preceeding year gave the name of their physician, who was contacted to confirm the diagnosis. This physician follow-up turned out to be very important because fully 69% of the people who claimed to have had skin cancer within the preceding year were mistaken—56% of these people were treated for skin conditions other than cancer and 12% were treated for skin cancer that occurred prior to the beginning of the 12-month index period of the study. Nevertheless, this means that nearly 1% of the sampled individuals had had skin cancer within the year preceding the study, which is an extraordinarily high disease incidence.

The incidence rate for skin cancer was dramatically higher among these Australians than is typical for the rest of the world.[72] For example, the rate of nonmelanoma skin cancer in Australia is 3.5-fold higher than in the United States, five-fold higher than in New Zealand, and nearly 30-fold higher than in Britain. Skin cancer risk increases depending upon the individual's reaction to the sun: a person who burns first and then tans is 1.8-fold more likely to get skin cancer than someone who just tans and never burns, while a person who burns and never tans is 2.9-fold more likely to get skin cancer than someone who just tans and never burns. A crude dose-response relationship was found between sun exposure and skin cancer, since the incidence of skin cancer was higher among persons living close to the equator; skin cancer was more than twice as common in Queensland (29°S latitude) as in Victoria (37°S latitude). The cancer rate was also higher in Australian men than in women, presumably because men are more likely to suffer extreme sun exposure. About 62% of all skin cancers reported were on the head or neck, which is consistent with sun exposure being causative of skin cancer. Unfortunately, this study did not attempt to measure sun exposure by the respondents, so it was not possible to determine whether there was a real dose-response relationship or to determine the relative risk from low levels of sun exposure.

On the basis of the incidence of skin cancer in Australia and the average cost of diagnosing and treating a skin cancer, it was possible to calculate the magnitude of the public health problem caused by sun exposure.[74] Roughly 140,000 people are diagnosed with nonmelanoma skin cancer each year in Australia. Considering the likelihood of diagnosing basal cell carcinoma or squamous cell carcinoma, and the cost of treating each cancer, scientists calculated that skin cancer cost the Australian government about fifty million Australian dollars each year. This is a staggering sum, especially since this calculation does not include lost wages or the cost of diagnosing and treating other skin conditions caused by sunlight exposure (e.g., solar keratosis). This cost to the taxpayer argues strongly that public health measures are required to moderate sun exposure, especially in fair-skinned persons who burn easily.

Scientists now believe that regular use of sunscreen with a sun-protection factor (SPF) value of 15 or greater during the first 18 years of life could reduce the incidence of non-melanoma skin cancer by as much as 78%.[75] However, it is not at all clear whether sunscreens can prevent melanoma. There is circumstantial evidence that UV light can cause melanoma, and no risk factors other than sunlight exposure and family history have ever been identified. In the absence of definitive evidence one way or the other, several recommendations can still be made about sunlight exposure. It is suggested that everyone minimize exposure to direct sunlight, with special care taken for children and those with a family history of melanoma or other skin cancer. In particular, prudent individuals should apply sunscreen, wear hats and other protective clothing, minimize sunlight exposure during the hours from 10:00 A.M. until 2:00 P.M. when UV light is at a peak, wear UV-opaque sunglasses, and avoid tanning salons.[46] These recommendations are especially timely, since very recent evidence suggests that ozone depletion is causing a significant increase in UV exposure even for persons living in Canada.[77]

STRESS, DEPRESSION, AND CANCER

The question of whether or not stress and depression can cause cancer is very controversial. It is a widely held belief in the lay public that stress and depression can cause a range of diseases, [78] but very little evidence supports this belief.[79] Those who work at the intersection between psychology and oncology often have strongly held beliefs, but this is an emotionally charged issue and the evidence is quite equivocal.

The most recent evidence suggests that cancer may be marginally more prevalent in clinically depressed persons.[80] This study utilized a computer database that was originally set up by a medical center in San Francisco to monitor reactions to drugs dispensed by the hospital pharmacy. Since depression diagnosed by a psychiatrist is almost always treated with one of a very few drugs, it was possible to separate clinically depressed persons from a cohort of 4,881 persons who filled prescriptions in the pharmacy between 1969 and 1973. In this cohort, a total of 923 patients with some form of depression was treated by the Psychiatry Clinic. Since the follow-up period was as long as 19 years, a total of 455 cancers were diagnosed in the cohort of 4,881 persons. There was a 1.2-fold higher risk of cancer among those who filled prescriptions for anti-depressants than among those who filled prescriptions for drugs unrelated to depression, and the elevation in risk among depressed persons was greatest for skin cancer. However, this study was unable to show a really convincing elevation in cancer risk among depressed persons, since there were too few cases of cancer to be sure, from a statistical standpoint, that depression is actually a risk factor. This result is consistent with several other similarly equivocal studies.

Another recent study analyzed the relationship between depression and cancer mortality in a group of 2,585 men and women who responded to a questionairre between 1971 and 1975.[81] This questionnaire characterized their mental state as either cheerful or depressed and assessed their level of general physical and psychological well-being. These subjects were then followed for eight to nine years to determine whether individuals scored as depressed were any more likely to die of cancer. At the end of the follow-up period, 7% of the depressed subjects had been diagnosed with cancer, but so had 7% of the nondepressed subjects. Depression, as measured by either one of two different psychological tests, was not significantly related to cancer diagnosis or mortality. Even when a high-risk (older) subgroup was followed for an additional four years, no evidence was found for depression causing cancer.

Whenever a scientific study fails to find a connection that was hypothesized to be important, the study is subject to criticism that it was improperly done. Perhaps if more subjects had been tested, or if a longer follow-up period had been used, or if a better measure of depression had been employed in the first place, then it might have been possible to show a relationship between cancer and depression. Negative results are seldom definitive and are often not even publishable, so there is a tendency to ignore these results and repeat the studies. Nevertheless, these two recent studies are consistent with some larger early studies of cancer and depression.

However, strikingly discrepant results have been reported recently by scientists who examined the connection between stressful life events and all-cause mortality.[82] In 1983 a random sample of 776 men, all 50 years old, was selected in Gothenburg, Sweden. Each of these men received a physical examination, and each answered a questionnaire that assessed smoking habits, physical activity during leisure time, psychological stress, and the strength of each man's social support network. This cohort of men was followed prospectively for seven years, at the end of which time there had been only 41 deaths— a mortality rate of just 5%. Because this mortality rate is low, showing a strong relationship between stressful life

TABLE 11-1
WEIGHTED RISK CALCULATIONS FOR LIFESTYLE RISK FACTORS

RISK FACTOR	RELATED CANCER	RELATIVE RISK	RELATIVE FREQUENCY	RISK WEIGHT
Heavy drinking × smoking	Larynx	330.3	2	660b
Heavy drinking × smoking	Oropharyngeal	37.7	3	113a
Late pregnancy × family cancer	Breast	5.8	5	29a
Heavy drinking (any alcohol)	Oropharyngeal	8.8	3	26a
Long-term drinking (vodka)	Larynx	9.0	2	18b
Heavy drinking (hard liquor)	Oropharyngeal	5.5	3	17a
Stressful life events (> 2)	All cancers	3.3	5	17c
Nulliparous × family cancer	Breast	3.0	5	15a
Heavy drinking (beer)	Oropharyngeal	4.7	3	14a
Obesity	Colon	2.4	5	12a
Obesity × family cancer	Breast	2.2	5	11a
Late pregnancy (≥ 30 years)	Breast	2.0	5	10a
Low activity (<1000 kcal/wk)	Colorectal	2.0	5	10b
Female obesity	Kidney	3.3	3	10c
No use of aspirin	Colon	1.7	5	9a
Alcohol (>4 drinks/day)	Colon	1.8	5	9c
Heavy drinking (wine)	Oropharyngeal	2.5	3	8a
Weight ≥ 175 pounds	Breast	1.6	5	8a
Body-mass index ≥ 30.7	Breast	1.5	5	8a
Low coffee consumption	Colon	1.6	5	8b

RISK FACTOR	RELATED CANCER	RELATIVE RISK	RELATIVE FREQUENCY	RISK WEIGHT
Low coffee consumption	Rectum	1.5	5	8c
Obesity	All cancers	1.5	5	8c
Male obesity	Kidney	2.5	3	8c
Sedentary occupation	Colon	1.6	5	8c
Air pollution	Lung	1.4	5	7a
Weight at 141–174 pounds	Breast	1.3	5	7a
Body-mass index, 27.4–30.7	Breast	1.3	5	7a
Nulliparous (no children)	Breast	1.3	5	7a
Pregnant but never lactated	Breast	1.3	5	7a
Alcohol (> 2 drinks/day)	Breast	1.4	5	7b
Living in an urban area	Breast	1.3	5	7b
Regular drinking × smoking	Liver	3.4	2	7c
No contraceptive tubal ligation	Ovary	3.0	2	6a
Clinical depression	All cancers	1.2	5	6b
Less than high school education	Prostate	1.3	4	5a
Moderate drinking (any alcohol)	Oropharyngeal	1.7	3	5a
Moderate drinking (beer)	Oropharyngeal	1.7	3	5a
Regular drinking	Liver	2.6	2	5c
High coffee consumption	Kidney	1.8	3	5c
No use of aspirin	Stomach	1.9	2	4a
Moderate drinking (hard liquor)	Oropharyngeal	1.3	3	4a

The relative importance of a risk factor is quantified by considering three factors: the relative risk associated with the factor; the relative frequency of the related cancer; and the statistical power of the study that linked the risk factor with the cancer. Body-mass index (BMI) is calculated by dividing body weight (in kilograms) by the square of the height (in meters).

events and mortality was difficult. However, when mortality rate was determined as a function of the number of recent stressful life events, those who experienced three or more recent stressful life events were more than three times as likely to have died from cancer. In addition, the mortality rate from coronary heart disease was twice as high for these men, the alcohol-related mortality rate was five times as high, and the mortality rate from all other causes was five times as high.

Stressful life events assessed by this study included a range of different things: serious illness or death of a family member; serious concern about a family member; divorce or separation; being forced to move or change jobs; feelings of insecurity at work; serious financial trouble; or legal prosecution for any reason.[83] Of these various stressful life events, legal prosecution seemed to be the worst; those who had been legally prosecuted within the last year were nearly eight-fold more likely to die than those who had not been. Being forced to move from a house or encountering serious financial trouble increased the risk of mortality approximately three-fold, while feelings of insecurity at work increased the risk of mortality more than two-fold. Overall, of the men who had experienced three or more of these life events during the past year, 10.9% had died, compared with 3.3% among those with no stressful life events. The association between recent stressful life events and mortality remained true even after correcting for smoking, occupation, and health.

Interestingly, there was strong evidence that a supportive family life could act to reduce the risk of mortality.[84] Those who experienced three or more stressful life events but who were buffered by an emotionally supportive family were only about 1.2-fold more likely to die than those who experienced no stressful life events. However, those who experienced three or more stressful life events but who were not buffered by an emotionally supportive family were 15-fold more likely to die than normal. Similarly, among those with three or more stressful life events, those with a high degree of social integration were only 2.5-fold more likely to die, while those with a low degree of social integration were seven-fold more likely to die. Reduced mortality from all causes was strongly associated with living in a family group, having a high degree of emotional support, and having many home activities. The only conclusion possible is that men who enjoy adequate emotional support are somewhat protected from the mortality that is often associated with highly stressful life events. Since most of the earlier studies on cancer and depression failed to adequately characterize social support, it may be that social support is actually the key—those with adequate social support may or may not be clinically depressed, but they are less likely to die anyway.

SUMMARY

Many of the cancer risk factors discussed in this chapter are really common sense and were well-known to our parents. Many of these risk factors can be summarized by saying that they relate to abuse or disuse. Since it is often relatively easy to avoid the pitfalls of abuse and disuse, the cancers discussed here are almost completely preventable. Our parents were right when they advised us to eat sparingly, to get plenty of exercise and fresh air, to drink alcohol and coffee in moderation, to get a good education, to avoid direct sunlight, and to get married and give them grandchildren soon. The difference is that there is now strong scientific evidence to support these views.

While it may be hard to take our parents advice, even now, ignoring common sense involves a certain amount of risk. It is certainly not healthful to be obsessed with cancer risk factors, but it is also not wise to ignore them. The rule of all things in moderation, including moderation itself, may be the best compromise between wisdom and impulse.

NOTES TO CHAPTER 11

1. I-M. Lee, J.E. Manson, C.H. Hennekens, R.S. Paffenbarger, "Body weight and mortality: A 27-year follow-up of middle-aged men," *J. Amer. Med. Assoc.* 270 (1993): 2823–2828.
2. *Ibid.*
3. *Ibid.*
4. I.M. Lee, R.S. Paffenbarger, C-C. Hsieh, "Physical activity and risk of developing colorectal cancer among college alumni," *J. Natl. Cancer Instit.* 83 (1991): 1324–1329.
5. B.E. Henderson, R. Ross, L. Bernstein, "Estrogens as a cause of human cancer," *Cancer Res.* 48 (1988): 246–253.
6. S. Tretli, "Height and weight in relation to breast cancer morbidity and mortality: A prospective study of 570,000 women in Norway," *Int. J. Cancer* 44 (1989): 23–30.
7. *Ibid.*
8. P.K. Mills, W.L. Beeson, R.L. Phillips, G.E. Fraser, "Dietary habits and breast cancer incidence among Seventh-day Adventists," *Cancer* 64 (1989): 582–590.
9. *Ibid.*
10. T.A. Sellers, L.H. Kushi, J.D. Potter, S.A. Kaye, C.L. Nelson, et al. "Effect of family history, body-fat distribution, and reproductive

factors on the risk of post-menopausal breast cancer," *N. Engl. J. Med.* 326 (1992): 1323–1329.

11. *Ibid.*
12.. M.C. Yu, T.M. Mack, R. Hanisch, C. Cicioni, B.E. Henderson, "Cigarette smoking, obesity, diuretic use, and coffee consumption as risk factors for renal cell carcinoma," *J. Natl. Cancer Instit.* 77 (1986): 351–356.
13. Lee, "Physical activity and risk of devloping colorectal cancer among college alumni," 1324–1329.
14. *Ibid.*
15. I.M. Lee, R.S. Paffenbarger, "Quetelet's index and risk of colon cancer in college alumni," *J. Natl. Cancer Instit.* 84 (1992): 1326–1331.
16. D.H. Garabrant, J.M. Peters, T.M. Mack, L. Bernstein, "Job activity and colon cancer risk," *Am. J. Epidemiol.* 119 (1984): 1005–1014.
17. *Ibid.*
18. *Ibid.*
19. S.D. Harlow, G.M. Matanoski, "The association between weight, physical activity, and stress and variation in the length of the menstrual cycle," *Am. J. Epidemiol.* 133 (1991): 38–49.
20. L. Bernstein, R.K. Ross, R.A. Lobo, R. Hanisch, M.D. Krailo, B.E. Henderson, "The effects of moderate physical activity on menstrual cycle patterns in adolescence: implications for breast cancer prevention," *Br. J. Cancer* 55 (1987) 681–685.
21. C.D. Sherman, K.C. Calman, S. Eckhardt, I. Elsebai, D. Firat, et al., "Aetiology," in *Manual of clincial oncology.* (New York: Springer-Verlag, 1987), 13–29.
22. S.I. Mufti, "Alcohol acts to promote incidence of tumors," *Cancer Detect. Prevent.* 16 (1992): 157–164.
23. W.J. Blot, J.K. McLaughlin, D.M. Winn, D.F. Austin, R.S. Greenberg, et al., "Smoking and drinking in relation to oral and pharyngeal cancer," *Cancer Res.* 48 (1988): 3282–3287.
24. *Ibid.*
25. *Ibid.*
26. *Ibid.*
27. *Ibid.*
28. G.L. Day, W.J. Blot, D.F. Austin, L. Bernstein, R.S. Greenberg, et al., "Racial differences in risk of oral and pharyngeal cancer: alcohol, tobacco, and other determinants," *J. Natl. Cancer Instit.* 85 (1993): 465–473.
29. *Ibid.*

30. W.H. Zatonski, H. Becher, J. Lissowska, J. Wahrendorf, "Tobacco, alcohol, and diet in the etiology of laryngeal cancer: a population-based case-control study," *Cancer Causes Control* 2 (1991) 3–10.
31. *Ibid.*
32. M.P. Longnecker, "A case-control study of alcoholic beverage consumption in relation to risk of cancer of the right colon and rectum in men," *Cancer Causes Control* 1 (1990): 5–14.
33. M.P. Longnecker, M.J. Orza, M.E. Adams, J. Vioque, T.C. Chalmers, "A meta-analysis of alcoholic beverage consumption in relation to risk of colorectal cancer," *Cancer Causes Control* 1 (1990): 59–68.
34. *Ibid.*
35. G.A. Kune, L. Vitetta, "Alcohol consumption and the etiology of colorectal cancer: a review of the scientific evidence from 1957 to 1991," *Nutr. Cancer*, 18 (1992): 97–111.
36. E. Giovannucci, M.J. Stampfer, G.A. Colditz, E.B. Rimm, D. Trichopoulos, et al., "Folate, methionine, and alcohol intake and risk of colorectal adenoma," *J. Natl. Cancer Instit.* 85 (1993): 875–884.
37. *Ibid.*
38. *Ibid.*
39. M.P. Longnecker, J.A. Berlin, M.J. Orza, T.C. Chalmers, "A meta-analysis of alcohol consumption in relation to risk of breast cancer," *J. Amer. Med. Assoc.* 260 (1988): 652–656.
40. *Ibid.*
41. M.E. Reichman, J.T. Judd, C. Longcope, A. Schatzkin, B.A. Clevidence, et al., "Effects of alcohol consumption on plasma and urinary hormone concentrations in premenopausal women," *J. Natl. Cancer Instit.* 85 (1993): 722–727.
42. *Ibid.*
43. H. Austin, E. Delzell, S. Grufferman, R. Levine, A.S. Morrison, et al., "A case-control study of hepatocellular carcinoma and the hepatitis B virus, cigarette smoking, and alcohol consumption," *Cancer Res.* 46 (1986): 962–966.
44. *Ibid.*
45. R.K. Ross, A. Paganini-Hill, J. Landolph, V. Gerkins, B.E. Henderson, "Analgesics, cigarette smoking, and other risk factors for cancer of the renal pelvis and ureter," *Cancer Res.* 49 (1989): 1045–1048.
46. *Ibid.*
47. C. La Vecchia, M. Ferraroni, E. Negri, B. D'Avanzo, A. Decarli, et al., "Coffee consumption and digestive tract cancers," *Cancer Res.* 49 (1989): 1049–1051.

48. Ross, "Analgesics, cigarette smoking, and other risk factors for cancer of the renal pelvis and ureter," 1045–1048.
49. M.J. Thun, M.M. Namboodiri, E.E. Calle, W.D. Flanders, C.W. Heath, "Aspirin use and risk of fatal cancer," *Cancer Res.* 53 (1993): 1322–1327.
50. *Ibid.*
51. *Ibid.*
52. G. Gridley, J.K. McLaughlin, A. Ekbom, L. Klareskog, H-O. Adami, et al., "Incidence of cancer among patients with rheumatoid arthritis," *J. Natl. Cancer Instit.* 85 (1993): 307–311.
53. *Ibid.*
54. E.R. Greenberg, J.A. Baron, D.H. Freeman, J.S. Mandel, R. Haile, "Reduced risk of large-bowel adenomas among aspirin users," *J. Natl. Cancer Instit.* 85 (1993): 912–916.
55. S.E. Hankinson, D.J. Hunter, G.A. Colditz, W.C. Willett, M.J. Stampfer, et al., "Tubal ligation, hysterectomy, and risk of ovarian cancer: A prospective study," *J. Amer. Med. Assoc.* 270 (1993): 2813–2818.
56. *Ibid.*
57. Mills, "Dietary habits and breast cancer incidence among Seventh-day Adventists," 582–590.
58. Sellers, "Effect of family history, body-fat distribution, and reproductive factors on the risk of post-menopausal breast cancer," 1323–1329.
59. *Ibid.*
60. M. Ewertz, S.W. Duffy, H-O. Adami, G. Kvale, E. Lund, et al., "Age at first birth, parity, and risk of breast cancer: A meta-analysis of 8 studies from the Nordic countries," *Int. J. Cancer* 46 (1990): 597–603.
61. E. White, "Projected changes in breast cancer incidence due to the trend toward delayed childbearing," *Am. J. Public Health* 77 (1987): 495–497.
62. P.A. Newcomb, B.E. Storer, M.P. Longnecker, R. Mittendorf, E.R. Greenberg, et al., "Lactation and a reduced risk of premenopausal breast cancer," *New Engl. J. Med.* 330 (1994): 81–87.
63. *Ibid.*
64. *Ibid.*
65. American Cancer Society, Cancer facts & figures—1992. (Atlanta: American Cancer Society, 1992), 30.
66. D.W. Dockery, C.A. Pope, X. Xu, J.D. Spengler, J.H. Ware, et al., "An association between air pollution and mortality in six U. S. cities," *New. Engl. J. Med.* 329 (1993): 1753–1759.

67. *Ibid.*
68. *Ibid.*
69. R.G. Ziegler, R.N. Hoover, M.C. Pike, A. Hildesheim, A.M.Y. Nomura, et al., "Migration patterns and breast cancer risk in Asian-American women," *J. Natl. Cancer Instit.* 85 (1993): 1819–1827.
70. *Ibid.*
71. P.K. Mills, W.L. Beeson, R.L. Phillips, G.E. Fraser, "Cohort study of diet, lifestyle, and prostate cancer in Adventist men," *Cancer* 64 (1989): 598–604.
72. G.G. Giles, R. Marks, P. Foley, "Incidence of non-melanocytic skin cancer treated in Australia," *Brit. Med. J.* 296 (1988): 13–17.
73. *Ibid.*
74. *Ibid.*
75. H.K. Koh, R.A. Lew, "Sunscreens and melanoma: implications for prevention," *J. Natl. Cancer Instit.* 86 (1994): 78–79.
76. *Ibid.*
77. J.B. Kerr, C.T. McElroy, "Evidence for large upward trends of ultraviolet-B radiation linked to ozone depletion," *Science* 262 (1993): 1032–1034.
78. P. Sterling, J. Eyer, "Biological basis of stress-related mortality," *Soc. Sci. Med.* 15E (1981): 3–42.
79. B.H. Fox, "Depressive symptoms and risk of cancer," *J. Amer. Med. Assoc.* 262 (1989): 1231.
80. G.D. Friedman, "Psychiatrically-diagnosed depression and subsequent cancer," *Cancer Epidemiol. Biomarkers Prev.* 3 (1994): 11–14.
81. A.B. Zonderman, P.T. Costa, R.R. McCrae, "Depression as a risk for cancer morbidity and mortality in a nationally representative sample," *J. Amer. Med. Assoc.* 262 (1989): 1191–1195.
82. A. Rosengren, K. Orth-Gomer, H. Wedel, L. Wilhelmsen, "Stressful life events, social support, and mortality in men born in 1933, *Br. Med. J.* 307 (1993): 1102–1105.
83. *Ibid.*
84. *Ibid.*

12

....

CANCER RISK AVOIDANCE

The preceding chapters have provided a comprehensive summary of the major cancer risk factors thus far identified. However, these chapters separated cancer risk into various categories, many of them somewhat arbitrary, and little effort was made to make explicit comparisons between categories. When so many data are presented in so many separate categories, it is difficult to achieve a coherent impression of the relative importance of cancer risk factors. Therefore, in this chapter, we will compile and rank the major cancer risk factors according to their calculated weighted risk (recollect that weighted risk is calculated by multiplying relative risk by relative frequency; see Chapter 1 for details). By so doing, we hope to put cancer risk factors into better perspective, so that personal choices and public policies can be directed to achieve the maximum possible reduction in cancer mortality.

A COMPILATION OF THE MAJOR CANCER RISK FACTORS

The Appendix contains a compilation of all cancer risk factors in this book that are associated with a weighted risk greater than 10. This master compilation will be abridged and edited here, in order to facilitate comprehension of the relative importance of the major risk factors.

The top 25 cancer risks are ranked (Table 12-1) in order, as determined by the magnitude of the weighted risk factor. Several surprises emerge from this analysis, some of which would probably not be anticipated even by someone familiar with the cancer literature:

1. 48% of the top 25 cancer risk factors involve lifestyle choices that can be changed or modified. This confirms that cancer is, in large part, a preventable disease, and that adult cancer is often a disease of abuse or disuse.

2. 44% of the top 25 cancer risk factors involve heritable susceptibility to one or several different cancers. Many susceptibility genes have been identified in the very recent past, which implies that more will be identified in the future. This finding is consistent with the impression of most physicians that cancer runs in families, but the extent to which heritable risk dominates this list is something of a surprise.

3. 40% of the top 25 cancer risk factors involve use of tobacco, which should not be a surprise. Tobacco is without question the single most important preventable cancer risk factor.

4. 28% of the top 25 cancer risk factors involve interactive risks, in which the risk associated with one risk factor is increased substantially by exposure to a second risk factor. Many of these interactive risks have also been identified in the very recent past, which implies that more will be identified in the future. Cancer susceptibility genes and interactive risk factors together account for 68% of the top 25 cancer risk factors, which suggests that these phenomena should become the focus of an increased research effort.

5. the first risk factor on this list that is neither heritable nor interactive is the hepatitis B virus, which is associated with a 223-fold increase in risk of liver cancer. This may misrepresent the situation in the United States somewhat, since HBV is not extremely common, and liver cancer induced by HBV is relatively rare. Yet this is a devastating cancer when diagnosed, and an inexpensive vaccine already exists for the virus associated with this cancer. Therefore, this is an attractive target if the goal is to reduce the public health burden of cancer.

The argument can be made that familial risk is overrepresented in Table 12-1, since familial cancers are not preventable by any means short of not having children. For those fortunate enough to be unaffected by the familial risks included in Table 12-2, this table is a misleading summary of risk. Therefore, in Table 12-2, the top 25 cancer risk factors are tabulated, with familial cancer risks specifically excluded. Again, several key findings emerge from this table:

1. 48% of the top 25 nonfamilial cancer risk factors involve exposure to chemicals (including tobacco smoke).

2. 48% of the top 25 nonfamilial cancer risk factors involve use of tobacco. This emphasizes strongly that cessation of tobacco use is not only a vitally important personal goal, it should become a greater focus of public health effort. The relatively ineffectual programs now in place need to be greatly strengthened to overcome the pervasive influence of the tobacco lobby.

TABLE 12-1
TOP 25 WEIGHTED RISK FACTORS

RISK FACTOR	RELATED CANCER	RELATIVE RISK	RELATIVE FREQUENCY	WEIGHTED RISK
Retinoblastoma (Rb) gene mutation	Retinoblastoma	28,500	1	28,500
Ataxia-telangiectasia (AT)	Leukemia	769	2	1,538
Xeroderma pigmentosum	Skin	1,000	1	1,000
High radon (mines) × tobacco	Lung	194	5	970
Tobacco × alcohol	Larynx	330.3	2	660
Breast cancer susceptibility gene	Ovary	300	2	600
Ataxia-telangiectasia (AT)	All cancers	100	5	500
Hepatitis B virus (HBV)	Liver	223	2	446
Tobacco (≥2 pks/day, 10 yrs)	Lung	81	5	406
Thoratrast infusion	Liver	126	2	252
Tobacco × asbestos	Lung	50	5	250
Lung cancer susceptibility × tobacco	Lung	42	5	210
High radon (home) × tobacco	Lung	32.5	5	163
Rb gene mutation	Brain	73.7	2	147
Tobacco smoke (>30 cigs/day)	Larynx	59.7	2	119
Rb gene mutation	Bladder	28.8	4	115
Tobacco × alcohol (40 cigs + 5 drinks/day)	Oral	38	3	114
Heavy drinking × smoking	Oropharyngeal	37.7	3	113
Tobacco smoke (men, any use)	Lung	22.4	5	112
Chronic immunosuppression	Lymphoma	35	3	105
HPV-16 or 18	Cervical	51.0	2	102
Familial adenomatous polyposis	Colon	20	5	100
DES (*in utero* exposure)	Vaginal	~100	1	~100
Rb gene mutation	Lung	16.4	5	82
Rb gene mutation	Skin (melanoma)	73.3	1	73

TABLE 12-2
TOP 25 NONFAMILIAL WEIGHTED RISK FACTORS

RISK FACTOR	RELATED CANCER	RELATIVE RISK	RELATIVE FREQUENCY	WEIGHTED RISK
High radon (mines) × tobacco	Lung	194	5	970
Tobacco × alcohol	Larynx	330	2	660
Hepatitis B virus (HBV)	Liver	223	2	446
Tobacco (≥2 pks/day, 10 yrs)	Lung	81	5	406
Thoratrast infusion	Liver	126	2	252
Tobacco × asbestos	Lung	50	5	250
High radon (home) × tobacco	Lung	32.5	5	163
Tobacco smoke (>30 cigs/dy)	Larynx	59.7	2	119
Tobacco × alcohol (40 cigs + 5 drinks/day)	Oral	38	3	114
Heavy drinking × tobacco	Oropharyngeal	37.7	3	113
Tobacco smoke (men, any use)	Lung	22.4	5	112
Chronic immunosuppression	Lymphoma	35	3	105
HPV-16 or 18	Cervical	51.0	2	102
DES (in utero exposure)	Vaginal	~100	1	~100
Human papilloma virus (HPV)	Cervical	33.6	2	67
HPV-31, 33, 35, or 39	Cervical	33.0	2	66
HPV-45, 51, or 52	Cervical	33.0	2	66
High radon (mines)	Lung	12.7	5	64
Average radon (home) × tobacco	Lung	11.6	5	58
Salted fish consumption	Nasopharynx	38	1	38
Saturated fat	Lung	6.1	5	31
Low intake of folate	Cervical	10	3	30
Tobacco smoke (10 yr. smoker)	Oral	8.9	3	27
Heavy drinking (any alcohol)	Oropharyngeal	8.8	3	26
Tobacco smoke	Larynx	10.3	2	21

3. 28% of the top 25 nonfamilial cancer risk factors involve interactive risks. In 100% of these cases of interactive risk, tobacco use forms half the risk.

4. 20% of the top 25 nonfamilial cancer risk factors involve exposure to viruses. In every one of these cases, either exposure to the virus can be minimized by simple lifestyle choices, or a vaccine exists against the virus, or both. Therefore these risk factor exposures are completely preventable. It may be a surprise that viral causes of cancer figure as prominently in this list as do dietary causes of cancer.

5. 12% of the top 25 nonfamilial cancer risk factors involve inadequate dietary sources of a critical nutrient or exposure to a dietary carcinogen (e.g. salted fish). It may be a surprise that diet is a relatively minor component of this list, since dietary choices are emphasized so heavily in media presentations about cancer prevention. However, modifying the diet is a relatively easy change to make, compared with other possiblities such as smoking cessation.

The inclusion of interactive risks in a compendium of cancer risk factors is likely to be controversial for several reasons. First, interactive risks are newly discovered, so relatively little time has elapsed to put these risks in scientific perspective. Second, since tobacco is involved in every single interactive risk in Table 12-2, smoking cessation would eliminate 10 of the top 25 nonfamilial cancer risk factors, meaning that other cancer risk factors may be underrepresented. Therefore, in Table 12-3, the top 25 cancer risk factors are tabulated with familial and interactive cancer risks specifically excluded. The key findings that emerge from this table are:

1. 64% of the top 25 nonfamilial, noninteractive cancer risk factors involve (nonoccupational) lifestyle choices. Poor lifestyle choices include smoking, improper diet, alcohol abuse, exposure to venereal viruses, and a "high-stress" lifestyle that de-emphasizes the family. Since all of these choices are modifiable, they should be considered preventable causes of cancer.

2. 20% of the top 25 nonfamilial, noninteractive cancer risk factors involve exposure to viruses. HPV exposure occurs through unprotected sex, so fully 80% of these viral causes of cancer could be eliminated through use of condoms.

3. 20% of the top 25 nonfamilial, noninteractive cancer risk factors are medically related (including Thoratrast, immunosuppression, and DES exposure). However, the only currently accepted medical practice is immunosuppression (for organ transplant patients), so this table may be

somewhat misleading. Nevertheless, medical mistakes and abuses have been a significant cause of cancer in the past.

4. 16% of the top 25 nonfamilial, noninteractive cancer risk factors involve dietary risk factors. It is a surprise that dietary factors remain a relatively minor cause of cancer even when both familial and interactive causes of cancer are excluded.

Several risk factors in Table 12-3 are included more than once (tobacco, HPV, alcohol), so that their impact is perhaps overemphasized at the expense of less damaging risk factors. In addition, several risk factors are included in this table even though their impact in the United States is minimal. Some of these risk factors have been minimized in the United States by changing medical practice (Thoratrast and DES exposure), or by rarity of exposure to the risk factor (chronic immunosuppression, high radon levels in mines, salted fish). Therefore, in Table 12-4, in addition to specifically excluding familial and interactive risk factors, those risk factors that were repeated more than once in Table 12-3 have been eliminated. Finally, those risk factors that are very rare, or are unlikely to be encountered within the United States, have been eliminated, so as to formulate a list of the top 25 completely preventable causes of cancer in the United States. The key findings from this compilation are:

1. About 84% of the top 25 preventable causes of cancer are lifestyle-related. Those few that are not clearly lifestyle-related (HBV infection, DDT exposure, infection with *Helicobacter pylori*, and second-hand smoke) nevertheless can have a significant component of lifestyle choice involved. For example, HBV infection is more prevalent among homosexual men who engage in anal sex, high-level DDT exposure is usually occupational and can be minimized through careful application of the pesticide, and second-hand smoke is often avoidable. Infection with *Helicobacter pylori* occurs by unknown means, but it is possible that this too, could be prevented.

2. At least 48% of the top 25 preventable causes of cancer are related to diet. This shows that the current emphasis on dietary prevention of cancer is not a misplaced effort, since diet is more easily changed than certain other lifestyle risk factors, such as tobacco use or obesity.

3. At least 28% of the top 25 preventable causes of cancer are specifically related to an inadequate intake of fruits and vegetables. This would seem to be a relatively easy dietary change to make, since modern farming and shipping practices make fresh fruits and vegetables available year-round to virtually everyone in the United States. Many cookbooks provide recipes that make vegetables more palatable, so all that may be

TABLE 12-3
TOP 25 NONFAMILIAL, NONINTERACTIVE WEIGHTED RISK FACTORS

RISK FACTOR	RELATED CANCER	RELATIVE RISK	RELATIVE FREQUENCY	WEIGHTED RISK
Hepatitis B virus (HBV)	Liver	223	2	446
Tobacco (≥2 pks/day, 10 yrs.)	Lung	81	5	406
Thoratrast infusion	Liver	126	2	252
Tobacco smoke (>30 cigs/day)	Larynx	59.7	2	119
Tobacco smoke (men, any use)	Lung	22.4	5	112
Chronic immunosuppression	Lymphoma	35	3	105
HPV-16 or 18	Cervical	51.0	2	102
DES (*in utero* exposure)	Vaginal	~100	1	~100
Human papilloma virus (HPV)	Cervical	33.6	2	67
HPV-31, 33, 35, or 39	Cervical	33.0	2	66
HPV-45, 51, or 52	Cervical	33.0	2	66
High radon (mines)	Lung	12.7	5	64
Salted fish consumption	Nasopharynx	38	1	38
Saturated fat	Lung	6.1	5	31
Low intake of folate	Cervical	10	3	30
Tobacco smoke (10 yr. smoker)	Oral	8.9	3	27
Heavy drinking (any alcohol)	Oropharyngeal	8.8	3	26
Tobacco smoke	Larynx	10.3	2	21
Thoratrast infusion	Leukemia	10	2	20
DDT in pesticides	Breast	3.5	5	18
Arylamines	Bladder	4.6	4	18
Frequent meat consumption	Colon	3.6	5	18
Hp infection (black Americans)	Stomach	9.0	2	18
Long-term drinking (vodka)	Larynx	9.0	2	18
Phenoxyacetic acid in pesticides	Lymphoma	5.5	3	17

TABLE 12-4
TOP 25 PREVENTABLE WEIGHTED RISK FACTORS

RISK FACTOR	RELATED CANCER	RELATIVE RISK	RELATIVE FREQUENCY	WEIGHTED RISK
Hepatitis B virus (HBV)	Liver	223	2	446
Tobacco (≥2 pks/day, 10 yrs.)	Lung	81	5	406
HPV-16 or 18	Cervical	51.0	2	102
Saturated fat	Lung	6.1	5	31
Low intake of folate	Cervical	10	3	30
Heavy drinking (any alcohol)	Oropharyngeal	8.8	3	26
DDT in pesticides	Breast	3.5	5	18
Frequent meat consumption	Colon	3.6	5	18
Hp infection (black Americans)	Stomach	9.0	2	18
Stressful life events (> 2)	All cancers	3.3	5	17
Low intake of vitamin E	Colon	3.1	5	16
Low intake of vitamin C	Cervical	5	3	15
OC use at 40–44 years age	Breast	2.7	5	14
Use of black hair dye	Lymphoma	4.4	3	13
Low intake raw fruits and vegetables	Lung	2.5	5	13
Obesity	Colon	2.4	5	12
Low carbohydrate intake	Colorectal	2.5	5	12
Second-hand smoke (>22 years)	Lung	2.4	5	12
Total caloric intake	Prostate	2.5	4	10
Low activity (<1000 kcal/week)	Colorectal	2.0	5	10
Low intake of selenium	Lung	2	5	10
Low fiber intake	Colorectal	1.9	5	10
Nulliparous (no children)	Breast	1.9	5	10
Low intake of peas and beans	Lung	1.9	5	10
Age at first birth > 30 yrs	Breast	1.9	5	10

Excluding familial and interactive risks, with repeats and unlikely risk factors (for the United States) eliminated.

required is the impetus to try these recipes. It is hoped that our analysis of cancer risk factors will provide such impetus.

4. 20% of the top 25 preventable causes of cancer are arguably stress-related, since stress can cause an increased intake of tobacco, alcohol, and total calories, and since many people respond to stress by becoming obese. Dealing productively with stress can therefore play a critical role in maintaining a healthy lifestyle and minimizing the risk of cancer. Perhaps the most effective way to deal with stress is to establish a regular routine of exercise.

5. 12% of the top 25 preventable causes of cancer involve largely voluntary contact with a carcinogenic chemical (tobacco smoke, hair dye, even DDT). Most members of the lay public recognize that chemicals can be potent carcinogens, yet many people still have voluntary contact with these chemicals. This suggests that psychological denial of personal risk will be a very difficult defense mechanism to overcome.

6. The most strongly weighted risk factor of all is the Hepatitis B virus, which is a completely preventable risk. A vaccine exists for this virus, and this vaccine is effective, easily administered, and inexpensive. Liver cancer killed more than 15,000 Americans in 1992—a compelling reason to routinely give this vaccine to all persons.

7. The second most strongly weighted risk factor is tobacco. The fact that this risk factor is only second on the list of preventable causes of cancer is actually an artifact of the way weighted risk was calculated. Each risk factor-cancer pair usually considers only a single type of cancer. While HBV is a powerful risk factor, it increases the risk of only one cancer, whereas tobacco is known to cause at least 85% of all lung cancers and up to 30% of all other cancers. Therefore, in the aggregate, tobacco is a vastly more important cause of preventable cancer than is HBV, even though this conclusion does not emerge from the way this table is structured.

8. The most strongly weighted risk factor that is a real surprise is DDT in pesticides, a risk factor for breast cancer. This conclusion is, however, based on very preliminary data, so this study badly needs to be repeated with a larger sample of women and a prospective study design. Breast cancer is the leading cancer killer in the United States and risk factors for this disease are poorly understood, so there is a compelling reason to pursue this finding very actively.

9. Certain cancers, such as lung, cervical, and colorectal cancer, are overrepresented in this list of preventable cancers, while other cancers, such as breast and prostate cancer or lymphoma, are under-represented. This simply demonstrates that identifying the risk factors for certain cancers has been easier than for other cancers. As an example, it is logical that colon cancer risk is related to diet, just as it is logical that breast cancer

risk is related to pregnancy, childbirth, and lactation. Diet actually explains a substantial proportion of all colon cancer cases, whereas pregnancy, childbirth, and lactation explain a relatively small proportion of breast cancer cases. Even heredity seems to explain a relatively small proportion of breast cancer cases, so the search for major breast cancer risk factors must continue.

10. The category of risk that has the greatest proportion of high weighted risk values are the familial risk factors, followed by viral and bacterial risk factors (Table 12-5). Although both of these risk categories have a potent effect on cancer risk, the reason that these categories of risk seem biased toward high weighted risk values may be that they have not been studied as extensively as nutrition or radiation. Because familial and viral risk factors are poorly known, only the very strong risk factors in these categories have been identified thus far.

11. Most cancer risk factors have a relatively small weighted risk value and a very small relative risk value. Of the 224 risk factor-cancer pairs listed in this book, Table 12-5 shows that 54% have a weighted risk value less than ten. In Table 12-4, the relative risk associated with the top 25 preventable cancer risk factors averages 17.5, but, if the top five risk factors are excluded, the average relative risk for a given risk factor drops to only 3.4. This is disheartening, because it shows that modifying personal behavior will not be enough to prevent cancer. Society as a whole must undertake various measures to reduce the incidence and mortality of cancer. The nature of these societal measures will form the focus of the remainder of this book.

ACTUAL CAUSES OF DEATH IN THE UNITED STATES

A recent study examined the actual causes of death in the United States, with the specific goal of identifying the major nongenetic factors that contribute to death.[1] Of the 2.1 million people who died in 1990, death certificates show that more than half a million people died of cancer, and that cancer was the second leading cause of death overall, after heart disease. But medical terms (e.g., cancer), used to describe the physical condition at death, do not reveal the actual root causes of death. In order to get at the root causes of death in the United States, a large number of separate studies were analyzed in a sort of meta-analysis. The actual (nongenetic) causes of death identified in this meta-analysis were, in descending order of importance: tobacco; diet and activity patterns; alcohol; microbial agents; toxic agents; firearms; sexual behavior; motor vehicles; and illicit use of drugs—together accounting for about 50% of all deaths in 1990.

TABLE 12-5
RISK FACTOR–CANCER PAIRS EVALUATED AND THE RELATIVE IMPORTANCE OF VARIOUS CATEGORIES OF RISK

CATEGORY OF RISK	NUMBER OF RISK FACTOR–CANCER PAIRS	NUMBER OF WEIGHTED RISKS ≥ 10	PROPORTION OF WEIGHTED RISKS ≥ 10
Hereditary	32	27	84%
Chemical	30	17	57
Dietary	15	9	60
Nutritional	24	9	38
Radiation	38	11	29
Hormonal	28	5	18
Viral/bacterial	16	10	63
Lifestyle	41	14	34
Total	224	102	46

Each category refers to a specific chapter in the book.

The major root cause of death identified in the United States was tobacco, which was calculated to be responsible for 400,000 deaths in 1990, or roughly 19% of all deaths in that year.[2] Tobacco is responsible for about 30% of all cancer deaths, 30% of all chronic lung disease deaths, 24% of all pneumonia and influenza deaths, 21% of all cardiovascular deaths, and a substantial fraction of deaths from cerebrovascular disease and diabetes. Without doubt, smoking is the most damaging carcinogen to which humans are regularly exposed.

Diet and activity patterns were the next most important root cause of death identified, as these factors were responsible for 300,000 deaths in 1990, or roughly 14% of all deaths in the United States annually.[3] Dietary factors are responsible for deaths from cardiovascular disease, cancer, and diabetes, while physical inactivity is responsible for deaths from heart disease and cancer. Together these factors account for at least 20% of all cancer deaths, 30% of all diabetes deaths, and 22% of all cardiovascular deaths.

The third most important root cause of death identified was alcohol, which was responsible for 100,000 deaths in 1990, or about 5% of all deaths in the United States.[4] An estimated 18 million people in the United States suffer from alcohol dependence, and 76 million are affected by alcohol abuse at some time during their lives. Alcohol abuse is responsible for at least 3% of all cancer deaths, 60% of all cirrhosis deaths, 40% of all motor vehicle fatalities, and 16% of all other injuries.

It is worth noting that more than 20 times as many people died from cancer in 1990 as died from acquired immune deficiency syndrome (AIDS).[5] Despite the public attention given to the human immunodeficiency virus (HIV), various other viruses were far more important as a cause of death in the United States in 1990. Viruses caused about six times as many deaths from cancer as from AIDS in 1990, and the death toll from virally induced cancer is rising at a rate comparable to the death toll from AIDS in the United States. Thus, cancer must remain a major focus of the medical research enterprise.

SUMMARY: TEN THINGS YOU CAN DO TO LESSEN YOUR RISK OF CANCER

1. Stop smoking. No rationale is possible for this devastating habit. Stop those you love from smoking or hound them senseless. Don't allow anyone to smoke in your house or your office, and make it as difficult as possible for smokers to abuse themselves. Smokeless tobacco is really no better than smoked tobacco— it just causes cancers that are somewhat less uniformly fatal than lung cancer.

2. Learn your familial risk factors and be especially vigilant about those cancers that seem to run in your family. Ask your older relatives for as full a description as possible of the cause of death of your deceased relatives, then specifically avoid the risk factors for these cancers.

3. Increase your consumption of fresh fruits and vegetables. A broad variety of each is best, with special emphasis on whatever is freshest in your produce department or store.

4. Decrease your consumption of red meat. This does not mean become a vegetarian, but rather place greater dietary emphasis on white meats, such as chicken and fish. An appropriate dietary modification might be as simple as having red meat fewer than four times per week, or having chicken or fish at least three times per week. Vegetarian dishes or dishes rich in complex carbohydrates (e.g., pasta) can also be substituted for red meat.

5. Exercise at least three times per week, for at least 20 minutes each time. This will help to maintain your weight at an appropriate level as well as conferring other benefits.

6. Get vaccinated against Hepatitis B virus if at all possible and avoid other viral exposures. This may mean using a condom, minimizing the number of different sexual partners, or avoiding intercourse with someone you suspect to be infected with human papilloma virus.

7. Practice moderation in all things. Overuse or abuse of alcohol, prescription drugs, and fast foods takes a very high toll in the modern world, as does overexposure to sunlight.

8. Make a yearly visit to a physician if you are over 40 years old, and make bi-annual visits if you are over 30 years old. This will certainly help to diagnose and treat current problems, but may also alert you to newly discovered cancer risk factors. In addition, there are several widely available cancer screening tests that should be used on the advice of your physician, including mammography, Pap test, fecal occult blood test, and prostate specific antigen screening.

9. Avoid unneccessary exposure to the hormones used in estrogen-replacement therapy.

10. Learn the 10 warning signs of cancer. These include: (a) a swelling, thickening, or lump in any soft tissue, but especially the breasts; (b) persistent or unexplained coughing or hoarseness; (c) a sore that does not heal or a mole that abruptly changes in size or color; (d) unexplained fatigue; (e) abrupt weight loss or loss of appetite; (f) changes in bowel habits, including pain or bleeding on defecation, narrow stools, or constipation; (g) changes in urinary function, particularly bleeding or difficulty in discharge; (h) changes in menstrual function, especially unexpected or excessive bleeding; (i) difficulty in swallowing or a feeling of bloat or fullness; and (j) pallor or abnormal bleeding.[6]

NOTES TO CHAPTER 12

1. J.M. McGinnis, W.H. Foege, "Actual causes of death in the United States," *J.Amer. Med. Assoc.* 270 (1993): 2207–2212.
2. *Ibid.*
3. *Ibid.*
4. *Ibid.*
5. *Ibid.*
6. H.B. Simon, *Staying well: your complete guide to disease prevention,*. (New York: Houghton Mifflin Co., 1992), 499.

13
·······································
PUBLIC HEALTH POLICY
AND CANCER PREVENTION

Many personal choices can affect cancer risk; a person careful to avoid exposure to known risk factors can substantially lessen his or her risk of developing cancer. But personal choices alone are not sufficient to reduce the incidence and mortality of cancer to a minimum. As we have seen, the incremental change in cancer risk from a given risk factor exposure is usually rather small. Even among the top 25 preventable risk factors for cancer (Chapter 12), when the top five risk factors are excluded, the average relative risk is only 3.4. A great many risk factors have a relative risk value of less than two, so that even the most prudent individual with the lowest possible exposure to the risk factor reduces their odds of that cancer by only half.

Thus, in addition to making tough personal choices, other measures must be undertaken to minimize the toll of cancer. These other measures fall into three broad categories, which will serve to focus the remaining chapters. The first measure is to modify public health policies, so that the government takes a more active role in educating the public about risk factors and in regulating public risk factor exposures. The second measure is to implement a broad range of cancer screening examinations, so that those cancers that have already become established can be detected while treatment is still likely to result in cure. The final measure is to actively intervene in the carcinogenic process, to reduce the likelihood that past or present exposure to a risk factor will result in cancer.

EDUCATIONAL PROGRAMS AS PUBLIC HEALTH POLICY

We are all familiar with the public health announcements that are occasionally broadcast on radio or television. Despite the fact that this familiarity can breed a certain amount of contempt, research shows that such announcements can have an effect on individual behaviors. When such announcements are part of a broad-spectrum educational effort, designed to publicize a particular risk factor, they can be highly effective.

In the relatively few years between 1973 and 1987, the mortality from cardiovascular disease declined dramatically.[1] Among white men aged less than 54 years, deaths from heart disease decreased by an astounding 42% in only 15 years. For white men between 55 and 84 years of age, cardiovascular mortality declined by 33% in the same period, while even for men more than 85 years old, heart attack mortality was down about 28%.[2] In the 37-year period between 1950 and 1987, there was a 55% decline overall in heart disease mortality.[3] Although several improvements were made in the treatment of heart disease during this period, this stunning decline in heart attack risk is largely due to a concerted program of risk factor reduction through education. Since 1950, the proportion of men who smoke has declined sharply (although a higher proportion of women smoke now than in 1950). A great deal of effort has also been devoted to detecting and treating hypertension—one of the most important early warning signs of heart disease. Finally, a great increase has been made in the awareness that diet plays an important role in heart disease risk, and that a diet low in cholesterol can significantly reduce the risk of heart disease. Thus, the decline in mortality from heart disease can serve as a model for the beneficial impact of a major disease prevention program.[4]

Another striking success story, in which a public education program produced an impressive decline in disease mortality, occurred in Queensland, Australia. The incidence of skin cancer in Australia is reported to be the highest in the world, probably because most of the population is of northern European origin, and the sunlight exposure is very intense.[5] A public awareness campaign was initiated in Queensland to educate people about warning signs and early symptoms of melanoma and other skin cancers. General awareness of skin cancer warning signs increased so much that now the cure rate for melanoma is 80%, even though melanoma incidence is largely unchanged. In fact, public awareness of skin cancer is so high that a substantial fraction of people mistakenly believed they had been cured of skin cancer in the previous 12 months.[6] While it may seem strange that many people thought they had skin cancer, when in fact they did not, this indicates a very high level of awareness of the problem.

A recent effort to promote dietary change in Sweden has illustrated the massive effort that a public education program can involve.[7] An ambitious program of cancer prevention was undertaken in 1982, part of which involved publicizing healthful dietary practices among the citizens of Stockholm. Explicit goals were set for this program: fat intake was to be reduced to 30% or less of total caloric intake, and fiber intake was to increase to 30 grams per day. The strategy to obtain these goals involved promoting the importance of several diet modifications:

1. Consumption of healthful foods should increase. Recommended food items included whole-grain breads, pasta, cereal, potatoes and other tubers, vegetables (especially dried peas and beans), fruits, and fish.
2. Consumption of high-fat foods should be reduced. High-fat foods such as meat, meat products, milk, cheese, and cream were to be exchanged for low-fat substitutes.
3. Consumption of sweets and salt should be reduced. These measures were more to avoid hypertension and heart disease than to avoid cancer, although obesity can have an impact on cancer risk.
4. Food preparation methods should emphasize cooking without fats and oils, and cooking fat should be replaced by margarine. In addition, cooking methods such as steaming, poaching, baking, and microwaving were to be substituted for frying whenever possible.

To foster these dietary modifications, the Stockholm Cancer Prevention Program (SCCP) office undertook a very comprehensive education program.[8] In order to reach the general population, SCCP sponsored exhibitions at local fairs, cooking courses, a Health Day Festival, and a health-related open house. The mass media were enlisted to publicize these activities and to publish articles relating to health issues. Informational material was printed for distribution through local food merchants, and the merchants themselves were informed and involved to ensure that a "Healthy Dietary Habits" week was successful. Restaurants and caterers were given information to assist in menu modification, and health care providers were enlisted in the process. Health information was disseminated to the public through the media, through public school programs, through health care providers, and through counseling sessions open to obese persons. Even pre-schoolers were targeted, through an open house specifically for supervisors of day care centers, through informational meetings for parents of pre-schoolers, through consultation with pre-school staff about food menus, and through staff educational programs. In addition, the SCCP published cookbooks for caterers and for families, sponsored a Food Fair that involved 60 different companies and organizations, collaborated with several large catering firms to offer healthful lunchs in company cafeterias, and worked with several occupational health services to help modify employee dietary habits.

This impressive effort to change dietary habits in Sweden demonstrates several important points about public education programs. First and most important, for to a program be effective, it must be well thought out and multifaceted, in order to reach all citizens with a consistent and fairly simple message. If the message is not consistent, confusion results, and if the message is not fairly simple, then people won't take the time to learn and incorporate it into their lives. Second, because human behavior is resistant to change, many years may be required before there is any observable effect of the program. Third, this sort of protracted and multifaceted campaign is very expensive and can only be accomplished when there is political consensus that the campaign's goals are both worthwhile and achievable. Fourth, even with time, effort, and money devoted to such an effort, success is not guaranteed. It is difficult to induce people to change old habits, even if these habits are proven to be harmful. Compliance is difficult to achieve even in a massive effort, and a less massive effort is probably doomed to failure. Finally, it is difficult or impossible to determine if an intervention is successful, because of the very long time lag between the intervention and any anticipated change in disease incidence. Because cancer usually occurs many years after an initial carcinogen exposure, no one will know whether the SCCP effort at diet modification has really been successful for at least two more decades.[9]

THE CAMPAIGN AGAINST TOBACCO USE IN THE UNITED STATES

For more than 20 years the United States has had a public education program to educate smokers about the risk of cancer associated with tobacco use. This program has met with some success, as the prevalence of smoking in the United States has dropped from 40% in 1965 to 29% in 1987.[10] There are strong indications that smoking cessation reduces cancer risk, even among people who have smoked for 40 years, or who are in their 60s when they quit.[11] Lung cancer rates are declining in men, and it has been calculated that about 800,000 deaths from tobacco-related causes have been delayed or averted by these efforts.

But smoking still causes up to 400,000 deaths per year and is responsible for at least 30% of all cancers.[12] About 50 million Americans still smoke, and teenagers start smoking at a rate that very nearly matches the rate at which adults quit. Between 1974 and 1985, approximately 1.3 million persons per year became non-smokers, but another one million people per year took up the habit. This is equivalent to an additional 3,000 new smokers every day.[13] If present trends continue, over 40 million

Americans, or 22% of the entire population, will still be smoking by the year 2000. The smoking habit is not expected to be evenly distributed among persons with different education levels. At least 30% of those who have not finished high school are expected to still be smoking, but less than 10% of college graduates will still smoke. New smokers are predominantly young and less well-educated, and smoking is increasingly a behavior of the socioeconomically disadvantaged.[14]

Among people with a high school education or less, only about 8% of smokers are able to quit.[15] This is an indication of how addictive smoking is and how difficult it can be to quit. Most people who try to quit smoking do not seek professional help; of those people who quit smoking for at least one day in the 1980s, only 10% sought help to make that effort successful. The low prevalence of help or support for smokers attempting to quit may contribute to the dismal success seen among poorly educated smokers.

The National Cancer Institute sponsors a free Cancer Information Service (CIS; telephone number: 1-(800)-4-CANCER) that has been available for 15 years and that has answered over five million calls. The CIS offers a telephone counseling service to smokers trying to quit that is occasionally publicized in television public service announcements. Recently a study examined whether these public service announcements were successful in promoting use of the CIS.[16] Information about the size of a particular audience exposed to television advertisements and on the frequency with which television "spots" were aired was used to determine how many people in a market were exposed to an anti-smoking message. Then the frequency of calls placed to the CIS was analyzed to determine whether television ads actually induced people to call for information on smoking cessation. Television spots caused the number of calls to the CIS to nearly double, at least transiently. Television spots were particularly effective in increasing the number of callers who were male, or who were under the age of 40, or who had received a high school education or less. Since this is an audience that is normally resistant to an anti-smoking message, this is a striking success. Therefore, television appears to be an effective medium for publicizing an anti-smoking message and for supporting smokers who are trying to quit. However, it is unknown whether speaking with a counselor at the CIS actually helped smokers to quit. More research is needed to identify the most effective strategies for utilizing the initial telephone contact to induce smoking cessation, for supporting the smoker during the quitting process, or for preventing smoking relapse.[17]

Several important lessons have been learned about smoking cessation in particular, and cancer prevention in general, from the CIS.[18] The most important lesson is that, if information or help or support is available, people will use it. During the past 15 years, the CIS has received more than 413,000 smoking-related calls, many from smokers interested in quitting. For many people, calling the CIS was the first positive step they took toward smoking cessation. Although it often seems that public service ad campaigns are not terribly successful, even hard-to-reach audiences can be approached with a targeted campaign. For example, blacks in the United States are chronically underserved by the health care system. Yet a National Minority Awareness Week campaign in California was able to increase the number of black callers to the CIS strikingly; normally the California office receives 9% of its calls from this target group, but during the campaign, this percentage rose to 26% of all callers. Thus, in some cases at least, people will hear what they need to hear, as well as what they want to hear.

A recent study examined the success of an anti-smoking campaign directed toward mothers with small children.[19] This particular target audience was chosen because a smoking mother places her children at risk of respiratory ailments by exposing them to second-hand smoke. Furthermore, the incidence of smoking in young women is increasing somewhat, while it is declining both in men and in older women. Tobacco companies have begun to target women with advertisements for cigarettes, so the CIS began to target the same audience with anti-smoking advertisements. A large anti-smoking campaign was begun across seven media markets in New York, Pennsylvania, and Delaware, and the response to this campaign was assessed by monitoring calls to the CIS offices in the same areas. A 46-week long media campaign resulted in a five-fold increase in the number of smoking-related calls to the CIS. The campaign was particularly successful in reaching the target audience of young mothers with children. Call logs inside the media market showed that 29% of all calls were from young mothers, while outside the media market only 10% of calls were from the same target audience. Anti-smoking ads were very successful, as 44% of all calls to the CIS occurred during a five week period when television spots were aired by the regional media.[20]

Although the prevalence of smoking declined from 40% in 1965 to 29% in 1987, the prevalence of smoking among blue collar workers in 1987 was estimated to be still about 37%.[21] Another study examined the success of an anti-smoking campaign that specifically targeted blue collar workers and that tried to incorporate the callers' stage in the smoking cessation process. Careful evaluation showed that about one-third of all callers to the CIS had already taken some step toward smoking cessation, whether setting a quit date, already attempting to quit, or actually quitting, while the remainder were thinking about quitting. In this group of people, nearly 19% were able to quit smoking successfully for at least a year. This compares favorably with the average of 5–8% of smokers able to quit for a year on their own or with minimal assistance. However, it was found that a program specifically tailored to blue collar workers that incorporated the smokers' stage in the smoking cessation process was no more successful than other smoking-cessation programs. This shows that, while any smoker is potentially able to quit, we know relatively little about the most effective strategies to foster smoking cessation.

When the cost and effectiveness of different smoking-cessation programs was evaluated, it became clear that cost-effectiveness is a very real consideration in determining the best program to use.[22] Three smoking cessation programs were assessed, in terms of total cost, ability to promote smoking cessation, amount of time required from participants, and overall cost-effectiveness. A formal smoking cessation class was compared with a self-help kit and with a contest with prize incentives to promote smoking cessation. The classroom approach was found to be most effective, but it required the most time from participants, had the highest total cost, and was the least cost-effective. The self-help kit had the lowest total cost, required the least time from participants, and was the most cost-effective, but it was also the least effective at promoting smoking cessation. The contest approach seemed to offer a good compromise, since it was intermediate in total cost, success rate, and cost-effectiveness. The smoking-cessation contest involved enrolling documented smokers at a community center, allowing a six-week period for smoking cessation, then randomly drawing the names of participants to receive prizes. To receive their prizes, these randomly chosen smokers had to prove they no longer smoked by submitting to a test of carbon monoxide in the bloodstream. This approach offers a substantial inducement to smokers to get through the most difficult period of tobacco withdrawal. At the end of the six-week period, those who quit may already perceive the health benefits to be obtained by long-term abstention.

Recent success has also been reported using a transdermal nicotine patch to help long-term smokers quit.[23] In a group of 1,070 smokers, aged 65 through 74 years, about 29% were able to quit smoking for six months or longer, which compares very favorably with the success rate using most other techniques. Most of those who had tried to quit previously reported that use of the transdermal patch made quitting easier. In general, frequent contact with physicians or pharmacists, and complete cessation of smoking at the initiation of patch use made success more likely. Another study compared the success of smoking cessation among those who used a transdermal nicotine patch and those who used a placebo.[24] Nearly 47% of those subjects treated with a patch containing nicotine were able to quit smoking for eight weeks, while only 20% of those treated with an inactive patch were able to quit for an equivalent period. One year later, nearly 28% of those treated with an active patch were still not smoking, while only 14% of those treated with an inactive patch were not smoking. Smoking cigarettes at all during the first few weeks of patch use was associated with very poor success at smoking cessation.[25] Among nicotine patch users who smoked during week two after quitting, only 7% had quit smoking six months later, while 43% of those who were able to abstain at week two were also able to abstain at six months. These new studies suggest strongly that the transdermal nicotine patch may be an effective aid to smoking cessation, although the patches cannot succeed without real effort and commitment on the part of the smoker.

Smoking cessation usually occurs in stages, and the likelihood of overall success is determined in part by the success with which a quitter can work through the whole process.[26] There appear to be four stages, with the following characteristics:

1. Pre-contemplation—in which people are not seriously thinking about changing, at least not in the next six months.
2. Contemplation—the period during which people are seriously thinking about changing an unhealthy behavior within the next six months.
3. Action—the six-month period following change of an unhealthy behavior.
4. Maintenance—the period from more than six months after an overt behavior change until the problem behavior is fully resolved. In fact, full resolution may never be reached.

Another study found that about 22% of smokers who were in the pre-contemplative stage prior to a smoking cessation program were able to remain smoke-free at six months after intervention.[27] Among those in the contemplative stage prior to intervention, the success rate for remaining smoke-free at six months increased to 44%, while those who were ready for action were 80% smoke-free at six months. While these success rates for smoking cessation at first seem very good, this study was conducted with smokers being treated for heart disease.[28] The fact that more of these smokers were unable to quit, even though they were at very high risk of further heart disease, shows how difficult it can be to quit smoking.

A study of smokers diagnosed with cancer of the head and neck has provided some insight into the psychology of the smoker, and into the motivational factors that are most effective in helping smokers to quit.[29] This is an important group to study because at least 80% of all head and neck cancer patients are heavy smokers and because these patients typically have a very difficult time with smoking cessation, even though the effects of continued smoking can be devastating. The three most common reasons these patients gave for smoking cessation were, in declining order: "effect on my health"; "doctor's advice"; and "knowledge of the dangers." By comparison, "pressure from others to quit," "effect my smoking has on others," "setting a good example for children" and "cost of cigarettes" were not rated as very important reasons to quit. The most effective inducements for addicted smokers to quit thus all involve an objective appraisal of health effects, whether these appraisals are self-appraisals or physician appraisals. Apparently even persons strongly addicted to smoking are able to make a balanced judgment about risk, although some were subsequently unable to respond effectively to their judgment. A comparison between smokers who tried to quit and smokers who made no such effort showed that those who tried to quit had greater confidence in their ability to quit and greater confidence that they would not be smoking in one year. But it is not clear whether greater self-confidence enabled these smokers to abstain, or whether abstaining increased the self-confidence of smokers. This is an important distinction, because it may help identify the strongest motivation for quitting.

Many studies have demonstrated convincingly the difficulty of changing human behavior, even if changes are made voluntarily. The average self-changer needs to make three or four serious attempts to quit smoking, spaced out over seven to 10 years, before actually achieving success.[30] Smokers (and other addicted persons), are often unwilling to admit that a problem even exists. One study, which was able to identify smokers objectively from chemical traces in the bloodstream, found that 2–3% of smokers actually deny having a smoking habit.[31] Because it is so difficult to quit smoking, the government must do everything in its power to motivate the smoker to quit and to prevent the non-smoker from ever starting. This is why it is especially bad that the government policy on smoking is so inconsistent. The existence of a tobacco subsidy directly counters the Public Health Service goal of encouraging smoking cessation and sends a mixed message to smokers.[32] There is a great deal of hypocrisy, and a certain amount of immorality, in this tacit endorsement of smoking. It seems quite likely that, in the near future, lawsuits will be brought to bear against the government, citing the government role in encouraging tobacco production and in causing the cancers that result from tobacco use.

PUBLICIZING CANCER RISK FACTORS

The American Cancer Society has done a very good job in increasing public awareness and understanding of cancer, and in publicizing cancer risk factors. But it is one agency, with a limited budget and limited staff, tackling a very large problem. Thus another authoritative, centralized source of information is needed to disseminate the latest findings in cancer prevention and cancer cure. A strong need also exists for a cancer referral service, so that newly diagnosed patients can know where to go for a second opinion, or how to become part of an established cancer treatment protocol. There is also a desperate need for a legally empowered agency to actively and forcefully expose some of the charlatans who, with the simple aim of getting rich quickly, sell expensive remedies and preventives that are often equivalent to snake oil. Finally, there is a real need for an authoritative source to correct some of the misinformation and disinformation that so often finds its way into the media.

These various needs might best be met by the National Cancer Institute (NCI) of the National Institutes of Health (NIH). While the NCI has done a fine job of performing vital research at the NIH, of funding promising basic reasearch at universities and medical schools across the country, of generating consensus among medical practioners, and of acting as an overseer of the research effort, it has done less well at acting as a liaison between the scientific community and the lay public. For this reason, basic research is often viewed with suspicion, taxpayers resent the relatively small amounts of money spent on cancer research, and scientists are occasionally accused of being part of a "cancer conspiracy" to hide a known cancer cure.

The media also need to report science fairly, with more objectivity and perspective than has been shown in the past. A recent Harris poll found that people think that science issues should be covered in the newspaper. In this poll, reported in *Science* magazine in 1993, 71% of a sample of 1,250 adults thought that "it makes no sense for the media to cut back on its coverage of science news." This same survey found that 67% of women and 52% of men were "very interested" in news of "AIDS research and treatment," and 67% of women and 32% of men were "very interested" in "women's health problems." This survey shows clearly there is a great interest in health science issues, which is not being adequately addressed by the media, presumably because of a shortage of good science writers.

Many newspaper reporters writing about science have not had experience in critically reviewing scientific data and so may be taken in by exaggerated claims for a new finding or a new treatment. Many stories in the press about cancer risk or cancer treatment are written by people with an inadequate science background and a poor understanding of the complexity of science. Science articles in the media typically focus on the scientists instead of the science. A newspaper article will often report a new and controversial finding before it has been adequately tested by other scientists. Other scientists may be interviewed, and many of them may express their reservations about the new finding, but these reservations never find their way into print. Instead, the finding may be reported as established fact or else may be reported as the result of a crusade by a lone scientist being suppressed as part of a mysterious conspiracy. Most of the reports we read about cancer in the popular press are only partly true, and many are completely false.

As an example of a shoddy job done reporting on medical science, a television news show in Seattle called *Evening Magazine* aired a story in 1989 about a new way of screening for early-stage cancer. This story concerned use of a technique called magnetic resonance spectroscopy (MRS) to detect changes in blood plasma that were supposed to be diagnostic of cancer. The story implied that this technique would have an immediate and important impact on diagnosis of cancer and featured a patient dying of breast cancer who lamented that the technique hadn't been available sooner. However, this technique had been completely discredited for at least two full years before *Evening Magazine* aired the story. The NCI had funded a large prospective study to evaluate the MRS screening test in 1987, but the study was terminated after only a month because early results resoundingly disproved the claim that MRS could screen for cancer. By 1989 there was probably not a single scientist in the field who still believed the claim, including the author of the original paper. Science progresses by building consensus, and consensus had been reached that this technique did not work as a cancer screening test. But the reporters who wrote the story never bothered to check their facts with scientists.

The media could play an important role in increasing public access to science. However, they will only succeed by avoiding sensationalism, countering alarmism, and refusing to permit science to be reported by press conference rather than published in traditional peer-reviewed journals. The media also have a responsibilty to report the news of advances in medicine in a way that does not raise false hopes among patients who may be very willing to grasp at straws. It seems fair to demand that the media should:[33]

1. Report science accurately.
2. Convey a balanced perspective, so that readers know where, in the scheme of things, the new result fits. This can only be achieved by interviewing other scientists with opposing views, and by reporting on the process of building consensus.
3. Monitor and publicize adverse health risks in a timely fashion. This does not mean that the speculation of scientists at the fringe

should be reported, but rather that reporters should report on those scientific developments that have already been peer-reviewed and published in scientific journals.

4. Influence public attitudes about risk factors, so as to minimize risk factor exposures.

5. Refuse to accept advertising for products such as tobacco, which are known to be in direct opposition to the public good.

REGULATING CANCER RISK FACTOR EXPOSURES

Governmental regulation of environmental exposure to carcinogens has been going on for many years. Many federal agencies, including the Environmental Protection Agency (EPA), the Food and Drug Administration (FDA), the National Institutes of Health (NIH), and the Occupational Safety and Health Administration (OSHA), regulate risk factor exposure. Although high-risk occupations remain,[34] the situation is generally much better now than it was 30 years ago. Because of the effectiveness of these regulatory agencies, pollution is not a major risk, except in isolated instances, and occupational exposure to carcinogens probably accounts for less than 4% of all cancers in the United States.[35] Generally, these agencies are quick to respond to a perceived public health risk, although the response may seem to be unguided by common sense or scientific data.

An example of questionable success in governmental regulation is seen in the recent effort to regulate exposure to asbestos fibers in the workplace. Asbestos has been used in construction, as fire retardant, insulation, and reinforcement, as well as in many consumer goods, and the opportunities were once legion for the public to be exposed to asbestos fibers. After asbestos fibers were recognized as a risk factor for a rare form of lung cancer known as mesothelioma, there was a great public outcry to abate asbestos exposure. Congress responded to this pressure by passing the Asbestos Hazard Emergency Response Act of 1986, which required that all public and private schools be inspected for the presence of asbestos and that immediate management efforts be undertaken to prevent further exposure.[36] In 1991, the EPA reported that 94% of the nation's school districts were in compliance with requirements, at a total cost estimated by the *Wall Street Journal* of at least $3.4 billion. The *Wall Street Journal* also reported that, if government, commercial, and residential buildings were similarly renovated, the price tag for all of these abatement efforts would grow to $100 billion to $150 billion. New York City alone is estimated to have asbestos in 67% of its buildings, meaning that 153,000 buildings might require abatement.

Yet building occupants are almost certainly at low risk, since the concentration of asbestos fibers in indoor air is comparable to fiber levels in outdoor air.[37] Furthermore, removal efforts release asbestos fibers, which could result in more cancers among the workmen than would have resulted among building occupants had the fibers been left in place.[38] By the Environmental Protection Agency's (EPA) own figures, a total asbestos ban would save the lives of 202 people over the course of 13 years, at a cost to taxpayers of $76 million to $106 million *per life*.[39] Fortunately in 1991, an Appeals Court overturned the EPA ban on asbestos, arguing that the EPA had failed to weigh financial costs against public health benefits when it banned the use of asbestos, despite the fact that the legislation upon which the ban was based (Toxic Substances Control Act of 1976) requires such a cost/benefit analysis. The court noted that, "Considering that many of the substances that the EPA itself concedes will be used in place of asbestos have known carcinogenic effects, the EPA not only cannot assure this court that it has taken the least burdensome alternative, but cannot even prove that its regulations will increase workplace safety."[40]

The asbestos abatement fiasco is a product of imperfect information, inadequate understanding, and media alarmism, and scientists are culpable because they failed to bring balance to the argument until it was too late. Almost certainly, the asbestos danger was initially overplayed, even though some asbestos miners, insulation workers, shipwrights, and pipe fitters actually were at an increased risk of mesothelioma. But on the basis of inconclusive epidemiologic information suggesting that many people might be at some level of risk, a storm of controversy was created that clouded the judgment of legislators and the public alike. Had the National Institutes of Health (NIH) held a consensus conference about the dangers of asbestos in the early 1980s, the EPA might have been better able to direct its regulatory efforts.[41] It is true the EPA did not mandate asbestos removal unless "building demolition or renovation activities threaten to release significant amounts of asbestos fibers into the air," and it is true that the EPA recommended that "if asbestos-containing material is in good condition and is unlikely to be disturbed, it is generally preferable to contain that material where it is rather than remove it."[42] But it is also true that the EPA failed to obtain accurate measures of indoor and outdoor asbestos fiber levels, failed to consider the costs as well as the benefits of remediation, failed to adequately differentiate risk from different types of asbestos, failed to fully consider what epidemiologic data there were, and instead fostered the view that a single asbestos fiber can cause cancer.[43]

The failure of the EPA with respect to asbestos abatement argues strongly that trained scientists need to become more involved in policy discussions, so that national policy can be based more on a careful analysis of the data and less on alarmism and hysteria. While the government clearly should have a strong role in regulating risk factor exposures, relatively little consensus exists about what form that role should take. The recent suggestion that the Federal Drug Administration (FDA) become involved in regulation of tobacco products is entirely appropriate, since nicotine is a highly addictive substance whose abuse has grave health consequences. In addition, it would be appropriate for the federal government to initiate additional regulatory efforts, perhaps including better regulation of food additives and pesticide use.

SUMMARY: TEN THINGS THE GOVERNMENT SHOULD DO TO HELP PREVENT CANCER

1. Foster a better public dialogue on health-related issues by using the Surgeon General's office to promote public health ideas and measures more effectively. Dr. C. Everett Koop is to be commended for his vigorous public service efforts while in this office.

2. Increase the excise tax on cigarettes to at least $2 per pack to reduce cigarette consumption. This is projected to reduce the number of American smokers by an estimated 7.6 million and would specifically reduce cigarette consumption by teenagers. This could prevent 1.9 million smoking-related deaths and would also raise $30 billion in additional revenue, even though cigarette consumption would fall. The excise tax should also be continually adjusted upward with inflation to maintain a steady pressure on smokers.[44]

3. End the Federal Tobacco Program immediately. This program amounts to a tobacco subsidy for farmers growing a crop that already costs the nation about $68 billion a year in health care costs and lost wages.[45] [27]. There is absolutely no reason why one of the most profitable businesses in the world should be further subsidized. The interests of a few thousand farmers should not be put ahead of the interests of millions of others in our society.

4. Aggressively promote smoking cessation programs aimed at adolescents, women, blue collar workers, minorities, and any other groups that are targeted by smoking advertisements.[46] According to the Federal Trade Commision, cigarette companies had spent a total of $2.1 billion dollars on tobacco advertising and promotion by 1984. Advertisements for cigarettes accounted for 22% of all billboard ads and 7% of all magazine ads in 1985, and the annual expenditure on such advertisments had grown seven-fold over the preceeding decade.[47] Cigarette companies spend vastly

more money in a year to promote their pro-smoking message than has ever been spent on anti-smoking ad campaigns. It should come as no surprise that these ads are having a strong effect on some people. This situation must change because the cost of smoking to our society is too high.

5. Initiate additional programs to increase cancer risk factor awareness. Programs that might be appropriate include raising public awareness about the need to increase consumption of dietary fiber or to undergo Pap screening examinations of the female cervix. There is a danger of dissipating force if too many such programs are initiated simultaneously, so care must be taken to plan a marketing strategy as carefully as any company would when marketing a new product. It is entirely appropriate to think of cancer prevention information as a new product being introduced to the public and to use the full range of marketing expertise of advertising firms. The tobacco companies have much to teach in this respect.

6. Fund more research into the most effective strategies of behavior modification.[48] Research should address all phases of intervention, including recruitment, retention, and relapse, and should be broad-based, so that behavior modifications other than smoking cessation are also studied.

7. Extend the charter of the National Cancer Institute to become a clearinghouse for dissemination of new findings on cancer prevention to the public. The American Cancer Society is already doing a fairly good job, but its budget is more limited and its level of authority is somewhat lower than the National Cancer Institute. A change in emphasis toward dissemination of information may already be happening—the NCI's Cancer Information Service is a qualified success, and the *Journal of the National Cancer Institute* has recently become the most frequently cited publication in cancer research. This journal contains well-written overview articles aimed at the nonscientist.

8. Implement new programs in public schools and in the workplace to foster a healthy lifestyle. In public schools, this could involve a federally mandated health education program to prevent smoking and drug abuse or to promote adequate diet and exercise. In the workplace, this could involve providing similar health education programs and seminars that could be given on-site in large companies, or it could involve a more extensive effort to alert individuals about their individual health risks.

9. Realign federal research spending in the health sciences to be more consistent with actual causes of death and, in all sciences, to be more in line with the public welfare. In 1990, about 21,000 deaths were caused by sexually transmitted human immunodeficiency virus (HIV), while about 505,000 deaths were caused by cancer.[49] In that same year, the National Institutes of Health spent about $744 million on AIDS research,[50] while the National Cancer Institute spent $1,631 million on cancer research.[51]

This means that, although cancer was responsible for killing more than 24 times as many people as were killed by AIDS, only about twice as much money was spent on cancer research. It is not clear that this relative allocation of funds best serves the public interest. Furthermore, in 1990, federal spending on the Strategic Defense Initiative (SDI) was $3,819 million, while the space station received $1,928 million.[52] Between 1980 and 1989, research and development sponsored by the Department of Defense increased 89% in real dollars, while research and development in domestic programs, including medical research, decreased by 9% in real dollars.[53] This allocation of money among various projects has since been reassessed, but continual reassessment of priorities in federal research spending is important. For example, in the 1995 federal budget for research and development, AIDS research is slated to receive $1,379 million, while breast cancer research is slated to receive only $383 million, despite a substantial recent increase in funding specifically for this cancer.[54]

10. Increase the equitability of health care distribution.[55] The American Cancer Society estimates that blacks have a 7% greater likelihood of developing cancer than whites, but they have a 27% greater likelihood of dying from cancer, probably because of limited access to adequate health care. The poor, the uninsured, and the underinsured have a higher risk of being diagnosed with an advanced stage cancer and of receiving inadequate treatment once that cancer has been diagnosed. Late diagnosis of cancer is frequently a consequence of inadequate routine health care; poor patients often do not have regular physicals and may postpone a visit to a physician until very serious symptoms are present. Even after these patients have been diagnosed, they have a significant chance of receiving inadequate health care. A recent study of women with breast cancer showed that women at small urban hospitals, which often serve a large population of poorly insured patients, are likely to receive inadequate cancer therapy at their neighborhood hospital and are ultimately more likely to die of their cancer.[56] Until health care access is equal for all people, the poor will continue to suffer needlessly and will often die of curable cancers.

NOTES TO CHAPTER 13

1. D.L. Davis, G.E. Dinse, D.G. Hoel, "Decreasing cardiovascular disease and increasing cancer among whites in the United States from 1973 through 1987," *J. Amer. Med. Assoc.* 271 (1994): 431–438.
2. *Ibid.*
3. B.E. Henderson, R.K. Ross, M.C. Pike, "Toward the primary prevention of cancer," *Science* 245 (1991): 1131–1138.

4. *Ibid.*
5. G.G. Giles, R. Marks, P. Foley. "Incidence of non-melanocytic skin cancer treated in Australia," *Brit. Med. J.* 296 (1988): 13–17.
6. *Ibid.*
7. L. Kanstrom, L-E. Holm, "Promoting dietary change in the Stockholm Cancer Prevention Program," *Cancer Detect. Prev.* 16 (1992): 203–210.
8. *Ibid.*
9. *Ibid.*
10. P. Cole, Y. Amoateng-Adjepong, "Cancer prevention: accomplishments and prospects," *Am. J. Pub. Health* 84 (1994): 8–10.
11. M.T. Halpern, , B.W. Gillespie, K.E. Warner, "Patterns of absolute risk of lung cancer mortality in former smokers," *J. Natl. Cancer Instit.* 85 (1993): 457–464.
12. J.M. McGinnis, W.H. Foege, "Actual causes of death in the United States," *J. Amer. Med. Assoc.* 270 (1993): 2207–2212.
13. J.P. Pierce, M.C. Fiore, T.E. Novotny, E.J. Hatziandreu, R.M. Davis, "Trends in cigarette smoking in the United States: Projections to the Year 2000," *J. Amer. Med. Assoc.* 216 (1989): 261–265.
14. *Ibid.*
15. J.P. Pierce, D.M. Anderson, R.M. Romano, H.I. Meissner, J.C. Odenkirchen, "Promoting smoking cessation in the United States: effect of public service announcements on the cancer information service telephone line," *J. Natl. Cancer Instit.* 84 (1992): 677–683.
16. *Ibid.*
17. *Ibid.*
18. M.E. Morra, .E.P Bettinghaus, A.C. Marcus, K.D. Mazan, E. O'D Nealon, J.P. Van Nevel, "The first 15 years: what has been learned about the Cancer Information Service and the implications for the future," *Monogr. Natl. Cancer Instit.* 14 (1993): 177–185.
19. K.M. Cummings, R. Sciandra, S. Davis, B.K. Rimer, "Results of an antismoking media campaign utilizing the Cancer Information Service," *Monogr. Natl. Cancer Instit.* 14 (1993): 113–118.
20. *Ibid.*
21. B. Thompson, S. Kinne, F.M. Lewis, J.A. Wooldridge, "Randomized telephone smoking-intervention trial initially directed at blue-collar workers," *Monogr. Natl. Cancer Instit,* 14 (1993): 105–112.
22. D.G. Altman, J.A. Flora, S.P. Fortmann, J.W. Farquhar, "The cost-effectiveness of three smoking cessation programs," *Am. J. Pub. Health,* 77 (1987): 162–165.
23. C.T. Orleans, N. Resch, E. Noll, M.K. Keintz, B.K. Rimer, et al., "Use of transdermal nicotine in a state-level prescription plan for the

elderly: A first look at 'real-world' patch users," *J. Amer. Med. Assoc.* 71 (1994): 601–607.

24. R.D. Hurt, L.C. Dale, P.A. Fredrickson, C.C. Caldwell, G.A. Lee, et al., "Nicotine patch therapy for smoking cessation combined with physician advice and nurse follow-up: One-year outcome and percentage of nicotine replacement," *J. Amer. Med. Assoc.* 271 (1994): 595–600.

25. S.L. Kenford, M.C. Fiore, D.E. Jorenby, S.S. Smith, D. Wteer, T.B. Baker, "Predicting smoking cessation: who will quit with and without the nicotine patch," *J. Amer. Med. Assoc.* 271 (1994): 589–594.

26. J.O. Prochaska, "Assessing how people change," *Cancer* 67 (1991): 805–807.

27. *Ibid.*

28. *Ibid.*

29. E.R. Gritz, C.R. Carr, D.A. Rapkin, C. Chang, J. Beumer, P.H. Ward. "A smoking cessation intervention for head and neck cancer patients: trial design, patient accrual, and characteristics," *Cancer Epidemiol. Biomarkers Prev.* 1 (1991): 67–73.

30. Prochaska, "Assessing how people change," 805–807.

31. E. Riboli, S. Preston-Martin, R. Saracci, N.J. Haley, D. Trichopoulos, et al., "Exposure of nonsmoking women to environmental tobacco smoke: a 10-country collaborative study," *Cancer Causes Control* 1 (1990): 243–252.

32. K.E. Warner, "The tobacco subsidy: does it matter?" *J. Natl. Cancer Instit.* 80 (1988): 81–83.

33. C.D. Sherman, K.C. Calman, S. Eckhardt, I. Elsebai, D. Firat, et al., "Prevention," in *Manual of Clinical Oncology* (New York: Springer-Verlag, 1987), 30–37.

34. C. La Vecchia, E. Negri, B. D'Avanzo, S. Franceschi, "Occupation and the risk of bladder cancer," *Int. J. Epidemiol.* 19 (1990): 264–268.

35. Henderson, "Toward the primary prevention of cancer," 1131–1138.

36. American Medical Assoc., Council on Scientific Affairs, "Asbestos removal, health hazards, and the EPA," *J. Amer. Med. Assoc.* 266 (1991): 696–697.

37. *Ibid.*

38. P.H. Abelson, "The asbestos removal fiasco," *Science* 247 (1990): 1017.

39. Editorial. "Common sense in the environment," *Nature* 353 (1991): 779–780.

40. *Ibid.*
41. American Medical Assoc., Council on Scientific Affairs, "Asbestos removal, health hasards, and the EPA," 696–697.
42. W.K. Reilly, "Asbestos removal," *Science* 248 (1990): 1063–1065.
43. Abelson, "The asbestos removal fiasco," 1017.
44. J. Flach, "NCI expert panel issues summary report on excise tax on cigarettes," *J. Natl. Cancer Instit.* 85 (1993): 1451–1452.
45. *Ibid.*
46. J.P. Pierce, L. Lee, E.A. Gilpin, "Smoking initiation by adolescent girls, 1944 through 1988. An association with targeted advertising," *J. Amer. Med. Assoc.* 271 (1994): 608–611.
47. R.M. Davis, "Current trends in cigarette advertising and marketing," *New. Engl. J. Med.* 316 (1987): 725–732.
48. S. Shiffman, B.R. Cassileth, B.L, Black, J. Buxbaum, D.D. Celentano, et al., "Needs and recommendations for behavior research in the prevention and early detection of cancer," *Cancer* 67 (1991): 800–804.
49. McGinnis, "Actual causes of death in the United States," 2270–2212.
50. C. Norman, "Bush budget highlights R&D," *Science* 247 (1990): 517–519.
51. A. Jacobs-Perkins, "President's budget request for NCI," *J. Natl. Cancer Instit.* 82 (1990): 351.
52. Norman, "Bush budget highlights R&D," *Science* 247 (1990): 517–519.
53. J.E. Ultmann, M. Donoghue, T.L. Lierman. "Government and cancer medicine," in *Cancer Medicine*, J.F. Holland, E. Frei III, R.C. Bast, D.W. Kufe, D.L. Morton, R.R. Weichselbaum, editors. (1992) 2481–2490.
54. J. Mervis, "R&D budget: growth in hard times," *Science* 263 (1994): 744–746.
55. R.G. Steen, *A conspiracy of cells: the basic science of cancer* (New York: Plenum Press, 1993), 427.
56. R. Hand, S. Sener, J. Imperato, J.S. Chmiel, J. Sylvester, A. Fremgen. "Hospital variables associated with quality of care for breast cancer patients," *J. Amer. Med. Assoc.* 266 (1991): 3429–3432.

14

CANCER SCREENING AND PUBLIC HEALTH POLICY

Cancer screening is the use of a medical tool or technique to examine a group of asymptomatic individuals for the presence of an undiagnosed cancer. Several cancer screening tests, such as Pap smears and mammograms, are currently applied broadly, as part of the national public health care program. But there are many more cancer screening tests which are available but are offered only to those who can afford them. One of the most most pressing and difficult issues in cancer medicine, which must be dealt with during implementation of a national health program, is whether or not these other screening tests should also be broadly available. While the ideal cancer screening test is inexpensive, easy to use, reliable, and accurate, no such screening test is available. Most tests are at least moderately expensive, difficult to use, and inaccurate, and there is often no good answer to the question of whether a particular screening test should be widely available. Only with a broad general dialogue, involving health care professionals, taxpayers, politicians, lawyers, and insurance companies, will these issues be resolved in a manner likely to actually benefit the health care consumer.

The American Cancer Society (ACS) has estimated that 100,000 people were likely to have been saved in 1992 had there been full implementation of all available screening tests.[1] According to the ACS, regular screening and self-examinations can detect cancers of the breast, tongue, mouth, colon, rectum, cervix, prostate, testis, and melanoma at an early stage, when treatment is likely to be successful. These sites account for nearly half of all new cancer cases, and about 67% of all newly diagnosed patients survive five years or more. However, with early detection, the ACS estimates that 89% of these people would survive for five years or more. This means that, of persons diagnosed with these cancers in 1992, about 100,000 additional people would have survived if their cancer had been detected early and treated aggressively. The actual cost of the cancer screening tests necessary would be about $4 billion.[2] Therefore, the cost of these screening tests per life saved would be about $40,000. Given the high cost of treating a dying cancer patient, this cost would seem to be low. However, this kind of cost/benefit decision must be made on an individual basis for each of the relevant cancer screening tests.

ROLE OF LARGE-SCALE SCREENING FOR CANCER IN THE GENERAL POPULATION

From a public health standpoint, it is very difficult to assess if a particular cancer screening effort is worthwhile, because several biases get in the way of an objective assessment of the worth of a particular screening test. These biases have confusing and even conflicting effects on cancer mortality, which are summarized below:[3]

1. Lead-time bias—if a cancer screening test is very effective, but treatment for the particular cancer is not effective, then a lethal cancer will simply be detected sooner. While this may give physicians more time to try different therapies, there is a chance that none of these therapies will be effective and overall cancer mortality will not be changed.
2. Length-time bias—if a cancer screening test is very effective, it can lead to detection of slow-growing less malignant tumors, so that treatment for the particular cancer is more effective. This can create a confusing picture, because it might appear that treatment for a particular cancer has improved, when in fact it is simply diagnosis that has improved.
3. Over-diagnosis bias—if a cancer screening test detects many tumors that are non-malignant and that would never be diagnosed otherwise, then it is, in effect, making a false-positive diagnosis of cancer. Again, this would make it appear that cancer treatment is more effective, although an untreated patient would not have died of the tumor anyway. This bias is a particular problem with prostate-specific antigen (PSA) detection of prostate cancer and, to a lesser extent, of mammographic detection of breast disease.
4. Selection bias—if a cancer screening test is thought to be effective, then it may not be possible to get an objective assessment of its utility. This is because the population of people who volunteer to be screened by the test during clinical trials is self-selected and often have good reasons for getting involved in a cancer screening effort. If a new screening test is applied to a

self-selected group with a higher-than-normal risk of cancer, then the new test may not be properly assessed. On the one hand, researchers might believe that the test is much more sensitive than it actually is, since it will detect many more cancers than expected in the test group. On the other hand, if overall mortality is measured as an endpoint, then researchers might believe that the test is ineffective in reducing overall cancer mortality.

In general, there is agreement that screening of certain high-risk individuals for certain cancers is worthwhile. However, disagreements tend to arise in determining whether a particular cancer screening test should be implemented for the general population. This is because the benefit is generally much lower or the test has a higher cost-to-benefit ratio when it is applied to persons at only moderate risk of cancer.

Clearly there is a role for large-scale cancer screening in the general population, because sometimes a relatively simple test can make an enormous difference in cancer mortality. For example, the Papanicolaou (or Pap) test, named for the physician who invented it, is a simple test for cervical cancer. This test relies upon microscopic examination of cells swabbed from the cervix and vagina to determine whether these cells show signs of cancerous transformation. The test is so sensitive that it can occasionally diagnose cancers of the ovary as well as the cervical cancers it was designed to detect, and it is a very accurate diagnostic tool for cervical cancer. An early study compared the Pap-smear history of 212 case patients with invasive cervical cancer and 1,060 age-matched controls free of disease.[4] In the five years preceeding the study, 56% of the controls had been screened by Pap smear, whereas only 32% of the cases had been screened. Overall, the relative risk of invasive cervical cancer was 2.7-fold higher in those women who were not screened. This difference in risk persisted even when the effects of age, income, education, marital history, smoking history, and access to medical care were factored in. Among women older than 60 years, the relative risk of invasive cervical cancer was 3.4-fold higher in women who were not screened in the preceeding five years.[5]

Another study examined the risk of cervical cancer as a function of time since the last Pap smear.[6] All cases of women in the northeast part of Scotland diagnosed with invasive cervical cancer during the years from 1968 to 1982 were identified. The screening history of each of these women was determined by consulting the records of the regional pathology laboratory; a total of 115 women were identified who had been screened at least once and who had subsequently been diagnosed with cervical cancer. These case patients were compared to a control group of 389 women who had also undergone at least one Pap test, but were free of cervical cancer. When the Pap screening histories of cases and controls were compared, 20% of the control women were found to have had a negative Pap test in the preceding two years, whereas less than 2% of the case women had undergone a recent test that gave negative results prior to the actual diagnosis. A negative Pap test in the preceding two years decreased the risk of a later positive Pap test nearly nine-fold. This is because, having obtained evidence that no cancer is present at the first test, the only way a cancer could be present at the second test is if it originated and grew rapidly or if the first test missed a cancer that was already present. Since the Pap test seems to be quite sensitive and since cervical cancers generally grow fairly slowly, a negative Pap test is a good indication that a woman will be free of cervical cancer for at least two years. In fact, a significantly reduced risk of cervical cancer was found up to three years after a Pap test, and a slight effect was observed for longer than that. If only deeply invasive cervical cancers are considered, then the Pap test is able to confer a protective effect that lasts up to 10 years. A negative test, even five years in the past, indicates that there has simply not been enough time to allow a cancer to become deeply invasive. Women who have had three or more negative Pap tests have a roughly five-fold lower lifetime risk of having invasive cervical cancer. In fact, the introduction of the Pap test to Scotland is thought to account for the roughly four-fold reduction in incidence of invasive cervical cancer that occurred between 1957 and 1981.[7]

Recent evidence has surfaced suggesting that the Pap test may cause overdiagnosis of cervical cancer in Sweden.[8] Thus, in some cases, cervical lesions may be diagnosed as precancerous or cancerous when, in fact, they are benign and would never have progressed in the absence of treatment. According to this study, the detection of an additional 100 precancerous lesions of the cervix will only lead to a reduction of one to five cases of invasive cervical cancer 10 years later. However, in Sweden, where this study was done, the incidence of invasive cervical cancer has fallen dramatically since the Pap test was introduced, and many lives are now saved that would otherwise have been lost.[9]

In the United States, the death rate from cervical cancer has declined by 70% over the last 40 years, almost solely as a result of the Pap test.[10] Now the majority of invasive cervical cancers occur in women who have not undergone a Pap test, and the most likely way to further reduce mortality from cervical cancer is to make the test available to more women. There is virtual unanimity that the Pap test has value as a screening test, and the major point of contention is in how often the test should be applied. From a public health perspective, annual screening has a 5% higher chance of diagnosing curable cancer than does screening every two to three years, but the cost is also two to three times higher. The National Cancer Institute (NCI) has recommended that three consecutive Pap tests be taken annually, which, if negative, can be followed by less frequent screening. Health care systems in England, Denmark, and Australia have opted to cover the cost of screening only once every three years. Probably screening every two years is sufficient for all women except those in known high-risk groups. Although the false negative rate of this test may be as high as 20% to 40%,[11] cervical cancers are somewhat indolent, and one missed diagnosis is probably not going to cause major additional mortality.

A recent study suggests that the Pap screening pattern of women is usually not based on a reasonable assessment of cervical cancer risk.[12] Research in the Netherlands has shown that the Pap smear detects 70% of all early stage cancerous conditions, that the rate of false positive test results is less than 1%, that roughly 60% of all early stage cancerous conditions regress spontaneously, and that the average length of time for an early stage cancerous condition to progress to an invasive cancer is about 15 years. These findings, together with information on population demographics, cervical cancer incidence, and cervical cancer survival, were used to mathematically determine the ideal Pap screening strategy. It was found that Pap screening should cover all women between the ages of 30 and at least 60 years, but that screening could occur at five-year intervals. With this approach, as many lives could be saved as are currently saved with the more arbitrary sort of testing intervals now used in the Netherlands. In addition, this type of coverage would cost half as much, and would reduce by 40% the number of unnecessary referrals and treatments for lesions that might have regressed anyway.[13] This sort of study badly needs to be done in each country, using data specific to that country, so that recommendations can be tailored to each populace. This study was especially instructive because it determined the years during which Pap smear screening should be used and because it identified those issues that need to be considered in developing a national screening policy for any cancer.

SCREENING FOR BREAST CANCER BY MAMMOGRAPHY

The benefits of mass screening for breast cancer by mammography are controversial, even though mammography is one of the most effective ways to detect early stage breast cancer.[14] The recommendations made for mammographic screening differ depending upon who is making them, and it is especially controversial whether women under age 40 should receive mammographic examinations at all. Most radiologists can read only 10 to 15 sets of mammographic films per day, spending between five and 30 minutes on each examination, before visual fatigue reduces efficiency. Careful analysis has shown that all but the most experienced radiologists will miss 20% to 25% of the potential signs of cancer. Even the most expert radiologists have a false negative rate of 10%. This means that, among women with breast cancer who had a recent mammogram, that mammogram will have been read as normal 10% of the time. The difficulty arises because breast tissue can be very dense in young women, so that virtually nothing can be seen, and because it is impossible to tell whether microcalcifications within the breast are benign or malignant by mammography alone. Nevertheless, screening by mammography appears to reduce breast cancer mortality by about 25%.[15] Although the mammogram is a flawed cancer screening test, the benefit is clear and there is really very little competition.

The sensitivity and specificity of mammography as a diagnostic tool was assessed by reviewing 2,266 cases of biopsy-proven breast disease in a single hospital.[16] Of these 2,266 cases, 69% were proven to be benign disease, while 31% were proven to be a malignancy. About 45% of the cancers could not be palpated and were first diagnosed by mammography; this ability to diagnose occult (inapparent) cancers has improved steadily. By 1986–1987, about 62% of the cancers diagnosed by mammography were clinically occult and could not be palpated. During the 15-year period from when mammography was first introduced at this hospital in 1974 until 1988, the average size of breast tumors at diagnosis decreased by about 65%, and there had been a five-fold increase in the frequency of diagnosing non-invasive cancers. The false-negative rate declined from 21% to 9% over the same period. This was partly the result of increased skill at reading mammograms, but major technical advances were also made during this time. In reviewing the entire 15-year period, mammography was found to give true-positive results 91% of the time, meaning that the test was sensitive to an existing cancer 91% of the time. The false-negative rate was only 9%, meaning that 9% of women who actually had breast cancer were falsely given a clean bill of health. In addition, 54% of women with benign breast disease were given a clean bill of health, meaning that the true-negative rate was 54%. The greatest problem with mammography was that the false-positive rate was 47%, meaning that 47% of women with benign breast disease were diagnosed as having a potentially malignant condition.[17] This is a very serious problem, because women who receive a false-positive diagnosis may forever be lost from the system in terms of future screening. A diagnosis of potential cancer is truly frightening, and a woman given a false-positive diagnosis of breast cancer may decide that it is better not to know than to be so frightened.

By contrast, the ability to detect breast cancer with a manual examination is considerably lower. As noted above, by 1987, a small community hospital was able to diagnose clinically occult cancers 62% of the time.[18] This means that mammography was able to detect cancers that could not be felt by a medical expert. Self-examination of the breasts is far less likely to detect breast cancer than an examination by a medical expert.[19] This is because breast self-examination is difficult to do properly, and the incentive to do it well may be lacking. The reward for doing an excellent job of breast self-examination is the identification of disease, while the reward for doing breast self-examination badly is a false sense of reassurance. Some studies have shown that women who attend a breast self-examination clinic are less likely to seek the immediate help of a physician if a lump is found than are women who have not attended such a clinic. Several studies suggest that breast self-examination leads to better overall breast cancer survival, but most studies have not confirmed this. A study with 18,242 participants was able to show that, by comparison with a medical expert, women were able to self-diagnose about 11% of all breast cancers. Nevertheless, 89% of women in this study reported that they intended to continue with breast self-examination. In the current context of empowerment of women, of responsibility for one's own health, and of health promotion in general, breast self-examination probably should not be ignored.[20] However, it is equally clear that breast self-examination should never be regarded as an adequate screening program for breast cancer.

The extent to which mammography is actually able to reduce cancer mortality has been estimated to be about 25%,[21] but this estimate is very contentious. A recent breast cancer screening trial in Sweden involved 282,777 women who were followed for an average of nine years.[22] Women were randomized, so that they were arbitrarily assigned to receive either a mammographic screening examination or no examination. In this huge group of women, there were a total of 843 deaths in which breast cancer was the "underlying cause of death," and another 882 deaths in which breast cancer was "present at death." Considering only those cases in which breast cancer was the "underlying cause of death," there was a 24% reduction in breast cancer mortality among those women who were screened by breast mammography. There was a 29% reduction in mortality in women who were between the ages of 50 and 69 at randomization, indicating that this age group benefits greatly from mammographic screening. Among women who were aged 40 to 49 at the beginning of the study, there was a slight reduction in breast cancer mortality, but the reduction was so small that it could have occurred by chance alone. Among women who were over the age of 69 at the beginning of the study, there was apparently no benefit from screening. No evidence suggested that mammographic screening itself was detrimental to any age group, and no breast cancers appeared to be induced by the radiation used in the screening test.[23]

These results are clearly in line with several other studies that show that women over age 50 benefit strongly from mammographic screening.[24] What is unusual about this study is that scientists were able to identify a slight protective effect of mammographic screening even in women under age 50. This protective effect did not become evident until nearly nine years into the study, and it did not become truly marked until 12 years into the study. Unfortunately, the study was unable to follow these younger women for any longer than 12 years, so it may be that the protective effect continued to increase with the passage of time. This would be a notable result, since it is a matter of great contention whether women under age 50 benefit significantly from mammographic screening.

The Canadian National Breast Cancer Screening Study is another recent study that followed a large group of women who were randomized to be screened either by annual mammography plus physical examination or annual physical examination only.[25,26] This study incorporated two separate study groups simultaneously: women between the ages of 40 and 49 and women between the ages of 50 and 59. A total of 50,430 women between the ages of 40 and 49 were enrolled in the study between 1980 and 1985, while another 39,405 women between the ages of 50 and 59 were enrolled during the same period. At enrollment, women were randomized to one of two screening groups, so that they were initially screened with mammography plus physical examination or with physical examination only, then the same screening test was performed annually for an average of 8.4 years. During the follow-up period, the number of breast cancers detected in each group was recorded, as well as the extent of disease at detection. Both groups of women displayed good adherence to the study guidelines, as more than 85% of the women in all groups were screened according to plan.

Among the younger women, a total of 265 breast cancers were detected over the course of the study, but just 23% of these cancers were detected in the group that received physical examination only.[27] This is not too surprising, since mammography should be more sensitive if it is a good screening test. What is quite surprising is that there were 29 deaths from breast cancer among women who were screened by mammography, while there were only 18 deaths from breast cancer among women who were screened by physical examination alone. That such a large discrepancy could exist in so large a group implies either that the mammograms may have actually induced breast cancer or that the women were not randomly allocated to each treatment group at the beginning of the experiment. Closer examination of the data shows that, at the time of enrollment in the study, 19 women were identified with advanced breast cancer in the mammography group, while only five women were identified with advanced breast cancer in the physical examination group.[28] Since advanced breast cancer, with involvement of four or more nodes at diagnosis, should be easily diagnosed by either type of screening, this implies that women were not randomly assigned to the two groups.[29] This calls into question the entire design of the study; in fact, the odds that this imbalance in assignment could arise by chance alone are 300 to one. While this does not prove that the study was biased deliberately, there is a bias nonetheless, which would tend to increase breast cancer mortality among the women receiving mammography.

The Canadian National Breast Cancer Screening Study was controversial from its inception, and several researchers who were initially involved actually withdrew from the study.[30] Another group of scientists has thoroughly evaluated the results of the Canadian study, and they have noted many serious flaws.[31] Most damaging is the apparent inappropriate assignment of women with breast cancer to the group scheduled to receive mammographic screening. In addition, the quality of mammographic images used in this study did not represent the state-of-the-art at the time and is much inferior to the image quality that is routinely available today. Mammography has advanced so rapidly that there were marked progressive improvements between 1985 and 1992. But most of the hospitals involved in this study used mammographic equipment that was purchased in 1980, and there was some delay in incorporating new technologic developments into the on-going study.

The Canadian National Breast Cancer Screening Study was designed to detect whether mammographic screening resulted in a substantial (40%) reduction in breast cancer mortality.[32] If mammography actually reduced the chances of dying from breast cancer by only 30%, the Canadian study could not have detected this difference in mortality, even if the expected number of deaths had occurred in the study group. Yet many fewer breast cancers were diagnosed than were expected, so the statistical power of the study was further reduced. Thus, a 30–40% reduction in breast cancer mortality from mammographic screening would have gone undetected by the Canadian study. In fact, the data shown in the Canadian study are compatible with a reduction in breast cancer mortality as large as 16% from mammographic screening. In short, the study was just too small, too flawed, and too short to determine whether mammographic screening is worthwhile. Perhaps longer follow-up of the same group of women will permit stronger conclusions to be made, but this is unclear.[33] It is worth noting that the Swedish study found that the benefits of mammography in women under age 50 did not become apparent until nearly nine years into the study, and did not become marked until 12 years into the study.[34]

The physical examination given women in the Canadian National Breast Cancer Screening Study may not be comparable to the normal physical examination given women outside the study.[35] This is because physicians involved in the study received special instruction in physical examination of the breasts. Thus, they may have been able to detect breast tumors that would escape notice by an untrained physician. This study may in fact be an important confirmation of the benefit to be obtained by careful physical examination of the breasts.

Recently, the National Cancer Institute convened an International Workshop on Screening for Breast Cancer to examine all available data on the benefits of screening mammography, with particular attention paid to benefits for women between the ages of 40 and 49.[36] A meta-analysis, or analysis of pooled data from eight separate studies, was conducted, with a combined number of subjects of nearly a half million women. Study subjects were 257,451 women who received regular mammographic examinations, and these women were compared with 224,299 control women of similar age who did not receive mammograms. About 83% of all the study women received mammograms at enrollment, so that incident cases of breast cancer could be identified before the studies began. Unfortunately, as always, it was difficult to specifically evaluate the benefits of mammography in the subgroup of women between 40 and 49 years of age. For women between the ages of 50 and 69, screening by mammography led to a reduction in breast cancer mortality of about 30% that became evident 10 to 12 years after enrollment in the study. For women between the ages of 40 and 49, no significant reduction in breast cancer mortality was seen among women screened by mammography, even 10 to 12 years after enrollment in the study. If all eight studies are averaged together, they showed less than a 10% reduction in breast cancer mortality among women aged 40 to 49 who were screened by mammography, and this reduction might have been illusory.[37]

However, contrary results were obtained by another study that specifically examined the benefits of mammographic screening to women less than 50 years of age.[38] This study identified 117 women under the age of 50 who were diagnosed with breast cancer on the basis of an abnormal mammogram alone. These women were compared with 928 control women who were diagnosed with breast cancer on the basis of a standard physical examination. Carcinoma *in situ*, an early-stage cancer with a favorable prognosis, was identified in 40% of the women who had received mammograms, but this early stage of disease was found in only 9% of women with palpable tumors. Therefore, mammography seemed to increase the likelihood of detecting treatable breast cancer even in younger women. Considering only invasive breast tumors, mammography alone was able to identify these tumors when 50% of them were still Stage I, while only 30% of the palpable tumors were Stage I. Five-year survival for all patients with breast tumors identified by mammography was 95%, whereas for women with palpable tumors the five-year survival was only 74%. This convincing study strongly suggests that women under age 50 who receive regular mammograms are more likely to survive breast cancer than women who receive only physical examination of the breasts.[39]

A recent study has found that the predictive value of screening mammography varies among women, depending upon their age and family history of breast cancer.[40] Positive predictive value is defined as the proportion of women with an abnormal mammogram who were later diagnosed as having breast cancer. If mammography is indeed a good screening test, then it should have a high positive predictive value, which translates into a low rate of false alarms. A total of 31,814 women aged 30 years or older were screened by a mobile mammography unit in the San Francisco area between 1985 and 1992. Those women who had an abnormal mammogram were followed over time to determine the outcome of the initial screening. Although women aged 50 years or older represented only 38% of all the women screened, 74% of all breast cancers were detected in this group. Among women aged 50 or more, 14.8 examinations were required to diagnose one cancer, while 48.3 examinations were required to diagnose one cancer among women less than 50 years old. The positive predictive value of mammographic screening increased progressively with age: it was 3% for women aged 30 to 39 years; 4% for women aged 40 to 49; 9% for women aged 50 to 59; 17% for women aged 60 to 69; and 19% for women aged 70 years old or older. Women over age 50 were more than seven-fold more likely to be diagnosed with invasive breast cancer than women under age 50. Furthermore, the positive predictive value was higher for women with a family history of breast cancer: it was 13% for women aged 40 to 49 with a family history of disease; and 22% for women aged 50 to 59 with a family history of disease. Thus, the largest positive predictive values for mammography were found among women aged 50 or older, or among women aged 40 or older with a family history of breast cancer. Thus, these two groups benefit most from mammographic screening and should be favored if screening availability is limited.[41]

Another recent study examined the effectiveness of breast cancer screening in different age groups of women in the Netherlands.[42] This could be a particularly informative study since the incidence of breast cancer in the Netherlands is perhaps the highest in the world. A total of 135,499 women were screened, of which 47,469 women were under 50 years old at screening. Some of these women have been followed for up to 15 years, although new study participants were added every two years. The proportion of women who agreed to participate in the study was quite high—75% of those women under age 50 who were invited to participate actually did attend a screening examination, while the attendance rate for women aged 50 to 69 years was 65%. For women younger than 50, mammographic screening detected 37% of all breast cancers, while in women aged 50 to 69, screening detected 48% of all breast cancers. In general, mammographic screening was able to detect smaller cancers than were detected by clinical examination; among women less than 50 years old, 89% of the cancers detected by mammography were 2 centimeters or less in diameter, while only 58% of the cancers detected by clinical examination were this size. However, in women under age 50, use of mammography did not lead to detection of more cancers before they spread to regional lymph nodes. Thus, in younger women, mammography did not catch cancers signficantly sooner than they would have been caught by clinical examination. Yet, in women older than 50, use of mammographic screening did lead to a substantial increase in diagnosis of early stage cancer. This shows that detecting early stage breast cancer in younger women is more difficult than in older women.[43]

Technical problems abound in any mammographic examination, and a reasoned consideration of mammography as a screening test must consider how these problems affect test utility. In general, the denseness of breast tissue can limit the utility of a mammographic examination.[44] It is very difficult to see a small, noncalcified tumor mass in women who have dense breast tissue. Older women tend to have breasts with more fatty tissue, but many older women still have dense breasts and some younger women have fatty breasts. About 80% of women have a dense breast pattern at age 30, while at age 40 about 70% of women, and at age 50 about 60% of women have dense breast tissue. By age 80, only 40% of women have dense breast tissue. Since mammography is much more effective in the fatty breast, this may help to explain why mammographic screening shows less benefit in younger women. The problem of breast denseness can be compensated for by using compression of the breast during filming, or by using longer film exposures. In addition, technical advances are on the horizon that may help in diagnosis of cancer in the dense breast.[45]

In addition to technical problems with mammographic examinations of women under age 50, social and ethical problems are associated with mammography in the younger woman. While the risk from radiation exposure during mammography is vanishingly small to all but a few,[46] there is a very real risk associated with incorrect results from a mammographic examination.[47] False-positive results, which are more common in younger women, can lead to further X-ray exposures, unnecessary biopsies, and possibly even unrequired surgery. False-negative results, which are also more common in younger women, can produce an unjustified sense of security that might cause a woman to ignore symptoms that would otherwise send her to a physician.[48] Since the prevalence of breast cancer is so much lower in young women, and the test is so much less sensitive in these women, the percentage of false interpretations is bound to be higher. With all these factors to consider, it is no wonder there is little consensus as to the appropriate age at which to begin mammographic screening.[49]

Nevertheless, recommendations for the frequency of mammographic examination must be made, since many women have been disturbed by the seeming lack of consensus among experts. Basically, there is unanimity that women over the age of 50 should be screened for breast cancer by mammography on a regular basis. The National Cancer Institute has recommended yearly mammographic exams for women over 50, together with yearly clinical breast examinations and monthly self-examinations.[50] The American Cancer Society, the American Academy of Family Practice, and the American College of Radiology all concur with these recommendations, while the U. S. Preventive Services Task Force recommends screening every one to two years. However, on the basis of a very recent review of data, the National Cancer Institute has indicated that screening every two years may be adequate for women over the age of 50. For women under the age of 50, the situation is even less clear. The National Cancer Institute recommends that each woman discuss the possible choices with her physician, and further recommends that family history play a role in the decision. The American Cancer Society and the American College of Radiology recommend screening every one to two years for women between the ages of 40 and 49, and the American Academy of Family Practice makes no specific recommendations for women under the age of 50.

Considering the way the positive predictive value of the mammographic examination varies with age,[51] we recommend that all women over the age of 50 receive yearly screening examinations, combined with yearly clinical breast examinations and monthly self-examinations. It seems premature to back away from recommending yearly mammograms for women over 50, given a false negative rate of nearly 10% in mammographic examinations.[52]

Women should receive a baseline mammogram at about the age of 40, at which point a lengthy discussion with a physician is appropriate. The technology involved in the mammographic examination is changing very rapidly, but not all hospitals have access to state-of-the-art equipment, so the image quality obtainable at the local mammographic center is critical. If there is a family history of breast cancer, or if the breasts are composed of fatty tissue permitting good quality mammograms, or if menopause occurs soon after age 40, then mammographic screening every one to two years until the age of 50 is appropriate. If there is no family history of breast cancer, if the breasts are composed of dense tissue that reduces mammographic image quality, and if menopause has not yet been reached, then a repeat examination at age 45 is probably more appropriate. Little or no benefit seems to accrue from mammographic examination of women under the age of 40, unless there is a very strong family history of breast cancer. Women over the age of 70 are similarly unlikely to benefit from screening, unless possible symptoms of disease are present. In general, women of any age with symptoms of breast cancer should obtain a mammographic examination as soon as possible.

These recommendations are consistent with studies that show relatively little benefit from breast mammography in women less than 50 years old,[53] and virtually no benefit in women less than 40 years old.[54] Our recommendations are also made in light of an analysis that strongly dissented with the conclusion that women under age 50 achieve no benefit from mammography.[55] This analysis correctly notes that there is very little ability to statistically determine the benefits of mammography for younger women, since only one study has ever been designed for this purpose. However, our recommendations were also strongly influenced by the study of differing disease outcome in women under 50, diagnosed either by mammography or by clinical examination.[56] Perhaps the best suggestion is that, before national policy is decided, another clinical trial of mammography for women under age 50 should be performed, and this trial should compute benefit by both age and menopausal status.[57]

Implementation of a mammographic screening program has several inherent difficulties. Surveys often reveal that compliance with current recommendations for breast mammography is quite poor.[58] As of 1992, at least 25% of women over the age of 50 had never had a mammogram. Although the prevalence of mammography increased between 1987 and 1991, 41% to 65% of white women aged 65 to 74 had not had a mammographic examination in the preceding year. The number of women who receive an annual clinical breast examination is actually declining. Although mammography utilization is increasing, change is slow and mass education has been difficult to achieve.[59] Community-based educational programs can be effective in increasing general awareness about the importance of mammography, but one three-year long program to increase mammography utilization still could only induce 55% of women to be screened. A pilot program in Australia found that recruiting women for a free mammographic examination was most cost-effective if a personal invitation letter was sent to each woman, but this strategy still only succeeded in recruiting 36% of the target women.[60] The best recruitment strategy, which cost nearly twice as much per woman to implement, was only able to recruit 44% of the target women. Another study that evaluated why women did not use a free mammography service found that 52% of women reported being too busy to attend,[61] while fully 29% of women were afraid of the radiation exposure involved.

The economics of large-scale mammographic screening have also been evaluated, and cost can be truly daunting. An early study concluded that annual screening for breast cancer by physical examination alone, in women over age 50, would cost $10,000 to $15,000 per year of life saved. This cost would increase to $20,000 to $90,000 per year of life saved if mammography was also performed. If 25% of the women in the United States between the ages of 40 and 75 were screened annually for 10 years by both mammography and physical examination, about 4,000 lives would be saved at a cost of approximately $1.3 billion, or $325,000 per life.[62] However, a more recent estimate projects considerably lower costs because of technical improvements.[63] The total cost per year of life saved is now estimated to be about $21,000 for women under 50, and about $2,500 for women over 50, which averages out to about $4,700 per year of life saved overall. This cost is roughly comparable to the cost per year of life saved for medical treatments such as coronary bypass surgery, bone marrow transplant, hypertension therapy, and kidney transplants, whose cost ranges from roughly $11,000 to $26,000 per year of life saved.[64] However, the economic value of a human life is a decision that must be reached by society as a whole.

CURRENT CANCER SCREENING EFFORTS IN THE UNITED STATES

Current cancer screening efforts in the United States tend to occur in a piecemeal fashion, given that there is no national health plan, no nationwide cancer registry, little or no consensus on which cancer screening efforts are appropriate, and seemingly little or no impetus to improve the situation. However, we all benefit from the efforts of those scientists who have ignored such difficulties to proceed with a rational analysis of available screening efforts.

Colorectal cancer is one of the leading cancer killers, and this cancer occurs disproportionately in the lowermost, or distal, portion of the bowel. Consequently, efforts have been made to screen for cancers of the distal bowel using an optical device called a colonoscope (or sigmoidoscope), which is inserted through the anus into the sigmoid colon. This test has never achieved much popularity because it is uncomfortable, relatively costly, and of unproven efficacy in reducing mortality from colorectal cancer.[65] A randomized trial of colonoscopy would require a large number of subjects, or a long time, or both, to detect a benefit, because mortality from this cancer can occur many years after the initial diagnosis. Therefore, in one study, a case-control approach was taken, in which case patients were paired retrospectively with control individuals to analyze the efficacy of colonoscopy.

Medical records were obtained from a California hospital for a group of 261 patients, all of whom had died of cancer of the distal bowel between 1971 and 1988.[66] These case patients were compared to a group of 868 healthy control subjects matched for age and sex. The use of screening by colonoscope was compared for cases and controls during the 10 years preceeding the diagnosis of cancer. It was found that only 9% of the case patients had ever undergone a colonoscopic examination, whereas 24% of the controls had submitted to this test. Examination by a colonoscope was associated with a 59% reduction in the chance of dying from a distal colorectal cancer. The protective effect of a colonoscopic examination was strong even when the colonoscopic examination had occurred eight to 10 years in the past. In fact, the average length of time between a colonoscopic "clean bill of health" and the development of a colon cancer was at least 10 years, on average. The success of colonoscopy in protecting specifically from distal colorectal cancer suggests that this screening test is very effective. Colonoscopy can thus reduce mortality from cancer of the distal colon, and screening once every 10 years may be nearly as effective as more frequent screening.[67] Yet, despite its effectiveness, this test will probably never achieve a great deal of popularity, so it is worthwhile to continue to search for other effective screening tests for this cancer. Given that the vast majority of people are screened by this technique no more than once, and given that the protective effect from screening may last up to 10 years, a balance of prudence and practicality would suggest that the first screening colonoscopic examination should occur at about age 50.

The fecal occult blood test is another approach to reducing mortality from colorectal cancer.[68] The test involves smearing small stool samples from three consecutive bowel movements onto a test card, which is then mailed in to a laboratory or physician. The stool samples are analyzed to detect occult or inapparent blood in the stool. The test costs only about

$20 to $40 to administer, in contrast with a colonoscopic examination, which often costs $700 to $900 to administer. While the fecal occult blood test is somewhat unpleasant to perform on oneself, most people prefer it to a colonoscopic examination. Therefore, if the efficacy of the test is comparable to a colonoscopic examination, the fecal occult blood test would be a very good cancer screening test.

To assess the efficacy of the fecal occult blood test, a total of 46,551 subjects aged 50 to 80 years were randomized to be screened every year, every two years, or not at all.[69] Subjects were followed prospectively for 13 years, to determine colorectal cancer mortality in each group. The cumulative mortality from colorectal cancer was 33% lower than normal among those people screened yearly, but only 6% lower among those screened every two years. Furthermore, among those diagnosed with colorectal cancer, survival was better for those who were screened annually, since cancers were diagnosed when they were less invasive. Biennial screening was not appreciably better than no screening at all, in terms of reducing mortality from colorectal cancer.

The major drawback of the fecal occult blood test is that test sensitivity is low if the test is not properly done, and the positive predictive value of the test is very low anyway.[70] The way the test is usually done (without rehydration of the stool samples), test sensitivity is 81%, meaning that 81% of the colorectal cancers present can be diagnosed. But, if the test is performed with a rehydration step in the analysis, sensitivity increases to 92%, which is comparable to most other medical tests. However, the positive predictive value of the test is only 2.2%, meaning that only about 2% of those who have an abnormal test result actually have colorectal cancer. False-positive results can be produced by a diet rich in meat, vitamin C, or aspirin-like drugs, and false-positive results are frequently obtained in those who have bleeding hemorrhoids. Nearly 10% of all persons screened have a positive test result for one reason or another, and the cost of follow-up for those with a positive result is high, since each must receive a screening colonoscopic examination. Nearly 98% of those with a positive test result were found to be clear of cancer after an expensive colonoscopic examination. Over the course of the study, 38% of those who were screened annually by the fecal occult blood test had to be further examined by a colonoscope.[71] There is, of course, a possibility that if 38% of a large group of people randomly received a colonoscopic examination, then colon cancer mortality would be reduced 33%, as in this study, but we really don't know.

The utility of the fecal occult blood test as a way to screen for colorectal cancer has now been confirmed.[72] The mortality rate of a group of persons offered colonoscopic screening alone was compared with the mortality rate of a group screened by both colonoscopy and fecal occult blood testing. A total of 21,756 people over the age of 40 were randomized to receive one of the two screening procedures, then these volunteers were followed for up to nine years. Mortality from colorectal cancer was about 43% lower in the group that was screened by fecal occult blood testing. Thus, a combination of colonoscopy and fecal occult blood testing is more effective at diagnosing early stage colorectal cancer than is colonoscopy alone.

While some data suggest that fecal occult blood testing is simply too insensitive to provide a useful marker for colorectal cancer,[73] one of the primary objections to this type of screening is that the final cost may be prohibitively high.[74] A study done in England compared the cost of treating colorectal cancer patients diagnosed as a result of fecal occult blood testing with the cost of treating patients diagnosed on the basis of symptoms. This comparison is of interest because it has been argued that early detection of colorectal cancer will not only save lives but will also increase the chances that low-cost endoscopic surgery (polypectomy) can be used instead of high-cost traditional surgery. In fact, the U. S. Office of Technology Assessment has estimated that treatment of early stage colorectal cancer costs about one-third less than treating late stage disease. But when the costs of screening, initial treatment, and treatment for disease recurrence are considered together, it turns out that fecal occult blood test screening leads to a savings of only 12% per patient in total cost.[75] However, this type of analysis fails to consider the emotional and financial cost of lives lost that could have been saved by screening. Although fecal occult blood testing is probably unlikely to provide substantial economies in the cost of treating colorectal cancer, this type of screening is nevertheless wholeheartedly endorsed on a humanitarian basis.

Prostate cancer is another major killer for which several screening tests exist. Although a great deal of interest has been generated by the prostate-specific antigen (PSA) test, there is an earlier, simpler test for prostate cancer known as the digital rectal examination. The digital rectal examination (DRE) simply involves insertion by the physician of a gloved finger into the rectum, so that the prostate gland can be palpated. Although the DRE is commonly thought to be an effective method of screening for prostatic cancer, this examination was never rigorously evaluated until recently.[76] To determine if the DRE is capable of preventing advanced prostate cancer, a group of 139 case patients with advanced, metastatic (stage D) prostatic cancer was compared with an equal number of matched control men free of disease. The number of DREs received by both cases and controls was determined from an evaluation of medical records going back an average of 23 years before the diagnosis of cancer. This extensive review of records was only possible because both cases and controls were members of a large health maintenance organization in northern California. In the 10 years preceding initial diagnosis, both cases and controls had the same average number of DREs, either for routine screening or to evaluate specific intestinal or rectal symptoms. The relative risk of metastatic prostatic cancer was not significantly lower among men who had received one or more screening DREs, as compared with men who had received none. Thus, prostate cancer screening by DRE appears to offer little if any benefit, in terms of preventing advanced prostatic cancer.[79] This is a very controversial finding, given that current recommendations by the National Cancer Institute include an annual DRE for every male over the age of 40, and it is not yet clear how to resolve the issue of which tests should be recommended.

Recent indications show that screening for prostate cancer using the prostate-specific antigen (PSA) test may be superior to the DRE.[78] To determine whether the PSA test could diagnose early-stage (treatable) prostate cancer, a prospective study was done in which 10,251 men aged 50 or older were enrolled and PSA levels were measured repeatedly for three years. Medical outcomes for these men were compared with medical outcomes in a small control group of 266 men who had symptoms of prostate cancer detected by DRE. Elevated levels of PSA were detected in about 9% of the large group of screened men. Prostate cancer was diagnosed in only about 42% of those men with elevated PSA levels, indicating that the PSA test has a moderately high rate of false-positives. However, there was a very significant difference in medical outcomes between those men diagnosed by PSA and those men diagnosed by DRE. Among those men diagnosed with prostate cancer by DRE, 57% were suffering from advanced disease, whereas only 29% of the men diagnosed with prostate cancer by serial PSA had advanced disease. The earlier diagnosis possible with serial PSA measurements was particularly important in men under age 70, as only 24% of these men had advanced disease when diagnosed with the PSA test. The generally recommended therapy for men under age 70 with early stage disease is surgery, and surgery provides surgical biopsy specimens for evaluation by a pathologist. When the extent of disease was evaluated by a pathologist, men who had been serially screened by PSA were found to be more than three times as likely to have nonmetastatic (organ-confined) disease as were men who had been diagnosed by DRE. This evidence strongly suggests that PSA screening can identify men with early stage prostate cancer who are likely to have a good response to surgery and a favorable long-term prognosis after surgery.[79]

Long-term serial evaluation of PSA levels is more likely to detect prostate cancer than is a one-time evaluation, since very early stage prostate cancer may be heralded by a small increase in PSA that would not be evident except by comparison with prior PSA values from the same person.[80] This conclusion is supported by the study described above, which found that serial PSA measurements are more than twice as likely to diagnose organ-confined prostate cancer as are one-time measurements of PSA level.[81] This argues strongly that PSA screening should be performed on a yearly basis, so that good baseline data can be developed for each man. On the other hand, prostate cancer is such a rare disease in men under age 60 that yearly screening of substantially younger men is unlikely to provide a significant benefit. A cancer registry that included seven million person-years of data has calculated that only 5% of all prostate cancer cases are diagnosed in men under age 60, while 15% are diagnosed in men under age 65.[82]

It has been argued that prostate cancer is normally such a slow-growing tumor that men are more likely to die with it than of it, and that the best treatment for prostate cancer may be no treatment, in some cases.[83] Nevertheless, this disease can behave very aggressively in some men, and most men, especially those under age 70, would be foolish to forgo treatment. While PSA screening has not been definitely proven to lead to a significant reduction in prostate cancer mortality, it has been endorsed by the American Cancer Society and the American Urological Society, and consensus seems to be emerging that the test is worthwhile.[84] We recommend a baseline series of PSA examinations for every man at about age 40, and an annual PSA test for every man over the age of 50. Use of the DRE test, which cannot be as fully endorsed, should be discussed with a physician.

Another cancer screening test that has established itself in certain parts of the country is a test for carcinoembroyonic antigen (CEA) in the bloodstream, which is used in follow-up monitoring of patients treated for colon cancer.[85] This test is too insensitive to be used as a mass screening test for colon cancer, but about 20% of those patients who undergo surgery for colon cancer develop recurrent disease. Even a test of low sensitivity that is able to predict some of these recurrences could reduce colon cancer mortality by as much as 5%. Therefore a study was undertaken to determine the effectiveness of CEA in monitoring for recurrence of surgically treatable colon cancer. A total of 1,017 patients with surgically resected colon cancer were monitored by CEA, and these patients were compared with a group of 199 patients with resected colon cancer who were not monitored by the CEA test. It was found that 59% of those patients with recurrent colon cancer had a preceeding elevation of CEA above 5 nannograms per milliliter, meaning that test sensitivity was 59%. But about 16% of patients without recurrence showed elevation of

CEA above 5 ng/mL, so the rate of false-positives was fairly high. If a CEA level of 10 ng/mL was accepted as being positive, then sensitivity of the test fell to 45%, but the rate of false-positives declined to only 4%. Elevation of CEA was best at predicting disease recurrence in the liver, which is one of the most common sites of recurrence for colon cancer. The CEA test was by far the cheapest of the available tests used to monitor for disease recurrence in these patients; the CEA test costs $55, while a physician evaluation costs $120, a magnetic resonance imaging (MRI) exam costs $300, and endoscopy costs $500. Since these patients will almost certainly be monitored for recurrence by some method, the CEA test seems preferable to any of the alternatives. However it is not clear that this monitoring actually produces a benefit in terms of disease survival, since the one-year disease-free survival rate was virtually identical in the group that was screened by the CEA test and the group that was unscreened.[86] This study does not provide convincing evidence that the CEA test actually saves lives among patients treated for colon cancer, but it does suggest that CEA should perhaps be re-evaluated as a mass screening test. A test sensitivity of 45% (for CEA > 10 ng/mL) is not inspiring, but colon cancer is a major killer and is far more curable if caught early.

Prior to 1980, the American Cancer Society recommended an annual chest X-ray as a screen for lung cancer among certain high-risk individuals, including smokers.[87] A study was initiated in which men over age 45, all of whom smoked at least a pack of cigarettes per day, were screened for lung cancer by X-ray.[88] In a group of 10,933 men, a total of 91 lung cancers were identified, showing that the prevalence of lung cancer among asymptomatic smokers is slightly less than 1%. The remaining men, who were judged healthy by the screening X-ray examination, were randomized into two study groups. The control group of men received the recommended yearly chest X-ray, together with a sputum test that was used to reveal abnormal cells in saliva. The experimental group of men received the same two screening tests, but the time interval between tests was reduced to only four months. Both these groups of men were followed for a total of six years. Frequent screening was found to lead to an increase in the proportion of men diagnosed with early stage lung cancer: 50% of the men receiving frequent screening tests were diagnosed with Stage I cancer, whereas only 33% of the men receiving annual screening tests were diagnosed with Stage I cancer. However, at the end of a seven-year follow-up period, there was no significant difference in mortality from lung cancer. This is because lung cancer responds very poorly to therapy, no matter at what stage it is diagnosed. Thus there is essentially no point to obtaining an early diagnosis since the outcome is the same anyway. If detection of early stage cancer was perfect, while the probability of cure remained the same, lung cancer mortality would be reduced by a maximum of 32%. Alternatively, if lung cancer detection was unchanged but treatment of early stage cancer was always effective, mortality would be reduced by no more than 37%. Therefore both detection and treatment must improve before lung cancer mortality can be significantly reduced.[89]

In spite of the ineffectiveness of chest X-rays as a screening test for lung cancer, 40% of physicians still recommend them for asymptomatic individuals over age 40.[90] Even the most favorable evaluation of lung cancer screening by chest X-ray estimates that an active screening program would reduce lung cancer mortality by about 10% annually, or about 14,000 lives per year. It has been estimated that lung cancer screening by chest X-ray is a $1.5 billion per year industry, which means that, even by the most favorable analysis, we are spending roughly $107,000 per life saved. A less sanguine analysis would note that long-term survival of lung cancer patients is very poor even among patients diagnosed with early stage cancer. Thus the cost per life saved is probably considerably higher than indicated, since lung cancer screening by chest X-ray may be useless. Since lung cancer is largely preventable by smoking cessation, this level of expenditure cannot be justified; in fact, money would be much better spent on programs to induce smoking cessation.

POSSIBLE FUTURE SCREENING EFFORTS IN THE UNITED STATES

Ovarian cancer is a very serious medical problem because, while fairly uncommon, it has a high mortality rate, making it the leading cause of death among the gynecologic cancers. Ovarian cancer is also very insidious, in that early stage treatable cancers often have no notable symptoms at all. Consequently, there is a strong impetus to develop a screening test that would be capable of identifying this cancer in asymptomatic women. A good deal of excitement has surrounded a blood test for ovarian cancer that relies upon detection of a blood protein known as serum CA-125.[91] This test is already being offered, in some parts of the United States, to women with a family history of ovarian cancer, even though there are little data on test efficacy.

About 80% of women with ovarian cancer have the serum CA-125 marker protein present in their bloodstream, and CA-125 is elevated in about 50% of women with early stage ovarian cancer.[92] Unfortunately, CA-125 is also elevated in various other conditions, including cancers of the lung, breast, gastrointestinal tract, and of the blood itself, and the test seems to give spontaneously high readings in nearly 1% of the cancer-free population. It has been proposed that serial evaluation of CA-125 may improve the specificity of the examination, much as serial examination of PSA is used to increase test specificity for prostate cancer. In addition, use of multiple markers has been proposed as a way to reduce the false-positive rate; a combination of CA-125, CA72, and CA15-3 may succeed in increasing test specificity for ovarian cancer.

A recent study evaluated the CA-125 test for ovarian cancer in a large population of women.[93] A total of 11,009 women over the age of 18 donated a blood sample during a large blood collection campaign in Washington County, Maryland, in 1974. During the 15-year period between 1974 and 1989, 37 of these women developed ovarian cancer. Frozen blood samples from these case women were compared to frozen blood samples from a control group of 73 healthy women selected from among the same original study participants. Cases and controls were matched on the basis of age, race, menopausal status, time since last menstrual period (at the time of blood donation), and time of day blood was collected. Serum levels of CA-125 were then measured in cases and controls, and a questionnaire answered at the time of blood collection was used to determine exposure to known risk factors for ovarian cancer. It was found that women who developed ovarian cancer within three years of serum collection had a serum level of CA-125 that was nearly four-fold higher than normal. Normal levels of CA-125 averaged less than 10 Units per milliliter (U/mL) of blood, but women who developed ovarian cancer within 12 years of screening had an average level of CA-125 higher than 12 U/mL of blood. Generally, the higher the level of CA-125, the greater the risk of ovarian cancer; levels of CA-125 higher than 10 U/mL were associated with a three-fold increase in cancer risk, but levels higher than 20 U/mL were associated with a near six-fold increase in risk. If a reference value of 35 U/mL is accepted as indicative of ovarian cancer, the sensitivity and specificity of the CA-125 test can be calculated. Considering only those cancers diagnosed within three years of blood collection, the sensitivity of the test was 57%, a level that is low by comparison to most other accepted cancer screening tests. This means that only slightly more than half of the ovarian cancers present among the case group were heralded by CA-125 levels that exceeded 35 U/mL. On the other had, none of the control subjects had CA-125 levels over 35 U/mL, so the specificity of the test is 100% (meaning that CA-125 levels were associated with ovarian cancer 100% of the time in this study). Sensitivity decreased rather sharply with increasing time to diagnosis, but specificity was higher than 95% even 15 years before the diagnosis. These results indicate that the CA-125 test is probably not sufficiently sensitive to be used alone as a screening test for ovarian cancer, particularly if a reference value of 35 U/mL is used. If a lower reference value is used, this will increase test sensitivity at the cost of generating many more false-positive test results and much more anxiety among those women who test positive.[94]

Thus an ideal test for ovarian cancer is clearly not yet available, although the CA-125 test is probably now preferable to most alternatives. The average cost of screening for ovarian cancer by the CA-125 test is about $50 per test, whereas the average cost of an ultrasound evaluation of the pelvis is about $300.[95] Since more than 43 million women are now over the age of 45 in the United States, it would cost nearly $11 billion dollars less to screen these women by the CA-125 test than by ultrasound. Given the cost of the CA-125 screening test and its relatively low sensitivity, the American College of Obstetrics and Gynecology has not endorsed routine screening by the CA-125 test, although it is probably appropriate for high-risk individuals or those with a family history of disease. On the other hand, we believe it is appropriate to consider application of the test every three-to-five years in women over the age of 45. While it is not clear that early diagnosis of ovarian cancer can significantly reduce the death rate from this cancer, the cost of the CA-125 test will probably decline to the point where routine screening would be hard to criticize in future.

Screening programs for liver cancer have been active for more than 20 years in some parts of the Orient, where liver cancer is the leading cause of cancer death. Large numbers of individuals have been screened to identify asymptomatic patients because surgical success and long-term prognosis is far better for small tumors. Because a large number of screened patients have been followed for a long period in China and Japan, some insight has been gained into the natural history of the disease. The best marker for primary liver cancer is an increase in blood levels of a protein called alpha-fetoprotein (AFP), which is present in 70–90% of all liver cancer patients. However, this protein is also present in patients with hepatitis, cirrhosis, bile duct obstruction, and alcoholic liver disease, so it is of somewhat limited utility in screening for liver cancer.[96] The interval between the first detectable rise in blood levels of AFP and the first appearance of cancer symptoms is about 14 months, at which point the tumor volume has grown five-fold.[97] After diagnosis, growth of the tumor is relentless and rapid, and death usually occurs within four months. Thus, by the time patients seek the care of a physician, the tumor is far advanced and the patient can deteriorate rapidly. The success of screening programs in Japan may indicate that such programs should be emulated in the United States, at least among certain high-risk populations.

Neuroblastoma is the most common solid tumor of young children, and screening of infants in Japan has shown that this cancer can be detected by a simple test for trace chemicals in the urine.[98] A mass screening test for neuroblastoma has been implemented in Japan, where disease incidence is comparable to the United States (roughly one case in 7,000 live births). A total of 282,000 children were screened, and less than 4% of these children had a positive initial test for neuroblastoma. Upon repeat screening, 264 infants were identified who had three consecutive positive tests. Among these 264 infants, a total of 16 cases of neuroblastoma were identified before these cases would have been diagnosed from clinical symptoms. The frequency of neuroblastoma is comparable to the frequency of other diseases that are already routinely screened for among infants in the United States, such as phenylketonuria or PKU (1 in 14,000 births), galactosemia (1 in 62,000 births), and congenital hypothyroidism (1 in 4,000). Therefore the question becomes, does neuroblastoma screening lead to improved disease survival or does it simply identify those who will die soon anyway? Among a small sample of patients in Japan, the answer seems to be that survival is improved for neuroblastoma patients identified by the screening test. This cancer has a tendency to metastasize early, and about 60% of patients have metastatic disease at diagnosis. However, among the 16 patients identified by screening in Japan, none had metastatic disease at diagnosis. Since prognosis is in large part determined by disease extent, this suggests that neuroblastoma screening may improve disease survival.

However, this conclusion has been disputed by the American Cancer Society, which convened a Workshop on Neuroblastoma Screening in 1990.[99] Workshop participants noted that neuroblastoma screening may miss some cases that have an unfavorable prognosis and overdiagnose other cases that would have spontaneously resolved. Furthermore, the mass screening program has not yet produced a significant decline in neuroblastoma mortality in Japan. For these reasons, Workshop participants did not endorse a neuroblastoma screening program in the United States. In contrast, we believe that it should be general policy to spare no expense for children; extraordinary measures are far more appropriate for children than for adults.

Very recently a new screening test was developed that appears to be sensitive to cancerous changes in lung tissue.[100] The test relies upon very sophisticated molecular biology techniques to detect genetic changes in lung cells shed in sputum. The test was applied to sputum samples collected from 15 patients, all of whom were diagnosed with adenocarcinoma of the lung several months after sputum collection. In this group of 15 patients, 10 had genetic mutations in their tumor, while five patients had no detectable tumor mutations. The sputum test was unable to detect any abnormality in those patients with no tumor mutations, but 80% of those patients with tumor mutations also had detectable sputum abnormalities. Sputum abnormalities were detected up to a year prior to clinical diagnosis of the lung tumor, with the average time between detection of sputum abnormalities and clinical detection of the tumor being three months. This advance warning can be significant, since patients with sputum abnormalities prior to diagnosis tended to have small tumors. Although this was a very small group of patients, the five-year survival rate after surgery was 60%, which is far better than the normal five-year survival rate of about 15% for patients with lung cancer.[101] Because the sputum test is easy to apply and relatively inexpensive it is very appealing, but extensive validation in prospective trials will be required before the test can be endorsed.

POLICY ISSUES RESULTING FROM EARLY DETECTION OF CANCER

Widespread application of effective cancer screening tests will have a profound impact on individual lives and on public health policies. Pre-emptive care will usually benefit the patient and lower the cost to society of disease,[102] but pre-emptive care is a completely different model of medical care than is in place presently. Many of the current cancer screening tests are so expensive that costs can exceed savings.[103] It has been estimated that screening for cervical cancer every three years costs about $22,000 per year of life gained. Increasing screening frequency to every two years increases the cost to $440,000 for every additional year of life gained, while annual screening costs $1.8 million for each additional year of life. Many women are screened annually or even more frequently for cervical cancer, which is an expensive and relatively ineffective approach to public health. Yet nearly 25% of women in the United States have not had a Pap test in the past three years. In neither case is the screening frequency determined by a consideration of wise medical practice or wise investment of health care dollars. It should be incumbent upon our health care system to assure two things: that the standard medical practice for a given condition be proven effective by scientific studies and that health care dollars be spent where they will do the most good.

However, the argument about health care policy cannot become focused solely on cost to the exclusion of all other considerations. Health care is already effectively rationed on the basis of cost, with many inequities in the distribution of health care. For example, the outcome of breast cancer therapy is often determined by income level, as the type of health insurance coverage has a strong effect on breast cancer survival.[104] In New Jersey, women who are covered by Medicaid are more than twice as likely to be diagnosed with metastatic breast cancer as are women who are privately insured. The relative risk of death from breast cancer is 40% higher in women covered by Medicaid, and 49% higher in uninsured women, compared to women with private health insurance. Thus, women without private health insurance would benefit from improved access to breast cancer screening and optimal breast cancer therapy.[105] While there is certainly an economic cost associated with extending optimal treatment to all patients, there is a moral cost associated with denying treatment to the poor.

Thorny ethical issues have been raised by the identification of persons at high risk of cancer.[106] Some of these issues were revealed by a program of genetic counseling that was implemented for women and families affected by an inherited susceptibility to breast and ovarian cancer. A gene known as BRCA1 is estimated to be present in one of every 200 to 400 women, and this gene confers a lifetime risk of breast cancer that approaches 85%. Genetic markers of cancer risk have been identified in several families in the Midwest, and genetic testing is now able to prospectively identify women at high risk of breast cancer within these particular families. When this information was provided, upon request, to members of one such family, several very difficult situations were created. For example, one 33-year-old woman, who was very concerned about her familial risk of breast cancer, had already requested bilateral mastectomy as a prophylactic measure. When counselors revealed to this woman that she was unlikely to be a carrier of the BRCA1 mutation, she promptly canceled the planned surgery, but was subsequently racked with guilt that she had been spared the disease that had already been diagnosed in three first-degree relatives. Another woman, the 40-year-old cousin of the first woman, learned that she was likely to be a carrier of the BRCA1 gene, so she immediately had a mammographic examination that she had been postponing for years. This examination revealed an early stage breast cancer that would almost certainly have gone undetected until it was far advanced, since the woman admitted that she had no plans for a regular program of breast screening. Another woman was told that she probably did not have the BRCA1 mutation five years after she had already undergone prophylactic bilateral mastectomy. This woman later came to accept her earlier decision as the best decision possible under the circumstances.[107] Finally, in a tragic case, a woman who was told she had a lifetime risk of breast cancer of 86% underwent prophylactic mastectomy, only to be diagnosed with advanced ovarian cancer within three months.[108] These stories illustrate some of the ethical quandaries that can be created by access to knowledge that was not only unavailable, but unthinkable, even a generation ago.

An evaluation of the psychological impact of screening for familial ovarian cancer has shown that, in any screening test, false-positive indications of cancer are likely to create the worst problems.[109] A group of 302 women, all of whom were at high risk of ovarian cancer and all of whom were enrolled in an experimental screening program for this cancer, were surveyed to determine their psychological state, coping style, and anxiety level about risk of cancer. After they completed the questionnaire, the women were screened by abdominal and vaginal ultrasound to identify changes in ovarian volume or tissue consistency. Women were informed of any abnormality immediately and were asked to return for an exhaustive screening test six weeks later. Those women with persistent abnormalities could elect to have a hysterectomy with bilateral removal of the ovaries. Women who were further screened were asked to fill out the same questionnaire again, after the second screening test and after any surgery. About 23% of the initial group of screened women were found to have ovarian abnormalities during the first examination, and about 7% of the women had two positive scans and elected to undergo surgery. However, none of the women were found to have ovarian cancer. Psychological distress and worries about cancer were considerably reduced among those women fortunate enough to have a negative screening result. Psychological responses to a positive screening result were determined in part by the physicians' evaluation of malignant potential at the time, but coping style may also play a role at this stage. Women with an information-seeking coping style tended to be more anxious, as were those women who were referred for surgery immediately. At follow-up, women who had two positive screening tests, but were negative for ovarian cancer, had returned to normal in terms of anxiety level. These findings show that false positive results can have a profound effect on psychological well-being, but that psychological effects are generally short-term rather than severe or persistent. Even women who had surgery, but did not have cancer, seemed to welcome the certainty that they could never develop ovarian cancer.[110]

Attitudes toward the predictive testing of disease susceptibility have also been carefully explored in a group of adults at risk of Huntingtons disease (HD).[111] A group of 250 participants in a study of HD responded to a questionnaire about whether or not they would be interested in a predictive test that could reveal to them their chances of developing HD. People were specifically asked whether they would take a predictive test that was either 100% accurate or only 99% accurate. It was found that about 72% of people would take a predictive test if it were 100% accurate, whereas only 58% would take the test if it were 99% accurate. In either case though, a significant minority would not take a predictive test, presumably because of fear of a positive test result. Persons who believed themselves to be at higher risk of HD were more likely to take a predictive test, even though there is no treatment known for HD. Overall, the major factor limiting acceptance of predictive testing was the feeling that there was no point in predicting the presence of an untreatable disease. Thus, while many would probably accept a predictive test for a treatable disease, acceptance of screening would diminish as the perception of disease treatability diminished.[112] These findings may have relevance for cancer screening as well, since certain cancers (e.g., lung cancer) are widely regarded as untreatable.

RECOMMENDATIONS FOR CANCER SCREENING PROGRAMS

A series of recommendations have been made by scientists involved with a program of predictive testing for mutations of the p53 gene, the most frequently mutated gene in human cancer.[113] While these recommendations were made specifically for a single type of screening test, they are broadly applicable and entirely appropriate for any new type of cancer screening test:

1. Protocols for application of the screening test, and for obtaining informed consent prior to application, should be carefully worked out before the test is offered. This should be done in collaboration with a Review Board, whose role is to act as patient advocate throughout the process.
2. Test centers should establish an Advisory Board to oversee and monitor the screening program, and this board should include "outside experts" from other institutions, as well as experts in medical ethics and medical genetics.
3. Testing should only be offered to competent adults who can understand the procedure to the extent required to give truly "informed consent." Since our understanding of the impact of testing on children is very poor, testing should probably not be offered to children. Prenatal testing for genetic mutations must be dealt with on a case-by-case basis.
4. Subjects should participate in some sort of psychological screening evaluation prior to testing, and should agree to participate in a long-term follow-up program of genetic counseling and psychological evaluation.

5. Subjects should provide a complete family and medical history, undergo a physical, and generally cooperate enough to become a part of a clinical trial of the new test.

6. Follow-up counseling should be available, so that those who learn they are at high risk of cancer can be advised about how to minimize their risk.

7. Cost of participation in the test should initially be borne by the test facility, since efficacy of the test is unknown, and since equal access to testing is important to validate the test.

8. All test results must be kept in strictest confidence, to eliminate the possibility that this information can be used to deny medical insurance coverage.

9. All test results and medical data from participants should be incorporated into a national registry, so that test efficacy can be determined as quickly as possible, and so that subject data can be used in future epidemiological studies. However, this must be done in a way that preserves patient confidentiality. Since any reduction in cancer mortality resulting from a new test will take many years to become evident, long-term follow-up is essential.

10. Subjects identified as being at high risk of a particular cancer are appropriate subjects for cancer prevention studies, so a mechanism must be in place to maintain subject privacy while still allowing medical personnel to contact potential subjects.[114] It is almost inevitable that, with our current health care system, the results of genetic testing will be used to deny medical coverage to those who need it most. Because there is a strong economic incentive for insurance companies to identify those individuals at high risk of cancer, large-scale trials of a cancer screening test will find it very difficult to preserve patient confidentiality. Therefore, it is unethical to offer cancer screening tests when such screening may substantially worsen the outcome for those who test positive. The only way out of this quandary is to nationalize the insurance industry, require universal participation in the health care system, and offer uniform access to quality health care for all persons.

SUMMARY

It is almost certainly foolish to make recommendations about which cancer screening tests are worthwhile and which are not. In most cases, too little is known about the test, or about the significance of positive test results.

Nevertheless, it is somewhat cowardly to shirk from summarizing what information is available. With the caveat that the following recommendations will almost certainly change as new information is obtained, the existing information about cancer screening tests can be summarized.

RECOMMENDED	NOT RECOMMENDED
Pap smear: baseline at age 30, then every two to three years except women at high risk of cervical cancer	**digital rectal examination:** for prostate cancer
mammography: baseline at age 40	**chest X-ray:** for lung cancer
yearly, if family history includes first-degree relative with breast cancer	**alpha fetoprotein:** for liver cancer

Pap smear: baseline at age 30, then every two to three years except women at high risk of cervical cancer

mammography: baseline at age 40
yearly, if family history includes first-degree relative with breast cancer
every two years, if no family history and if image quality good (i.e., low-density breasts)
repeat in five years, if no family history and if image quality poor (i.e., high-density breasts)
yearly, for women between 50 and 70 years
monthly self-examination may be useful
mammograms should be combined with clinical breast examinations

colonoscopy: baseline at age 50
consult with physician, but screening frequency greater than once every five years unnecessary

fecal occult blood test: yearly, after age 40

prostate specific antigen (PSA): baseline series at age 40, yearly after age 50

carcinoembryonic antigen (CEA): recommended for recurrent colon cancer, consult physician for use as screening test

serum CA-125: every three to five years, baseline at about age 45, more frequent if family history of ovarian cancer

Urine catecholamines: once for newborns to screen for neuroblastoma susceptibility

digital rectal examination: for prostate cancer
chest X-ray: for lung cancer
alpha fetoprotein: for liver cancer

NOTES TO CHAPTER 14

1. American Cancer Society, *Cancer Facts & Figures–1992*. (Atlanta, American Cancer Society), 1992.
2. *Ibid.*
3. J.R. Harris, M.E. Lippman, U. Veronesi, W. Willett, "Breast cancer" (Part 1), *N. Engl. J. Med.*, 327 (1992): 319–328.
4. E.A. Clarke, T.W. Anderson, "Does screening by Pap smears help prevent cervical cancer? A case-control study," *Lancet* 2 (1979): 1–4.
5. *Ibid.*
6. E. MacGregor, S.M. Moss, D.M. Parkin, N.E. Day, "A case-control study of cervical cancer screening in north-east Scotland," *Brit. Med. J.* 290 (1985): 1543–1546.
7. *Ibid.*
8. R. Bergstrom, H.O. Adami, L. Gustafsson, J. Ponten, P. Sparen, "Detection of preinvasive cancer of the cervix and the subsequent reduction in invasive cancer," *J. Natl. Cancer Instit.* 85 (1993): 1050–1057.
9. *Ibid.*
10. D. Solomon, "Screening for cervical cancer: prospects for the future," *J. Natl. Cancer Instit.* 85 (1993): 1018–1019.
11. *Ibid.*
12. M. van Ballegooijen, J.D.F. Habbema, G.J. van Oortmarssen, M.A. Koopmanschap, J.T.N. Lubbe, H.M.E. van Agt, "Preventive Pap-smears: balancing costs, risks and benefits," *Brit. J. Cancer* 65 (1992): p. 930–933.
13. *Ibid.*
14. Harris, "Breast cancer," 319–328.
15. *Ibid.*
16. F.R. Margolin, "Detecting early breast cancer: experience in a community hospital," *Cancer* 64 (1989): 2702–2705.
17. *Ibid.*
18. *Ibid.*
19. C.J. Baines, "Breast self-examination," *Cancer (Suppl)* 64 (1989): 2661–2663.
20. *Ibid.*
21. Harris, "Breast cancer," 319–328.
22. L. Nystrom, L.E. Rutqvist, S. Wall, A. Lindgren, M. Lindqvist, et al., "Breast cancer screening with mammography: overview of Swedish randomised trials," *Lancet* 341 (1993): 973–978.
23. *Ibid.*
24. *Ibid.*

25. A.B. Miller, , C.J. Baines, T. To, C. Wall, "Canadian National Breast Screening Study: 1. Breast cancer detection and death rates among women aged 40 to 49 years," *Can. Med. Assoc. J.* 147 (1992): 1459–1476.
26. A.B. Miller, C.J. Baines, T. To, C. Wall, "Canadian National Breast Screening Study: 2. Breast cancer detection and death rates among women aged 50 to 59 years," *Can Med. Assoc. J.* 147 (1992): 1477–1488.
27. Miller, "Canadian National Breast Screening Study: 1," 1459–1476.
28. *Ibid.*
29. N.F. Boyd, R.A. Jong, M.J. Yaffe, D. Tritchler, G. Lockwood, C.J. Zylak, "A critical appraisal of the Canadian National Breast Cancer Screening Study," *Radiology* 189 (1993): 661–663.
30. K. Smigel, "New data suggest fewer mammograms for younger, older women," *J. Natl. Cancer Instit.* 84 (1992): 1860–1862.
31. Boyd, "A critical appraisal of the Canadian National Breast Cancer Screening Study," 661–663.
32. *Ibid.*
33. *Ibid.*
34. Nystrom, "Breast cancer screening with mammography," 973–978.
35. Smigel, "New data suggest fewer mammograms for younger, older women," 1860–1862.
36. S.W. Fletcher, W. Black, R. Harris, B.K. Rimer, S. Shapiro, "Report of the International Workshop on Screening for Breast Cancer," *J. Natl. Cancer Instit.* 85 (1993): 1644–1656.
37. *Ibid.*
38. A. Stacey-Clear, K.A. McCarthy, D.A. Hall, E. Pile-Spellman, G. White, et al., "Breast cancer survival among women under age 50: is mammography detrimental?," *Lancet* 340 (1992): 991–994.
39. *Ibid.*
40. K. Kerlikowske, D. Grady, J. Barclay, E.A. Sickles, A. Eaton, V. Ernster, "Positive predictive value of screening mammography by age and family history of breast cancer," *J. Amer. Med. Assoc.* 270 (1993): 2444–2450.
41. *Ibid.*
42. P.G.M. Peer, R. Holland, J.H.C.L. Hendriks, M. Mravunac, A.L.M. Verbeek, "Age-specific effectiveness of the Nijmegen population-based breast cancer-screening program: assessment of early indicators of screening effectiveness," *J. Natl. Cancer Instit.* 86 (1994) 436–441.
43. *Ibid.*

44. L. D'Agincourt, "Technique is everything when breast is dense," *Diag. Imaging* Sept. (1993): 57–61.

45. *Ibid.*

46. M. Swift, D. Morrell, R.B. Massey, C.L. Chase, "Incidence of cancer in 161 families affected by ataxia-telangiectasia," *N. Engl. J. Med.* 325 (1991): p. 1831–1836.

47. W.R. Hendee, "Reexamine screening of women under age 50," *Diag. Imaging* Sept. (1993): 27–30.

48. *Ibid.*

49. S.W. Fletcher, R.H. Fletcher, "The breast is close to the heart," *Ann. Internal Med.* 117 (1992): 969–971.

50. K. Smigel, "NCI proposes new breast cancer screening guidelines," *J. Natl. Cancer Instit.* 85 (1993): 1626–1628.

51. Kerlikowske, "Positive predictive value of screening mammography," 2444–2450.

52. Margolin, "Detecting early breast cancer," 2702–2705.

53. Fletcher, "The breast is close to the heart," 969–971.

54. Fletcher, "Report of the International Workshop on Screening for Breast Cancer," 1644–1656.

55. E.A. Sickles, D.B. Kopans, "Deficiencies in the analysis of breast cancer screening data," *J. Natl. Cancer Instit.* 85 (1993): 1621–1624.

56. Stacey-Clear, "Breast cancer survival among women under age 50," 991–994.

57. T.C. Chalmers, "Screening for breast cancer: What should national health policy be?," *J. Natl. Cancer Instit.* 85 (1993): 1619–1620.

58. Fletcher, "The breast is close to the heart," 969–971.

59. S.W. Fletcher, R.P. Harris, J.J. Gonzalez, D. Degnan, D.R. Lannin, et al., "Increasing mammography utilization: a controlled study," *J. Natl. Cancer Instit.* 85 (1993): 112–120.

60. S.F. Hurley, D.J. Jolley, P.M. Livingston, D. Reading, J. Cockburn, D. Flint-Richter, "Effectiveness, costs, and cost-effectiveness of recruitment strategies for a mammographic screening program to detect breast cancer," *J. Natl. Cancer Instit.* 84 (1992): 855–863.

61. A.C. Marcus, R. Bastani, K. Reardon, S. Karlins, I.P. Das, et al., "Proactive screening mammography counseling within the Cancer Information Service: results from a randomized trial," *Monogr. Natl. Cancer Instit.* 14 (1993): 119–129.

62. Harris, "Breast cancer" (Part 1), 319–328.

63. D'Agincourt, "Technique is everything when breast is dense," 57–61.

64. *Ibid.*

65. J.V. Selby, G.D. Friedman, C.P. Quesenberry, N.S. Weiss, "A case-control study of screening sigmoidoscopy and mortality from colorectal cancer," *N. Engl. J. Med.* 326 (1992): 653–657.
66. *Ibid.*
67. *Ibid.*
68. J.S. Mandel, J.H, Bond, T.R. Church, D.C. Snover, G.M. Bradley, et al., "Reducing mortality from colorectal cancer by screening for fecal occult blood," *N. Engl. J. Med.* 328 (1993): 1365–1371.
69. *Ibid.*
70. *Ibid.*
71. *Ibid.*
72. S.J. Winawer, B.J. Flehinger, D. Schottenfeld, D.G. Miller, "Screening for colorectal cancer with fecal occult blood testing and sigmoidoscopy," *J. Natl. Cancer Instit.* 85 (1993): 1311–1318.
73. D.A. Ahlquist, H.S. Wieand, C.G. Moertel, D.B. McGill, C.L. Loprinzi, et al., "Accuracy of fecal occult blood screening for colorectal neoplasia: A prospective study using Hemoccult and HemoQuant tests," *J. Amer. Med. Assoc.* 269 (1993): 1262–1267.
74. D.K. Whynes, A.R. Walker, J.O. Chamberlain, J.D. Hardcastle, "Screening and the costs of treating colorectal cancer," *Brit. J. Cancer* 68 (1993): 965–968.
75. *Ibid.*
76. G.D. Friedman, R.A. Hiatt, C.P. Quesenberry, J.V. Selby, "Case-control study of screening for prostatic cancer by digital rectal examinations," *Lancet* 337 (1991): 1526–1529.
77. *Ibid.*
78. W.J. Catalona, D.S. Smith, T.L. Ratliff, J.W. Basler, "Detection of organ-confined prostate cancer is increased through prostate-specific antigen-based screening," *J. Amer. Med. Assoc.* 270 (1993): 948–954.
79. *Ibid.*
80. H.B. Carter, J.D. Pearson, E.J. Metter, L.J. Brant, D.W. Chan, et al, "Longitudinal evaluation of prostate-specific antigen levels in men with and without prostate disease," *J. Amer. Med. Assoc.* 267 (1992): 2215–2220.
81. Catalona, "Detection of organ-confined prostate cancer," 948–954.
82. C.S. Haines, J.M. Tonita, P. Wang, "Forty-two year prostatic cancer incidence trends in a defined population of one million served by a reimbursement-linked cancer registry," *J. Natl. Cancer Instit.* 86 (1994): 230–231.

83. H.M. Pollack, M.I. Resnick, "Prostate-specific antigen and screening for prostate cancer: much ado about something?," *Radiology* 189 (1993): 353–356.

84. *Ibid.*

85. C.G. Moertel, T.R. Fleming, J.S. Macdonald, D.G. Haller, J.A. Laurie, C. Tangen, "An evaluation of the carcinoembryonic antigen (CEA) test for monitoring patients with resected colon cancer," *J. Amer. Med. Assoc.* 270 (1993): 943–947.

86. *Ibid.*

87. C.R. Smart, "Annual screening using chest X-ray examination for the diagnosis of lung cancer," *Cancer* 229 (1993): 2295–2298.

88. B.J. Flehinger, M. Kimmel, T. Polyak, M.R. Melamed, "Screening for lung cancer: The Mayo Lung Project revisited," *Cancer* 72 (1993): 1573–1580.

89. *Ibid.*

90. Smart, "Annual screening using chest x-ray examination," 2295–2298.

91. C.D. Runowicz, "Advances in the screening and treatment of ovarian cancer," *Ca—A Cancer Journal for Clinicians* 42 (1992): 327–349.

92. *Ibid.*

93. K.J. Helzlsouer, T.L. Bush, A.J. Alberg, K. Miller-Bass, H. Zacur, G.W. Comstock, "Prospective study of serum CA-125 levels as markers of ovarian cancer," *J. Amer. Med. Assoc.* 269 (1993): 1123–1126.

94. *Ibid.*

95. Runowicz, "Advances in the screening and treatment of ovarian cancer," 327–349.

96. G. Klose, W. Schmiegel, "Laboratory investigations in hepatobiliary and pancreatic malignancies: the role of tumor markers" in *Hepatobiliary and pancreatic malignancies: diagnosis, medical and surgical management*, N.J. Lygidakis, G.N.J. Tytgat, editors. (New York: Thieme Medical Publishers, 1989), 257–261.

97. T.K. Choi, J. Wong, "Expectations and possibilities of liver resection in the management of hepatocellular carcinoma" in *Hepatobiliary and pancreatic malignancies: diagnosis, medical and surgical management*, N.J. Lygidakis, G.N.J. Tytgat, editors. (New York: Thieme Medical Publishers, 1989), 179–182.

98. M. Tuchman, W.G. Woods, "The scientific basis for neuroblastoma screening: facts and hypotheses" in *Neuroblastoma: tumor biology and therapy*, C. Pochedly, editor. (Boston: CRC Press, 1990), 349–366.

99. S.B. Murphy, R.P. Castleberry, S.L. Cohn, H.L. Levy, A.W.

Craft, et al., "Consensus statement from the American Cancer Society Workshop on neuroblastoma screening: Do children benefit from mass screening for neuroblastoma?," *Ca–A Cancer J. Clin.* 41 (1991): 227–230.

100. L. Mao, R.H. Hruban, J.O. Boyle, M. Tockman, D. Sidransky, "Detection of oncogene mutations in sputum precedes diagnosis of lung cancer," *Cancer Res.* 54 (1994): 1634–1637.

101. *Ibid.*

102. C.T. Caskey, "Presymptomatic diagnosis: a first step toward genetic health care," *Science* 262 (1993): 48–49.

103. L.B. Russell, "The role of prevention in health reform," *New Engl. J. Med.* 329 (1993): 352–354.

104. J.Z. Ayanian, B.A. Kohler, T. Abe, A.M. Epstein, "The relation between health insurance coverage and clinical outcomes among women with breast cancer," *New Engl. J. Med.* 329 (1993): 326–331.

105. *Ibid.*

106. B.B. Biesecker, M. Boehnke, K. Calzone, D.S. Markel, J.E. Garber, et al., "Genetic counseling for families with inherited susceptibility to breast and ovarian cancer," *J. Amer. Med. Assoc.* 269 (1993): 1970–1974.

107. *Ibid.*

108. M-C. King, S. Rowell, S.M. Love, "Inherited breast ovarian cancer: What are the risks? What are the choices?," *J. Amer. Med. Assoc.* 269 (1993): 1975–1980.

109. F.J. Wardle, W. Collins, A.L. Pernet, M.I. Whitehead, T.H. Bourne, S. Campbell, "Psychological impact of screening for familial ovarian cancer," *J. Natl. Cancer Instit.* 85 (1993): 653–657.

110. *Ibid.*

111. R. Babul, S. Adam, B. Kremer, S. Dufrasne, S. Wiggins, et al., "Attitudes toward direct predictive testing for the Huntington disease gene: relevance for other adult-onset disorders," *J. Amer. Med. Assoc.* 270 (1993): 2321–2325.

112. *Ibid.*

113. F.P. Li, J.E. Garber, S.H. Friend, L.C. Strong, A.F. Patenaude, et al., "Recommendations on predictive testing for germ line p53 mutations among cancer-prone individuals," *J. Natl. Cancer Instit.* 84 (1992): 1156–1160.

114. *Ibid.*

15

NUTRITIONAL AND
CHEMICAL CANCER
PREVENTION

This chapter is devoted to the range of different nutritional and chemical interventions that can potentially result in a reduction in cancer incidence or mortality. Nutritional intervention is defined as supplementation of the diet with concentrated forms of the same vitamins and minerals that are present in a balanced diet. These nutritional supplements are in the same, or at least a very similar, chemical form as naturally occurring vitamins and minerals. Chemical intervention is defined as administration of chemicals that are not closely related to the vitamins and minerals present in a balanced diet. In many cases, chemical intervention involves chemicals that are completely unrelated to normal dietary elements. Much of the work with chemical prevention of cancer is still in the early stages of experimentation and has not progressed beyond tests in cultured cells or in experimental animals. While this work is fascinating and may hold great promise for the future, our discussion will largely be limited to agents that have already been tried in humans. In many cases, little is known of the efficacy of even those chemopreventive agents that are already in clinical trials, so our discussion will necessarily be somewhat brief.

NUTRITIONAL INTERVENTION AND
CANCER PREVENTION

If the availability of vitamins and minerals in the diet is truly capable of protecting one from cancer, then reducing the risk of cancer should be possible by deliberate supplementation of the diet. Very recently, several studies have described an effort to reduce the incidence of esophageal and stomach cancer in Linxian Province, China. This study was undertaken for several reasons. Most important is the extremely high incidence of esophageal cancer in Linxian—the mortality rate from esophageal cancer in this county is 10-fold higher than the national average in China, and more than 100-fold higher than the mortality rate for whites in the United States. This discrepancy has been studied for many years, so a great deal of information is available on cancer incidence and cancer risk factors in China. Furthermore, people in Linxian Province tend to have a rather poor nutritional status, so that nutritional interventions are more likely to have a clear effect on the average diet. In addition, because the Chinese people themselves are very aware of the prevalence of esophageal cancer, they are more likely to be compliant and to closely follow dietary instructions. Finally, because the Chinese government is also keenly aware of the high incidence of esophageal cancer, getting official approval to do this study was relatively easy. Thus, a massive study of the efficacy of nutritional intervention was initiated in Linxian County in 1985.

Epidemiological studies have thus far failed to reveal the causes of the extraordinarily high incidence of esophageal and stomach cancer in Linxian, China.[1] Nevertheless, evidence from elsewhere in the world suggests that consumption of fresh vegetables and fruit protects from these cancers. It is unknown what particular component of vegetables and fruits is actually protective, but researchers have suspected that vitamin C and beta-carotene might be the active agents. In Linxian, food availability is limited and intake of fresh fruits and meat is particularly low. Dietary staples are corn, millet, sweet potatoes, and wheat, and consequently, blood levels of retinol, beta-carotene, riboflavin, vitamin C, and vitamin E are consistently low by Western standards. Vitamin and mineral supplements were given daily to 29,584 healthy adults between the ages of 40 and 69, and these people were followed for more than five years. Most of these people did not smoke tobacco or drink alcohol, but 68% had a family history of esophageal or stomach cancer. People were randomly assigned to one of four different groups, so that four different combinations of vitamins and minerals could be tried. The four different supplements given were: retinol and zinc; the B vitamins riboflavin and niacin; vitamin C and molybdenum; and beta-carotene, vitamin E, and selenium. Doses of these vitamins and minerals ranged from one to two times the Recommended Daily Allowance in the United States.[2]

A total of 2,127 persons died during the course of the study in Linxian. Cancer was the leading cause of death, and 32% of all deaths were due to esophageal or stomach cancer. Most of the vitamin and mineral supplements were found to have no effect on cancer mortality, but the combination of beta-carotene, vitamin E, and selenium was found to be moderately protective. Individuals receiving this combination were 9% less likely to die of any cause, 13% less likely to die of cancer, and 21% less likely to die of stomach cancer. Interestingly, incidence of fatal strokes was also reduced by this regimen of vitamins and minerals. However, the incidence of esophageal cancer was not significantly reduced among people receiving this regimen, and the reduction in stomach cancer incidence did not become apparent until more than two years into the study.[3]

While these results convincingly show that dietary intervention can reduce the incidence of stomach cancer in Linxian, caution needs to be exercised in extending these results to people elsewhere in the world. The population of Linxian is marginally deficient in many micronutrients, and it is possible that dietary intervention will only work in a population that is similarly deficient. The incidence of stomach and esophageal cancer in Linxian is so extraordinarily high that hereditary susceptibilities to these cancers are implied. If this is true, then dietary intervention may overcome some inborn error of vitamin metabolism, and people without a similar inborn error of metabolism might not achieve the same benefit from vitamin supplements. Finally, the experimental design used for this study was very ambitious—it attempted to test four different vitamin supplements in eight different combinations in order to extract information on many different combinations of vitamins and minerals. Because many different treatments were studied simultaneously, the statistical power of the experiment was low, meaning that the ability to identify effective combinations of vitamins and minerals was rather limited. If a particular vitamin or mineral had a very powerful effect on cancer incidence, then this study design would have been appropriate. But since all of the vitamins and minerals seemed to have a rather small effect on cancer incidence, researchers were stuck with a study design that was not very sensitive.

Another major study of the efficacy of nutritional intervention was conducted in Linxian, China, at the same time as the study described above. This second study tested the ability of vitamin and mineral supplements to reduce the incidence of esophageal cancer among people who were already diagnosed with a condition known to be a precursor to this cancer.[4] The precursor condition, called esophageal dysplasia, affects over 20% of the adults in Linxian, and a high proportion of people with esophageal dysplasia progress to cancer over their lifetimes. A group of 3,318 people with esophageal dysplasia was selected, with the criteria that they were between 40 and 69 years of age, were free of cancer at the beginning of the study, and were not taking any other vitamin or mineral supplements. These people were given either daily pills containing 14 vitamins and 12 minerals, or else identical pills that contained no active ingredients (i.e., placebo). Persons receiving supplementation were at a dose level two to three times higher than the Recommended Daily

Allowance in the United States. These two groups of people were followed for a total of more than six years to determine whether esophageal cancer incidence was lower in persons receiving supplementation than in persons receiving placebo. Over the course of the study, a total of 324 deaths occurred, and cancer was responsible for 54% of all deaths. Persons receiving supplementation were found to be 8% less likely to develop esophageal cancer than persons receiving placebo, but this difference was not large enough to be significant. In fact, cumulative cancer rates and cumulative death rates did not differ between the two groups. This discouraging result means that no effect of supplementation on survival could be seen in this high-risk population. However, it is possible that the benefits of supplementation will not become obvious until more time has passed; in fact, the death rate from cancer in the two study groups began to diverge three years into the study, although the death rates never diverged very much. It is certainly possible that differences in death rate between the two groups will become manifest at some point in the future. Researchers will continue to follow these two groups to determine whether there is a long term benefit to supplementation with vitamins and minerals. However, the results so far have been very disappointing.[5]

Several clinical trials have also tested the ability of beta-carotene to prevent new or recurrent oral cancers in patients already diagnosed with an oral cancer.[6] This is potentially a very important application because oral cancers are rather common, because the rate of death from local tumor recurrence can be 60%, and because up to 40% of patients cured of their initial tumor nevertheless die of a second primary oral tumor. Because most oral cancers arise from small white patches on the oral surface known as leukoplakias, cancer preventive efforts have focused on causing regression of leukoplakias. Several studies have used supplementation with beta-carotene or vitamin A, together with measurements of patch size, to determine whether oral cancer recurrence can be prevented. In one study, a 57% remission rate and complete suppression of new oral lesions was experienced by a group receiving Vitamin A, compared with a 3% remission rate and a 21% rate of new lesions in a group receiving placebo. Several serious side effects of treatment were reported during these trials, including conjunctivitis in most patients, yet these side effects are certainly preferable to tumor recurrence. These results are encouraging because both beta-carotene and vitamin A are inexpensive and easily administered.[7]

Another clinical trial tested the ability of beta-carotene to prevent skin cancer recurrence in patients already diagnosed with nonmelanoma skin cancer.[8] This is potentially a worthwhile intervention, because persons diagnosed with one nonmelanoma skin cancer are at high risk of developing a second skin cancer, and because persons with a high intake of fruits and vegetables have a reduced cancer risk. A group of 1,805 patients were randomly assigned to receive either an active pill containing 50 milligrams of beta-carotene, or a placebo pill containing no active ingredients. Because the pills were physically indistinguishable, neither the patients nor their physicians knew whether a given patient was receiving beta-carotene or placebo. Blood tests revealed that compliance with the pill-taking regimen was good, even a year after the study began. Patients who were taking the active pill had nearly nine-fold more beta-carotene in their blood serum than did patients taking the placebo pill. Yet, even after five years of follow-up, there was no difference in skin cancer incidence between beta-carotene- and placebo-treated patients. Approximately 40% of these patients developed a second skin cancer, whether or not they were taking supplemental beta-carotene. Further analysis of sub-groups in the study showed that beta-carotene was also not protective for smokers or for persons in the lowest quartile of dietary beta-carotene consumption.[9]

Further striking evidence that beta-carotene is unable to protect cigarette smokers from lung cancer has recently been presented.[10] A large randomized and double blind clinical trial of beta-carotene was reported from Finland, involving 29,133 male smokers, 50 to 69 years of age. Smokers were randomized to receive either beta-carotene alone (20 mg/day), vitamin E alone (α-tocopherol, 50 mg/day), beta-carotene in combination with vitamin E, or placebo. Each volunteer was followed for five to eight years, during which a total of 876 cases of lung cancer were diagnosed. Neither beta-carotene nor α-tocopherol alone was associated with a reduced risk of lung cancer, nor was there evidence of a protective interaction between the two agents. In fact, men who took supplementary beta-carotene were actually 18% more likely to develop lung cancer—a statistically significant increase in risk. Supplementary beta-carotene was also unable to reduce the risk of any other cancers in this population of smokers. This very surprising finding raises the possibility that beta-carotene is actually harmful to smokers,[11] but care must be taken in interpreting these data. The lung cancer risk of smokers is so much higher than that of non-smokers that these findings may say nothing at all about the effect of beta-carotene on lung cancer risk in non-smokers. Further-more, the increased risk associated with beta-carotene supplementation was small, despite the fact that the number of smokers enrolled in the study was very large. These results are so surprising that they must be replicated before any reputable scientist would feel comfortable giving a final interpretation of the relationship between beta-carotene supplementation and lung cancer risk.

Fortunately, another large clinical trial was begun recently to determine whether a combination of beta-carotene and retinol can decrease the incidence of lung cancer in at-risk populations.[12] The trial is often referred to as CARET, which stands for the beta-Carotene And Retinol Efficacy Trial. These two agents were chosen because beta-carotene is an antioxidant, which may prevent formation of chemicals containing activated oxygen, while retinol is thought to be a tumor suppressor. The populations chosen for this study are men and women age 50–69 years with a history of at least 20 pack-years of cigarette smoking and men age 45–69 years with evidence of extensive occupational exposure to asbestos plus a history of smoking. A total of 14,420 smokers and 4,010 asbestos-exposed workers will be accrued and randomized to receive either placebo or beta-carotene (30 mg/day) plus retinyl palmitate (25,000 Units/day). Preliminary studies have shown that these dose levels increase the plasma level of beta-carotene roughly 12-fold and the plasma level of retinol about four-fold. Volunteers are generally willing and able to stay with the program; about 80% of the participants in a pilot study are still active in the clinical study six years after recruitment. All volunteers will be followed until 1998, at which point there will have been about 114,100 person-years of follow-up. This study is large enough that it should be able to detect a 23% reduction in lung cancer incidence caused by nutritional intervention. However, a smaller reduction in lung cancer incidence may be difficult or impossible to detect with the CARET design. This shows just how difficult it is to do meaningful clinical trials; a larger clinical trial would be more sensitive but much more expensive, while a smaller trial would be less expensive but unlikely to detect an effect even if the effect was fairly large.

The Nurses Health Study recently reported on the effect of various antioxidant vitamins on the risk of breast cancer.[13] In this study, a total of 89,494 women between 34 and 59 years of age were followed for eight years, during which time 1,439 women developed breast cancer. Women in the highest quintile (20%) of intake of foods rich in vitamin A precursors were about 16% less likely to get breast cancer than women in the lowest quintile of intake. The protective effect of vitamin A was generally stronger when vitamin A was obtained from the diet than when obtained from multivitamin pills. However, intake of supplemental vitamin A reduced breast cancer risk by 20% with respect to women in the lowest quintile of intake. To be in the highest quintile of total vitamin A a woman needed to consume nearly 18,000 Internation Units (IUs) of vitamin A each day, so vitamin pills containing only a few hundred IUs were not significantly protective. Yet for women with a relatively low dietary intake of vitamin A, those multivitamins that supply several thousand IUs of preformed vitamin A were significantly protective.

However, it is premature to suggest that vitamin pills be used as a source of preformed vitamin A, except for those women in the lowest category of vegetable intake. Even nutritionally deficient women would probably be better served by increasing their vegetable consumption than by taking multivitamins.[14]

Vitamin A has also been found to decrease the risk of colon cancer in women.[15] A four-year prospective study of 35,215 Iowa women showed clearly that supplemental vitamin A, but not dietary vitamin A, could reduce the risk of colon cancer. Women who used more than 5,000 IU of vitamin A reduced their colon cancer risk by about 53% with respect to women who did not use a vitamin A supplement.

The ability of supplemental vitamin B12 and folate to reverse the harmful effects of smoking was tested in a small group of long-term smokers.[16] This study was undertaken because experiments had suggested that tobacco smoke might specifically induce a deficit of folate in cells lining the airways of the lung. A large group of men who had smoked for at least 20 years was screened for precancerous lung changes using a sputum test. A group of 73 men was identified, all of whom scored as abnormal in repeated sputum tests. These men were then randomly assigned to receive either a placebo or a daily supplement of folate (10 milligrams) and vitamin B12 (0.5 milligrams), using a prospective study design. Since these men were randomly assigned to receive either placebo or supplement, neither the men nor their physicians knew which agents the men were receiving until after the study was over. Four months after treatment began, the men again donated sputum samples, which were tested for cellular abnormalities. Men who received supplements of vitamin B12 and folate were found to be less likely to have an abnormal sputum test than men who received the placebo. This suggests that supplements of these vitamins may be able to reverse the carcinogenic process caused by tobacco.[17] However, a great deal of caution must be used in interpreting this study. The small number of men in the study, the very short follow-up period, the relatively small changes observed, and the high levels of vitamins used, all show that these results are preliminary. Furthermore, in the six years since this study was published, no other study has confirmed these findings, which may mean that other researchers have been unable to duplicate the results. Thus there is no reason for a smoker to use this regimen in order to try to reverse the effects of smoking; it is far more effective to just stop smoking.

The Iowa Women's Health Study discussed above also found a reduced risk of colon cancer in women with a high intake of vitamin E (α-tocopherol).[18] The study found that dietary sources of vitamin E reduced risk somewhat, but that dietary and supplemental sources combined reduced colon cancer risk substantially. Women in the highest quintile of total vitamin E intake enjoyed a 68% reduction in risk of colon cancer, compared to women in the lowest quintile of intake. Women who used vitamin E supplements of more than 30 International Units (IU)/day were at a 56% lower risk of colon cancer, no matter what their level of dietary vitamin E, but women with a high dietary intake of vitamin E did not have a reduced incidence of colon cancer unless they also used vitamin E supplements. Vitamin E supplements provided a strong protective effect from colon cancer, even for women with a low dietary intake of vitamin E. The vitamin E effect on colon cancer risk was stronger and more significant than any other nutritional effect, especially in women under the age of 65. This is a strong argument in favor of multivitamin pills with vitamin E.[19]

Women in the highest quintile of intake of vitamin E from food sources are apparently also at a reduced risk of breast cancer.[20] High dietary intake of vitamin E put these women at a level of risk 60% lower than women in the lowest quintile. Vitamin E obtained from dietary supplements was not as effective at reducing breast cancer risk, as women in the highest quintile of supplementary vitamin E intake were only 30% less likely to suffer breast cancer. There was a fairly large discrepancy between the efficacy of vitamin E as a dietary component and the efficacy of vitamin E as a supplement. This suggests either that supplemental vitamin E is not available in the biologically most active form, or that the protective effect is conferred by some other ingredient of fruits and vegetables.[21]

Vitamin E has also been tested as a way to reverse oral leukoplakia.[22] A group of 43 patients with symptomatic leukoplakias were treated with oral vitamin E (400 IU) twice daily for 24 weeks. Follow-up examinations were performed at six, 12, and 24 weeks after starting treatment, to assess whether there had been regression of the lesions and to determine whether the patient was suffering any ill effect from treatment with the vitamin supplement. Patient compliance with the regimen of vitamin supplementation was evidently quite good, as the average blood level of vitamin E more than doubled over the 24 weeks of the study. In this group of patients, a total of 46% showed a clinical response to the supplements, as evidenced by regression in size of the lesions. No significant side effects of supplementation with vitamin E were observed. However, this study also suffered from a small sample size, an inadequate follow-up period, and results that were perhaps not as strong as one would like.[23] Yet the frequency of precancerous cellular changes was substantially reduced among individuals receiving the vitamin E supplement, which suggests that vitamin E may be able to reverse cancerous changes in cells[24].

Despite the apparent ability of vitamin E to reduce risk of certain cancers, the study in Finland discussed earlier has shown that vitamin E is apparently unable to reduce the risk of lung cancer in long-term smokers.[25] A group of 29,133 male smokers was randomized to receive α-tocopherol (50 mg/day) in various combinations with beta-carotene, in order to determine whether such supplementation could reduce the incidence of lung cancer in this at-risk population. It was found that α-tocopherol had no effect on lung cancer risk, nor was there any protective interaction between α-tocopherol and beta-carotene. However, some evidence suggested that α-tocopherol had a protective effect from another cancer, as men who received α-tocopherol were about 34% less likely to develop prostate cancer.[26] However, this study was not designed to measure the effect of α-tocopherol or beta-carotene on any cancers other than lung cancer, so the idea that α-tocopherol protects from prostate cancer should be regarded with some suspicion.

Multivitamin supplements have also been tested as a way to reduce the incidence of colon cancer in patients known to be prone to develop colon tumors.[27] A group of 41 patients, all of whom had undergone surgery to remove colonic polyps, was entered into a protocol in which they received either a combined supplement of vitamins A, C, and E or placebo. Patients were randomly assigned to one of the two protocols, so that the researchers were blinded with respect to which treatment each patient was receiving. Patients who were given supplements received vitamin A (30,000 IU), vitamin C (1,000 milligrams of ascorbic acid), and vitamin E (70 mg of α-tocopherol), combined in a single tablet. At the beginning of the study, each patient underwent a procedure in which a tiny biopsy sample of the intestine was used to measure the rate of growth of cells of the intestine. At the end of three and six months, patients again underwent the biopsy procedure, so that the rate of intestinal cell growth could be again measured. A slight reduction in the growth rate of intestinal cells was found among those receiving the multivitamin supplement. This suggests that a combination of several vitamins was able to reverse the tendency to progress toward cancer among a group of people diagnosed with a precancerous condition. While this small, preliminary study does not prove that multivitamins will have a role in colon cancer prevention, the results are certainly encouraging.

CHEMICAL INTERVENTION AND CANCER PREVENTION

A range of chemical agents are known that may be able to interfere with carcinogenesis, the process by which cells are induced to become cancerous and form a tumor. This process of interference in cancer causation has been called chemoprevention, more in hope for the future than in description of the present. Already about 22 different chemopreventive drugs or drug combinations are in various phases of development in the United States (Table 15-1); the phase of drug testing for each is indicated as of early 1994.[28]

Drugs are selected for testing as chemopreventive agents if there is reason to believe these agents might be effective in reducing cancer

TABLE 15-1
CHEMOPREVENTIVE AGENTS IN VARIOUS PHASES OF DEVELOPMENT AS OF EARLY 1994[57]

CHEMOPREVENTIVE AGENT	TOXICOLOGY TESTS COMPLETED	CLINICAL TRIAL PHASE		
		PHASE I	PHASE II	PHASE III
First generation				
Retinoids				
Isotretinoin	+		+	+
Fenretinide	+	+	+	+
Finasteride	+			+
Sulindac	+		+	
Aspirin	+	+	+	
Calcium	+	+	+	
Second generation				
DFMO	+	+		
Piroxicam	+	+		
Oltipraz	+	+		
N-acetyl-l-cysteine	+	+		
Ibuprofen	+	+		
Carbenoxolone	+	+		
18β-glycyrrhetinic acid	+	+		
DFMO + Piroxicam	+	+		
S-Allyl-l-cysteine	+	+		
Third generation				
Phenhexyl isothiocyanate	+			
Curcumin	+			
Ellagic acid	+			
Fumaric acid	+			
Fluasterone	+			
Fenretinide + Oltipraz	+			
Fenretinide + Tamoxifen	+			

Two retinoids related to vitamin A are currently under development: isotretinoin, which is the common name for 13-*cis*-retinoic acid, and fenretinide, which is the common name for all-*trans*-N-(4-hydroxyphenyl) retinamide.

incidence, but each drug is carefully tested and validated before being approved for use. The procedure used to validate a new chemopreventive agent is similar to that used to validate any new drug: a carefully defined clinical trial, with each phase of the trial designed to answer a specific set of questions.[29] A clinical trial proceeds from Phase I to Phase III in a process that can take years to complete. Phase I is a pilot study, often done with a small test population at increased risk of a particular cancer. A Phase I study can be designed to answer one of several different questions: maximum dose of a drug that can be tolerated; toxicity of the drug that may limit drug use; or the pharmacokinetics of drug in the bloodstream. Once these critical questions have been satisfactorily answered, the drug may move into Phase II clinical trials. Phase II tests involve a larger at-risk study population and are designed to determine the actual chemopreventive effect of the drug and to determine the degree of normal organ toxicity in relationship to drug efficacy. Phase III tests are designed to fit a new chemopreventive agent into a broader clinical context and to examine chemopreventive effects in a normal population. Phase III can be thought of as an experimental public health intervention. The discussion following will primarily focus on first generation agents, which are now involved in Phase II or Phase III testing. Second-generation agents are those agents that are currently in Phase I testing, while third-generation agents have completed preclinical toxicology tests, but have not yet entered a clinical trial.

The mode of action of chemopreventive agents is generally not well understood, but it has been proposed that these agents fall into one of several categories (diagramed in Table 15-2).[30] The boundary between agents used for cancer prevention and agents used for cancer treatment is beginning to disappear. In fact, agents such as the retinoids and DFMO (diflouoromethyl ornithine) are already being used for both purposes. It is quite likely that, as the state-of-the-art in cancer treatment advances, drugs will be found that are capable of inducing cancerous cells to cease growing and differentiate into more-normal cells. The ultimate therapeutic agent would be capable of inducing cancerous cells to differentiate and become completely normal again and would be able to maintain these cells in a normal state permanently. At that point, all distinction between cancer prevention and cancer therapy will vanish.

FIRST GENERATION CHEMOPREVENTIVE AGENTS

Retinoids, which are chemically similar to vitamin A, have been studied as chemopreventive agents for many years and can have chemopreventive

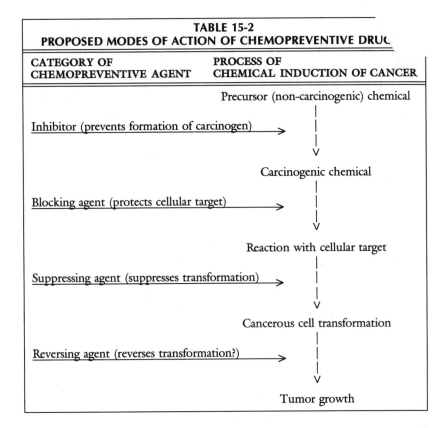

TABLE 15-2
PROPOSED MODES OF ACTION OF CHEMOPREVENTIVE DRUC

CATEGORY OF CHEMOPREVENTIVE AGENT	PROCESS OF CHEMICAL INDUCTION OF CANCER
	Precursor (non-carcinogenic) chemical
Inhibitor (prevents formation of carcinogen) →	
	Carcinogenic chemical
Blocking agent (protects cellular target) →	
	Reaction with cellular target
Suppressing agent (suppresses transformation) →	
	Cancerous cell transformation
Reversing agent (reverses transformation?) →	
	Tumor growth

activity in the skin, lung, breast, and bladder in animal models of cancer.[31] Vitamin A and its analogues, the retinoids, inhibit several cellular activities associated with cancerous transformation and can even induce redifferentiation of some cancerous cells. The retinoids can also increase cell-to-cell communication and stimulate the immune system. Unfortunately, they can also be fairly toxic, as vitamin A and many of the retinoids can cause liver damage, eye damage, and birth defects. Because of this toxicity, most clinical testing of retinoids has been limited to patients with previous cancers and to those at high risk of cancer.

Retinoids have undergone extensive testing as chemopreventive agents for cancers of the mouth. Oral cancers frequently arise from pre-malignant lesions in the mouth that are either white (leukoplakia) or raised red (erythroplasia) spots.[32] Since persistent oral lesions progress to cancer fairly frequently, progression or regression of these spots is often used as a short-term predictor of long-term success in preventing oral cancer. In one study, 44 patients with oral leukoplakia were randomized to receive either high-dose isotretinoin (13-*cis*-retinoic acid) or an inactive placebo drug. Over a three-month treatment period, 67% of the patients receiving isotretinoin showed regression of their lesions, while only 10% of the patients receiving a placebo showed spontaneous regression of their lesions. However, the toxicity of the isotretinoin was unacceptably high, and more than 50% of the responding patients relapsed within a few months after treatment ended. Nevertheless, this study served as a "proof of principle," by establishing that isotretinoin can induce remission of pre-cancerous oral lesions.

A later-generation study was done to determine whether patients who showed regression of oral leukoplakia following high-dose isotretinoin could be maintained in the regressed state with low-dose therapy.[33] Patients who responded to high-dose isotretinoin were randomized to receive low-dose maintenance therapy for nine months, with either isotretinoin or beta-carotene. Following the maintenance phase, only 8% of the patients who received isotretinoin showed progression of their lesions, whereas 55% of the patients receiving beta-carotene showed progression. Some lesions continued to regress during maintenance with isotretinoin, and the toxic effects of this treatment were fairly mild (e.g., dry skin and conjunctivitis). However, caution is appropriate in evaluating these results.[34] Although oral leukoplakia frequently progresses to cancer, it is not known whether regression of these lesions means that the risk of oral cancer has been reduced. The optimal choice and dose of retinoid is not known, and quite possibly there is a better agent for oral cancer prevention than isotretinoin. Finally, surgery or laser treatment is frequently successful in treating oral leukoplakia, and it is not known whether chemoprevention should replace or merely supplement these other treatments.

Isotretinoin has also been tried as an agent to prevent cancers of the head and neck among persons at high risk of these cancers.[35] Long-term smokers, especially those who drink hard liquor, frequently develop cancers of the nasal and oral cavities, the larynx, the pharynx, and the esophagus. Those who have had one primary cancer of the head and neck are at very high risk of recurrence of the original tumor, or of falling victim to a second primary cancer of the head and neck. People with a primary cancer of the head and neck develop a second primary cancer at a rate of about 5% to 7% per year, presumably because the tissues of the head and neck have been exposed to high doses of carcinogens, often for long periods. Those who have been treated for a primary cancer of the head and neck are thus a particularly good group to involve in chemoprevention trials, since their cancer risk is much higher than normal.

A group of 103 patients who were treated for a primary cancer of the head and neck was randomized to receive either isotretinoin or an inactive placebo drug in an effort to prevent tumor recurrence or the development of a second primary cancer.[36] This study was done prospectively, and used patients who were judged free of disease after surgery or radiation therapy for their first tumor. Patients received either the active or the inactive drug daily for 12 months, then their response was evaluated by a physician who had no knowledge of which drug the patient had received. Isotretinoin was found to have no effect on recurrence of the primary tumor, but those who received isotretinoin were at lower risk of developing a second primary cancer. After an average follow-up period of 32 months, only 4% of the isotretinoin group had developed a second primary cancer, whereas 24% of the placebo-treated patients had developed a second primary tumor. In fact, 8% of the placebo-treated group developed multiple second primary cancers, whereas none of the isotretinoin-treated patients had multiple cancers. These results indicate that daily treatment with isotretinoin is effective in reducing the incidence of second primary tumors of the head and neck, even though it cannot prevent recurrence of the original primary.

Unfortunately, long-term follow-up of the same group of patients has shown that the early protective effect of isotretinoin was partially lost over time.[37] After an average follow-up of 55 months (instead of the 32 months reported earlier), isotretinoin still showed no protective effect from recurrence of the primary tumor, and the protective effect from a second primary cancer was lessened. There was still a slight protective effect from developing a second primary cancer of the head, neck, and lungs, but several of the isotretinoin-treated patients developed second primary cancers elsewhere. Overall, there was no difference in survival between the isotretinoin-treated patients and the controls, perhaps because of the high drop-out rate from the experimental group due to side effects of therapy. This result is quite discouraging.

Another recent study examined the ability of isotretinoin to prevent basal cell carcinoma of the skin.[38] This is a potentially worthwhile application because, although better than 95% of basal cell skin carcinomas are curable, more than 480,000 new cases of this cancer are diagnosed each year. A group of 981 patients with two or more previous cases of basal cell skin carcinoma was randomized to receive either low-dose isotretinoin or placebo, and these patients were followed for an average of 36 months. Each patient was monitored at six-month intervals, both for new skin cancers and for toxic effects of therapy. After the three-year follow-up there was no difference in cancer incidence between patients who received isotretinoin and patients who received placebo. However, the group receiving isotretinoin reported very significant side effects of treatment, including skeletal changes. Isotretinoin was completely unsuccessful in reducing the incidence of this particular cancer, although the study was not designed to determine whether the drug could reduce the incidence of other types of cancer.

The effect of retinoids on lung cancer risk has also been studied, with retinoids administered as either vitamin A or isotretinoin, and with results similar to those achieved with oral cancer patients.[39] In both oral cancer and lung cancer, about 70% of all second primary tumors occur among cells exposed to tobacco smoke, suggesting that smoke exposure makes exposed cells vulnerable to cancerous transformation. When smoke-exposed lung cancer patients were treated with high-dose retinoids, the rate of primary tumor recurrence was unchanged, as was the rate of recurrence of oral cancer. In addition, neither study was able to find any difference between control and retinoid-treated patients in terms of overall survival. However, in both experiments, isotretinoin was able to increase the average length of time until the occurrence of a second primary tumor.[40]

Retinoids have been successful in reducing the incidence of breast cancer in animal models of cancer, so there is a great deal of interest in the retinoids as a chemopreventive agent for breast cancer. A relatively nontoxic retinoid, known as fenretinide, has been synthesized, and the effectiveness of this analogue is being evaluated in breast cancer patients in a large clinical trial.[41] This chemical is unusual in that it actually accumulates in breast tissue, and animal studies have shown that it can inhibit breast tumor growth. A clinical trial in Milan, Italy, was set up for early stage breast cancer patients to determine whether fenretinide could reduce the likelihood of cancer in the opposite breast. This is an important issue because history has shown that about 8% of women with curable breast cancer will go on to develop cancer in the contralateral breast within 10 years. As of mid-1993, 2,969 women with Stage I breast cancer have been enrolled and randomized to receive either fenretinide or no treatment. Women will receive the drug for five years and will be followed for an additional two years to determine whether fenretinide is able to reduce the incidence of contralateral breast cancer.

Fenretinide has been in a second clinical trial in Milan, to determine whether it can reduce the rate of recurrence in patients treated for oral leukoplakia.[42] This clinical trial has thus far enrolled 153 patients, half of whom receive fenretinide for one year and half of whom are untreated. All patients undergo frequent examination of the lesion site and receive counseling designed to help them to stop smoking and drinking. After a follow-up of one year, preliminary results show that 30% of the control patients relapse, whereas only 6% of the fenretinide-treated patients relapse or develop new leukoplakias. The drug is well-tolerated, and the only side effect reported was a mild-to-moderate loss of ability to dark-adapt the eyes, which affected 49% of patients. However, this symptom promptly reversed upon discontinuation of drug use.

Another drug, known as finasteramide or Proscar, has been tested as a chemopreventive agent for benign disease of the prostate, in hope that this agent might eventually also be used to reduce the incidence of prostate cancer.[43] This drug blocks the action of testosterone within the prostate, yet it appears to have no effect on male libido, potency, musculature, or other secondary sexual characteristics. Finasteramide was tested as a treatment for benign prostatic hyperplasia, a disease which is characterized by painless enlargement of the prostate gland with urinary obstruction.[44] A group of 895 men with prostatic hyperplasia was enrolled in a double-blind study, which means that neither the patients nor the physicians knew which drug each patient received until the study was over. Finasteramide was tested against inactive placebo in these men, with drugs administered daily, and the men were followed prospectively for a year. During the study period, urinary symptoms, urinary flow rate, prostatic volume, and blood concentrations of testosterone and prostate-specific antigen (PSA) were measured periodically. Men treated with finasteramide (5 milligrams/day) had a significant decrease in urinary tract symptoms, a 22% increase in urinary flow rate, and a 19% decrease in prostate volume. Men treated with placebo had no change in symptoms and only a 3% decrease in prostate volume. However, finasteramide treatment was also associated with about a 3% higher incidence of impotence, decreased sex drive, and ejaculatory disorders. These side effects were less severe at low doses of finasteramide (1 mg/day), a dose level that was still able to decrease prostate volume about 18%. Levels of PSA also declined about 50% during finasteramide treatment.[45] This could potentially cause some confusion if PSA is used to screen for cancer in men with prostatic hyperplasia. A small fraction of men progressed to prostate cancer while receiving finasteramide, and these men tended to show less change in PSA levels during treatment.

Finasteramide can thus induce regression of benign prostatic hyperplasia, but it is not yet clear whether this translates into a decreased risk of prostate cancer. To address this question, a large prostate cancer prevention trial was launched in the fall of 1993.[46] Researchers plan to enroll 18,000 men, aged 55 and older, in 40 states across the United States, at a total cost of $60 million. Participants will receive either finasteramide (5 mg/day) or placebo daily for seven years, and prostate cancer incidence will be compared in the two groups at the end of the study. This study will also evaluate the prostate-specific antigen (PSA) test and the digital rectal examination as screening tests for prostate cancer.

Another drug that has received recent attention as a potential chemo-preventive agent is sulindac (also called Clinoril), which may protect against colon cancer.[47] This drug is able to induce the regression of precancerous lesions of the colon, called polyps, which are benign growths on the wall of the intestine that tend to become malignant. A hereditary condition known as familial adenomatous polyposis (FAP) is characterized by the formation of hundreds of colorectal polyps in young adults, and virtually all patients with FAP develop colorectal cancer by their 50s unless they undergo prophylactic surgery to remove their colon. Because FAP has such a strong tendency to progress to colorectal cancer at a relatively young age, FAP patients are good candidates for a colorectal cancer prevention effort. A group of 22 young patients with FAP was randomized to receive either sulindac or inactive placebo daily for nine months, during which time the number and size of polyps were monitored at regular intervals. Sulindac treatment was found to cause a significant reduction in polyp number and size; among treated patients, the number of polyps decreased by 56%, the size of the polyps decreased by an average of 65%, and no side effects were noted. However, no patient was cured of polyps by sulindac treatment, and three months after treatment was stopped, the number and size of polyps had increased, although they had not returned to pretreat-ment values. Therefore, sulindac cannot replace surgical removal of the colon as primary therapy for FAP, but it could perhaps find a role in colorectal cancer prevention in persons who do not have FAP.[48] It is worth noting that sulindac is a nonsteroidal anti-inflammatory drug, as is aspirin.

Frequent aspirin use may be associated with a substantial reduction in mortality from cancers of the esophagus, stomach, colon, and rectum.[49] Death rates were approximately 40% lower for each of these cancers among persons who used aspirin regularly (at least 16 times a month for a year), compared to persons who used no aspirin. Persons with rheumatoid arthritis, who frequently use aspirin to control joint pain, have also been noted to have about a 33% lower risk of colorectal cancer.[50] Aspirin is thought also to reduce the death rate from cardiovascular disease, so a prospective study of aspirin use and heart disease was undertaken in 1982, and data from this study have been used to examine the relationship between aspirin use and cancer.[51] A group of 22,071 male physicians, aged 40 to 84 in 1982, was enrolled in the Physicians Health Study and they were randomized to receive either low-dose aspirin, beta-carotene, both, or neither, with appropriate placebos so that the study was double-blinded. Individuals were kept on their respective treatment for five years, then the incidence of cancer was evaluated from medical records. No significant difference was found between aspirin-treated and placebo-treated men, in terms of either advanced colorectal cancer or early stage colorectal cancer. This result suggests that aspirin, at a low-dose rate adequate to prevent myocardial infarction, does not prevent colorectal cancer.

However, this study was criticized because the period of follow-up was fairly short, given that colorectal cancer is believed to be a rather slow-growing tumor.[52] Any colorectal tumors detected during the first few years of the study were almost certainly present when the study began, therefore aspirin use could not possibly have prevented these cancers. Therefore a longer follow-up period is required to determine whether aspirin can actually prevent colorectal cancer. Furthermore, aspirin was found to cause gastrointestinal bleeding in some men. Colorectal cancers would be more likely to be detected in these men because they would be fully evaluated for gastrointestinal disease. Therefore, aspirin use may introduce a detection bias, so that incident cancer would be diagnosed more often in aspirin-users than among placebo-users. While the Physicians Health Study can provide no evidence of a protective effect from aspirin, it would be premature to discount this effect, given that epidemiological studies show a profound protective effect from aspirin use.[53]

The last chemopreventive agent about which much is known, from a clinical standpoint, is calcium, which is believed to be protective from colon cancer risk.[54] Early evidence suggested that elemental calcium could reduce the rate of colon cell growth in certain persons at high familial risk of colon cancer. However, a recent randomized, double-blind, placebo-controlled clinical trial was unable to confirm that calcium has any effect on the rate of colon cell growth.[55] A small group of 21 subjects was randomized to receive either supplemental calcium (1.2 gram/day) or an inactive placebo drug, and neither patient nor physician was aware of which drug each volunteer took until the experiment was over. Each case and control patient was treated for eight weeks, then the rate of growth of cells in the colon was measured in both cases and controls. This study found no significant decrease in the rate of cell growth associated with calcium treatment; in fact, calcium seemed to have the opposite effect, but the change was not large enough to be significant. While we have intriguing experimental data showing that calcium depresses the rate of colon cell growth in rats, this recent study does not suggest that calcium has any effect in humans. However, it may be that the dose of calcium used was simply too low, as a recent review suggests that calcium can be administered at a dose of 2 grams per day, without any significant toxicity to humans.[56]

SUMMARY

It is not yet clear whether nutritional intervention, using supplements of naturally occurring vitamins and minerals, will be effective in reducing cancer incidence. The relative lack of efficacy in numerous studies could occur for many reasons, but an obvious possibility is that we simply have an inadequate understanding of dietary risk factors and dietary protective factors. Another possibility is that the chemical form of vitamins and minerals in vitamin supplements may be incorrect, so that the supplements are not as effective as the naturally occurring vitamin or mineral. For example, perhaps some carotenoid other than beta-carotene is most effective in reducing cancer incidence. Epidemiological studies have shown that high levels of dietary beta-carotene are associated with protection from cancer, but perhaps beta-carotene is simply a marker for another, more effective, dietary component that we haven't yet discovered. Alternatively, the beta-carotene given in vitamin supplements may not be well-absorbed because of the absence of some other nutrient, or it may be broken down during digestion unless it is somehow protected. In short, we have a great deal to learn about vitamins and minerals. In the absence of sure knowledge, it is wise to consume vitamins and minerals in the form we know them to be effective: fresh fruits and vegetables.

Chemoprevention studies have been a tantalizing topic of investigation for many years. Yet a growing number of agents has been identified that are effective in experimental animals but ineffective in humans. This may mean that animal models of cancer are not always an adequate indicator of drug efficacy in humans, or that our normal exposure to carcinogens is so frequent and so extreme that minor chemopreventive effects are completely camouflaged. For example, calcium protects from colon cancer in laboratory rats, but lab rats are typically fed a balanced diet low in saturated fats. Perhaps, if rats were fed a diet that more closely reflects the average human diet, high in saturated fats and fatty acids, any protective effect of calcium would be overwhelmed. Thus, while no clinical trial of a chemopreventive agent can yet claim major success, it would be premature to stop research in chemoprevention.

NOTES TO CHAPTER 15

1. W.J. Blot, J-Y. Li, P.R. Taylor, W. Guo, S. Dawsey, et al., "Nutritional intervention trials in Linxian, China: Supplementation

with specific vitamin/mineral combinations, cancer incidence, and disease-specific mortality in the general population," *J. Natl. Cancer Instit.* 85 (1993): 1483–1491.

2. *Ibid.*
3. *Ibid.*
4. J-Y. Li, P.R. Taylor, B. Li, S. Dawsey, G-Q. Wang, et al., "Nutritional intervention trials in Linxian, China: Multiple vitamin/mineral supplementation, cancer incidence, and disease-specific mortality among adults with esophageal dysplasia," *J. Natl. Cancer Instit.* 85 (1993): 1492–1498.
5. *Ibid.*
6. H.S. Garewal, F. Meyskens, "Retinoids and carotenoids in the prevention of oral cancer: a critical appraisal," *Cancer Epidemiol. Biomarkers Prev.* 1 (1992): 155–159.
7. *Ibid.*
8. E.R. Greenberg, J.A. Baron, T.A. Stukel, M.M. Stevens, J.S. Mandel, et al,. "A clinical trial of beta carotene to prevent basal-cell and squamous-cell cancers of the skin," *N. Engl. J. Med.* 323 (1990): 789–795.
9. *Ibid.*
10. O.P. Heinonen, D. Albanes, and the Alpha-tocopherol Beta-carotene Cancer Prevention Study Group, "The effect of Vitamin E and beta-carotene on the incidence of lung cancer and other cancers in male smokers," *N. Engl. J. Med.* 330 (1994): 1029–1035.
11. *Ibid.*
12. G.S. Omenn, G. Goodman, M. Thornquist, J. Grizzle, L. Rosenstock, et al., "The beta-carotene and retinol efficacy trial (CARET) for chemoprevention of lung cancer in high risk populations: smokers and asbestos-exposed workers," *Cancer Res.* 54 (1994): 2038s–2043s.
13. D.J. Hunter, J.E. Manson, G.A. Colditz, M.J. Stampfer, B. Rosner, et al., "A prospective study of the intake of vitamins C, E, and A on the risk of breast cancer," *New Engl. J. Med.* 329 (1993): 234–240.
14. *Ibid.*
15. R.M. Bostick, J.D. Potter, D.R. McKenzie, T.A. Sellers, L.H. Kushi, et al., "Reduced risk of colon cancer with high intake of Vitamin E: The Iowa Women's Health Study," *Cancer Res.* 53 (1993): 4230–4237.
16. D.C. Heimburger, C.B. Alexander, R. Birch, C.E. Butterworth, W.C. Bailey, C.L. Krumdieck, "Improvement in bronchial squamous metaplasia in smokers treated with folate and Vitamin B12," *J. Amer. Med. Assoc.* 259 (1988): 1525–1530.

17. *Ibid.*
18. Bostick, "Reduced risk of colon cancer with high intake Vitamin E," 4230–4237.
19. *Ibid.*
20. S.J. London, E.A. Stein, I.C. Henderson, M.J. Stampfer, W.C. Wood, et al., "Carotenoids, retinol, and vitamin E and risk of proliferative benign breast disease and breast cancer," *Cancer Causes Control* 3 (1992): 503–512.
21. *Ibid.*
22. S.E. Benner, R.J. Winn, S.M. Lippman, J. Poland, K.S. Hansen, et al., "Regression of oral leukoplakia with alpha-tocopherol: a Community Clinical Oncology Program chemoprevention study," *J. Natl. Cancer Instit.* 85 (1993): 44–47.
23. *Ibid.*
24. S.E. Benner, M.J. Wargovich, S.M. Lippman, R. Fisher, M. Velasco, et al., "Reduction in oral mucosa micronuclei frequency following alpha-tocopherol treatment of oral leukoplakia," *Cancer Epidemiol. Biomarkers Prev.* 3 (1994): 73–76.
25. Heinonen, "The effect of Vitamin E and beta-carotene on the incidence of lung cancer and other cancers in male smokers," 1029–1035.
26. *Ibid.*
27. G.M. Paganelli, G. Biasco, G. Brandi, R. Santucci, G. Gizzi, et al., "Effect of vitamin A, C, and E supplementation in rectal cell proliferation in patients with colorectal adenomas," *J. Natl. Cancer Instit.* 84 (1992): 47–51.
28. G.J. Kelloff, C.W. Boone, J.A. Crowell, V.E. Steele, R. Lubet, C.C. Sigman. "Chemopreventive drug development: perspectives and progress," *Cancer Epidemiol. Biomarkers Prev.* 3 (1994): 85–98.
29. T. Ohnuma, J.F. Holland, "Chemotherapy from animals to man" in *Fundamental aspects of Cancer*, R.H. Goldfarb, editor. (Boston: Kluwer Academic Publishers, 1989) 171–191.
30. L.W. Wattenberg, "Prevention-therapy-basic science and the resolution of the cancer problem," *Cancer Res.* 53 (1993): 5890–5896.
31. Kelloff, "Chemopreventive drug development," 85–98.
32. W.K. Hong, S.M. Lippman, G.T. Wolf, "Recent advances in head and neck cancer—Larynx preservation and cancer chemoprevention," *Cancer Res.* 53 (1993): 5113–5120.
33. S.M. Lippman, J.G. Batsakis, B.B. Toth, R.S. Weber, J.J. Lee, et al., "Comparison of low-dose isotretinoin with beta carotene to prevent oral carcinogenesis," *N. Engl. J. Med.* 328 (1993): 15–20.
34. Hong, "Recent advances in head and neck cancer," 5113–5120.

35. W.K. Hong, S.M. Lippman, L.M. Itri, D.D. Karp, J.S. Lee, et al., "Prevention of second primary tumors with isotretinoin in squamous-cell carcinoma of the head and neck," *N. Engl. J. Med.* 323 (1990): 795–801.

36. *Ibid.*

37. S.E. Benner, T.F. Pajak, S.M, Lippman, C. Earley, W.K. Hong, "Prevention of second primary tumors with isotretinoin in patients with squamous cell carcinoma of the head and neck: long-term follow-up," *J. Natl. Cancer Instit.* 86 (1994): 140–141.

38. J.A. Tangrea, B.K. Edwards, P.R. Taylor, A.M. Hartman, G.L. Peck, et al., "Long-term therapy with low-dose isotretinoin for prevention of basal cell carcinoma: a multicenter clinical trial," *J. Natl. Cancer Instit.* 84 (1992): 328–332.

39. Hong, "Recent advances in head and neck cancer," 5113–5120.

40. S.M. Lippman, W.K. Hong, "Not yet standard: retinoids versus second primary tumors," *J. Clin. Oncol.* 11 (1993): 1204–1207.

41. A. Costa, F. Formelli, F. Chiesa, A. Decensi, G. De Palo, U. Veronesi, "Prospects of chemoprevention of human cancers with the synthetic retinoid fenretinide," *Cancer Res.* 53 (1994): 2032s–2037s.

42. *Ibid.*

43. R.S. Rittmaster, "Finasteride," *N. Engl. J. Med.* 330 (1994): 120–125.

44. G.J. Gormley, E. Stoner, R.C. Bruskewitz, J. Imperato-McGinley, P.C. Walsh, et al., "The effect of finasteride in men with benign prostatic hyperplasia," *N. Engl. J. Med.* 327 (1992): 1185–1191.

45. H.A. Guess, J.F. Heyse, G.J. Gormley, "The effect of finasteride on prostate-specific antigen in men with benign prostatic hyperplasia," *Prostate* 22 (1993): 31–37.

46. T. Reynolds, "Prostate cancer prevention trial launched," *J. Natl. Cancer Instit.* 85 (1993): 1633–1634.

47. F.M. Giardello, S.R. Hamilton, A.J. Krush, S. Piantodosi, L.M. Hylind, et al., "Treatment of colonic and rectal adenomas with sulindac in familial adenomatous polyposis," *N. Engl. J. Med.* 328 (1993): 1313–1316.

48. *Ibid.*

49. M.J. Thun, M.M. Namboodiri, E.E. Calle, W.D. Flanders, C.W. Heath, "Aspirin use and risk of fatal cancer," *Cancer Res.* 53 1(993): 1322–1327.

50. G. Gridley, J.K. McLaughlin, A. Ekbom, L. Klareskog, H-O. Adami, et al., "Incidence of cancer among patients with rheumatoid arthritis," *J. Natl. Cancer Instit.* 85 (1993): 307–311.

51. P.H. Gann, J.E. Manson, R.J. Glynn, J.E. Buring, C.H. Hennekens, "Low-dose aspirin and incidence of colorectal tumors in a randomized trial," *J. Natl. Cancer Instit.* 85 (1993) 1220–1224.
52. E.R. Greenberg, J.A. Baron, "Prospects for preventing colorectal cancer death," *J. Natl. Cancer Instit.* 85 (1993): 1182–1183.
53. Thun, "Asprin use and risk of fatal cancer," 1322–1327.
54. Kelloff, "Chemopreventive drug development," 85–98.
55. R.M. Bostick, J.D. Potter, L. Fosdick, P. Grambsch, J.W. Lampe, et al., "Calcium and colorectal epithelial cell proliferation: a preliminary randomized, double-blinded, placebo-controlled, clinical trial," *J. Natl. Cancer Instit.* 85 (1993): 132–141.
56. Kelloff, "Chemopreventive drug development," 85–98.
57. *Ibid.*
58. Wattenberg, "Preventive-therapy-basic science and the resolution of the cancer problem," 5890–5896.

16

HORMONAL AND
OTHER METHODS OF
CANCER PREVENTION

The preceding chapter discussed some fairly controversial approaches to cancer prevention, all of which remain unproven and many of which are considered extreme or very aggressive by some people. This chapter will consider several other unconventional approaches to cancer prevention that are likely to be considered extreme or aggressive even by comparison with the preceding approaches. However, it should be remembered that certain cancers are strongly familial, and this can create a crushing burden of anxiety and dread in otherwise healthy people. A person who has been aware of his or her own heightened risk of cancer for their entire adult life may view some of the following measures as less extreme than one who has not felt the same burden of anxiety.

HORMONAL PREVENTION OF CANCER

There is a clear association between exposure to estrogen and risk of breast cancer, which argues strongly that the female hormones have a profound effect on breast cancer risk. Therefore, manipulation of hormonal levels by the administration of drugs would be expected to reduce the incidence of breast cancer.[1] This is not as extreme an approach as it might seem, since women have been undergoing pharmacological manipulation of their hormones for a long time as a way to block conception. Since hormones are a risk factor for breast and many other cancers, hormonal manipulation is simply a way to reduce risk factor exposure. The validity of this approach is shown by the fact that women who take currently available oral contraceptives for more than five years reduce their risk of uterine and ovarian cancer roughly by half.

But oral contraceptives or oral hormone supplements can be formulated to further reduce the risk of those cancers that are hormone dependent,

355

including cancers of the breast, uterine endometrium, ovary, and even the prostate.[2] In fact, a number of hormonal cancer preventive agents are already in clinical trials (Table 16-1). Finasteride, discussed in the preceding chapter, could legitimately by included in this discussion, since it reduces the effect of testosterone on the prostate. However, it does this indirectly, by inhibiting an enzyme, rather than directly, by blocking a hormone receptor or some similar mechanism.

The effect of currently available oral contraceptive (OC) use on the risk of ovarian and endometrial cancer has already been discussed (Chapter 9), and that discussion will not be repeated. However, long-term OC use does give substantial protection from cancer of the uterine endometrium, the ovary, and perhaps the breast. When one compares the incidence and mortality rate for three hormone-related cancers in 1973–1974, and in 1986–1987 (Table 16-2), a decline in both incidence and mortality becomes apparent.[3] This comparison has been adjusted to show specifically cancer incidence and mortality for women under age 50, because women of this age in 1973–1974 could not have used OCs during most of their childbearing years (OCs did not become available until 1962). By contrast, women who were under age 50 in 1986–1987 would have had access to OCs for most of their reproductive life, since OCs became available when these women were in their early 20s. In fact, about 60% of women under age 50 in 1986–1987 used OCs for at least five years.[4] Therefore, reduction in cancer incidence may well be due to widespread use of OCs.

This chapter will focus primarily on new formulations or combinations of oral hormones that may be able to modulate hormonal risk factor exposure; it is almost incidental that most such new formulations will also act as contraceptives. Most contraceptives currently available in the United

TABLE 16-1
HORMONAL AGENTS THAT PREVENT CANCER AND THAT ARE
ALREADY IN CLINICAL TRIALS[52]

HORMONAL AGENT	PROTECTED SITE	MECHANISM OF ACTION
Oral contraceptives	Uterine endometrium	Block estrogen effect
	Ovary	Inhibit ovulation
Gonadotropin-releasing hormone blocker	Breast, endometrium	Inhibit ovarian hormone synthesis
	Ovary	Inhibit ovulation
Hormone replacement therapy with progestogens	Endometrium	Block estrogen effect
Tamoxifen	Breast	Block estrogen effect

TABLE 16-2 AGE-ADJUSTED INCIDENCE AND MORTALITY RATE (PER 1,000 WOMEN UNDER 50 YEARS OF AGE) FOR SEVERAL HORMONE-RELATED CANCERS					
	INCIDENCE RATE Average			MORTALITY RATE Average		
Cancer site	1973–1974	1986–1987	Change	1973–1974	1986–1987	Change
Ovary	4.8	3.9	−20%	1.9	1.2	−37%
Endometrium	5.1	3.7	−28%	0.5	0.3	−44%
Breast	30.6	33.6	+10%	6.9	6.4	−8%

Most cancers have shown a decline in incidence and all have shown a decline in mortality that may be correlated with widespread use of OCs.

States are combination contraceptives, containing both an estrogen component and a high-dose progestogen, so that cells are exposed to "unopposed" estrogen only during the menstrual portion of the ovulatory cycle, when OCs are not taken. Scientists believe that the protective effect of OCs arises because estrogen is usually opposed by progestogen, so that estrogen-stimulated growth of tumor cells is minimized. However, it is also possible to make an OC that contains very little estrogen, that uses instead a gonadotropin-releasing hormone (GnRH) blocker to achieve the same effect by inhibiting ovulation and reducing the production of ovarian hormones.

Recently a small clinical trial of a GnRH blocker was reported, in which a GnRH blocker was combined with other hormones in a specific formulation designed to reduce the risk of breast cancer as well as the risk of endometrial and ovarian cancer.[5] This trial involved only 18 women, all of whom had at least a five-fold higher risk of breast cancer because of family history. This was not a double-blind study; women were randomly assigned, so that experimental subjects received the prototype contraceptive (with GnRH, estrogen, and progestogen components), while control subjects received no medication. Women were treated for an average of four months, although some were treated for as long as one year. During this time, several important parameters were monitored including: tolerance of, and compliance with, the somewhat complicated hormone regimen, and the effect of hormones on the the pattern of vaginal bleeding, bone density, and lipid metabolism.

Women who were treated with the GnRH blocker reported fewer unpleasant menstrual symptoms than usual, due to elimination of most of the symptoms of premenstrual syndrome.[6] The pattern of menstrual flow was largely maintained during treatment, and there was also a beneficial rise in high-density lipoprotein (HDL) cholesterol, which could potentially protect against heart disease. However, women who received the GnRH blocker also suffered a loss of about 2% of their bone density per year, which could cumulatively become important as a risk factor for osteoporosis. In addition, about 18% of women reported a slight diminution of sex drive. Overall, this study showed that women tolerated the GnRH blocker very well, although there may have been some unanticipated costs as well as benefits. But this study did not attempt to answer the question of whether or not a GnRH blocker regimen could actually reduce the risk of breast cancer. This could only be determined from a clinical trial that enrolled a much larger number of women, followed them for a much longer time in a prospective manner, and was blinded so that neither the subjects nor their physicians knew who was receiving the treatment. The current work should be regarded as a Phase I trial, which now makes it possible to begin Phase II and Phase III testing.

A clinical trial of a GnRH blocker seems warranted at this point, because the theory suggesting a protective effect from breast cancer is fairly strong and because side effects of treatment are rather minimal.[7] It has been estimated that this hormone regimen could reduce lifetime breast cancer risk by 31% if used for five years, 47% if used for 10 years, and 70% if used for 15 years. The protection offered against ovarian cancer by a GnRH blocker should be similar to that of current OCs, or about a 41% reduction in risk with five years use, 65% reduction if used for 10 years, and 79% if used for 15 years. Finally, the GnRH blocker should also protect against uterine endometrial cancer, reducing risk about 18% if used for five years, 33% if used for ten years, and 45% if used for 15 years. This is a lower level of protection than afforded by current OCs, but because endometrial cancer has a low mortality rate, this may be an acceptable trade-off for a reduced risk of breast cancer. However, much work remains to be done; a more convenient formulation is required that involves oral (not injectable) hormone supplementation, and, more important, these preliminary results must be confirmed in a real clinical trial.

Hormone replacement therapy (HRT) has been used in the past to reduce menopausal symptoms and to protect from the consequences of estrogen deficiency (e.g., heart disease, osteoporosis). However, it is becoming clear that HRT could also be used to reduce the risk of endometrial cancer, although this is not a simple matter.[8] HRT with estrogen alone is thought to be responsible for an increase in the incidence of endometrial cancer in the 1960s and 1970s. When progestogen was added to estrogen, in a newer formulation for HRT, the incidence of endometrial cancer declined, but the incidence of breast cancer actually increased. This complicated picture of changing risks makes it impossible to recommend HRT for long-term therapy of post-menopausal women. Although HRT with estrogen can reduce all-cause mortality by as much as 20% (largely due to a decrease in cardiovascular disease deaths), the increase in risk of breast cancer appears to be substantial (about 2% higher risk per year of HRT use).

Hormonal prevention of cancer may also become possible using a drug called tamoxifen, which is an anti-estrogen agent that blocks cellular responses to estrogen. Tamoxifen has achieved striking success in the treatment of breast cancer, and it is possible that it could also reduce the risk of breast cancer in healthy women.[9] The most convincing argument for using tamoxifen to prevent breast cancer has come from a study of breast cancer risk in women who were already being treated for breast cancer.[10] A meta-analysis, which pooled the results of many separate studies, surveyed a total of 4,975 women with breast cancer who received tamoxifen as treatment, and compared them to a total of 4,971 women who did not receive tamoxifen. Analysis of the incidence of cancer in the opposite breast showed that women treated with tamoxifen had a 35% lower incidence of a second breast tumor. Tamoxifen treatment was well tolerated, as there were minimal harmful side effects during the study and several good ones. Tamoxifen preserved bone density, which should reduce the risk of osteoporosis, and it lowered serum cholesterol by about 20%, which might reduce the risk of death from coronary heart disease by as much as 40%. Furthermore, it also seemed to decrease the incidence of cancers of the ovary, urinary tract, and respiratory system. However, there was an increase in risk of endometrial cancer, in symptoms of menopause, and in risk of thrombophlebitis. Especially for those women who are at an elevated risk of breast cancer due to family history, the risks of tamoxifen may be negligible compared to the benefits.[11]

A very strong interest has been expressed in tamoxifen as a breast cancer preventive agent, because it seems to be protective against a major killer for which few other preventive measures are known.[12] The "Clinical Trial to Determine the Worth of Tamoxifen for Preventing Breast Cancer" was initiated in 1992, as a part of the Women's Health Initiative. This clinical trial is scheduled to enroll a total of 16,000 women, to randomize these women to receive either tamoxifen or a placebo, and to follow case and control women for five years. Although women at relatively high risk of breast cancer are to be preferentially enrolled, this study has still been very controversial because of the various side effects of tamoxifen treatment. Tamoxifen treatment of healthy post-menopausal women is predicted to reduce breast cancer risk by 2% per year of treatment.[13] However, very recently[14] several new objections were raised to this trial. Tamoxifen may increase the risk of endometrial cancer about three-fold, which is more than was previously known, and tamoxifen-induced cancers may also be more aggressive than normal. Nevertheless, breast cancer prevention is such a compelling goal that tamoxifen may be judged worthwhile as an intervention even if the risk of endometrial cancer is substantially higher. This is particularly true given that tamoxifen is also protective against heart disease.

SURGICAL PREVENTION OF CANCER

Surgery in a very aggressive approach to cancer prevention, which can only be justified under very special circumstances. Yet the medical need for surgical prevention of colon cancer is well-accepted in some cases, even though surgical prevention can involve prophylactic removal of the entire colon and much of the rectum. This is because a hereditary condition, called familial adenomatous polyposis (FAP), very strongly predisposes an afflicted individual to develop colorectal cancer. FAP is characterized by the presence of huge numbers of polyps (mushroom-like stalked growths) throughout the colon. These begin to grow early in childhood and often 1,000 or more polyps have developed by adulthood. Each polyp is initially benign, but the sheer number of polyps means that transformation from benign to malignant is almost certain to occur in one or more polyps. The probability of colon cancer occurring in affected individuals approaches 100% by the age of 40. In addition, sporadic cases of FAP are occasionally diagnosed with no family history of the disease, showing that this condition can arise spontaneously. The only reliable way for affected individuals to avoid colon cancer is to undergo total colectomy and ileostomy, or the surgical excision of the entire colon and rectum, together with establishment of an artificial opening through which intestinal contents are emptied. Because the risk of colorectal cancer is so high in patients with FAP, colectomy is the only established treatment for the disease.

Prophylactic mastectomy as a surgical preventive measure for breast cancer is considerably more controversial than is colectomy. Again, the rationale for surgery is that certain women are at a greatly elevated risk of breast cancer because of a family history of disease. For example, a gene known as BRCA1 was recently identified that, when mutated, confers a lifetime risk of breast cancer that approaches 85%.[15] This means that 85% of women with the BRCA1 mutation will develop breast cancer during their lifetime, a level of risk that is nearly eight-fold higher than normal. Many women identified with the BRCA1 mutation find that living with this level of anxiety is intolerable, and several have opted for a prophylactic bilateral mastectomy. This can only be justified when there is a greatly elevated risk of disease and when fear of the disease is becoming disabling, and this measure is more justifiable if breast tissue is dense and therefore difficult to image during a mammographic examination.

For women who elect to have prophylactic bilateral mastectomy, the type of mastectomy to have is also controversial.[16] Subcutaneous mastectomy, which preserves the nipple and areolus, does not remove all breast tissue and so does not prevent the development of breast cancer. The risk of breast cancer after this surgery is unknown, since this question is relevant to a small number of women and there has never been adequate follow-up of those patients who chose this operation. Most surgeons prefer total or radical mastectomy, with cosmetic reconstruction of the breast done simultaneously or subsequently. A woman weighing these alternatives must consider the balance between living with extremely high cancer risk versus living with relatively low cancer risk but personal and physical consequences of surgery. While reconstructive surgery is often very good at hiding the trauma of mastectomy, the cosmetic results are not always satisfactory.

Prophylactic ovariectomy, or surgical removal of the ovaries, is a very controversial preventive measure for ovarian cancer.[17] The factors that weigh in favor of prophylactic surgery are compelling—the risk of ovarian cancer is elevated about 20-fold for women with a close relative with this cancer, yet it is a very difficult cancer to diagnose, and those screening tests that are currently available are relatively ineffective. Ovarian cancer is usually diagnosed in a relatively late stage when the chances of cure are poor. Yet several major factors weigh against prophylactic ovariectomy. For pre-menopausal women, ovariectomy without estrogen replacement therapy will lead to the abrupt onset of menopausal symptoms, including decreased secondary sex characteristics and increased risk of heart disease and osteoporosis. Furthermore, estrogen replacement therapy can increase the relative risk of breast cancer. Finally, there are reports of women who believed they had undergone ovariectomy but who developed ovarian cancer nonetheless, either because the surgery was incomplete or because cancer developed in "developmentally misplaced" ovarian tissue. In women past childbearing who have an elevated familial risk of ovarian cancer, prophylactic ovariectomy may be worth considering. Although bilateral ovariectomy may reduce the risk of breast cancer substantially, it is also possible that the same results could be achieved by hormonal treatments.[18]

A much less radical surgical alternative that also leads to a significant reduction in ovarian cancer risk is tubal ligation.[19] A recent prospective study that involved 121,700 women found that tubal ligation, which is usually used for contraception, also led to a 67% reduction in risk of ovarian cancer. Tubal ligation was more effective than hysterectomy in reducing ovarian cancer risk, as hysterectomy only reduced ovarian cancer risk by 33%. While ovariectomy should reduce ovarian cancer risk by close to 100%, this is a fairly invasive procedure compared to tubal ligation. It is unknown why tubal ligation should have such a profound effect on the risk of ovarian cancer, but this study was large, well-designed, and prospective, so the results can presumably be trusted. Thus, tubal ligation may provide a very attractive alternative for a woman worried about her risk of ovarian cancer. Since about 21 million women have already undergone tubal ligation, this may explain why the incidence of this cancer has declined slightly in recent years. Tubal ligation, or more properly tubal sterilization, is easily performed during a Caesarian section or during any other operation when the abdomen is opened. In addition, tubal sterilization can also be performed by laparoscopic surgery ("video surgery"), so that hospital expenses, convalescence, and surgical scarring are all minimized.

VACCINE PREVENTION OF CANCER

Vaccine prevention of cancer is a concept that would have seemed ridiculous only a few years ago. But several recent conceptual and technical developments make this strategy seem much more reasonable now than before. One of the foremost considerations is that vaccines have been more successful than antiviral therapy in lessening the harmful effect of viruses. This is because vaccination is often effective in preventing viral infection, while therapies are very rarely effective in controlling an established infection. To the extent that human cancers are caused by viruses, antiviral vaccination will probably have good success at cancer prevention.

Most likely, the first successful vaccine against cancer will be a vaccine that has been developed against the hepatitis B virus (HBV), one of the major causes of liver cancer in the Far East and in Africa.[20] Particularly in China, chronic HBV infection occurs at birth, as 90% of infants born to an HBV-positive mother will become infected. Intervention at this point is critical, because once a chronic infection is established, it persists for life. After an average of 20 years, HBV infection produces cirrhosis in 40% of patients, with symptoms of progressive loss of liver function. A substantial fraction of patients with cirrhosis go on to develop hepatocellular carcinoma, or liver cancer, beginning in their 40s. In Taiwan, it has been estimated that as many as 50% of men infected with HBV will die of either cirrhosis or liver cancer.

Vaccination against HBV can prevent transmission of the virus from infected mother to child, so that the incidence of chronic HBV infection is reduced as much as 85%.[21] Currently, 47 countries have instituted national immunization policies that include HBV vaccination of infants. One of the first such programs, instituted in Taiwan in 1984, involved vaccination of all infants and children, and the incidence of HBV infection dropped from more than 10% to less than 2% in only nine years. Data are being collected from mothers and vaccinated children to determine whether HBV vaccination is actually able to reduce the incidence of liver cancer. If so, this would be the first time in history that a mass vaccination program was able to prevent human cancer.[22] The Gambia was the first African nation to institute a mass vaccination program for HBV, and this effort has been rewarded with a stunning decline in the rate of HBV infection.[23] A group of 720 children aged three to four who received the HBV vaccine was compared to a group of 816 children who did not receive the vaccination. It was found that 29% of children who did not receive the vaccine became infected with HBV, while only 5% of vaccinated children became infected. The vaccine was 84% effective against transient viral infection and 94% effective in preventing the development of chronic infection. This offers real hope for the prevention of liver cancer in adulthood, since virtually all cases of liver cancer begin with HBV infection.

Another potential target for a mass vaccination effort is the human papilloma virus (HPV), which is a major cause of cervical cancer. One study concluded that HPV infection accounted for at least 76% of all cases of cervical cancer in the United States.[24] HPV infection probably occurs during sexual intercourse, but most women are infected by the time they reach 15 to 19 years old, so HPV vaccination should occur at a young age.[25] No large-scale vaccination efforts for HPV have yet been reported, but efforts may well be under way to develop such a vaccine.

Infection with a bacterium known as *Heliocobacter pylori* is thought to be responsible for up to 60% of all stomach cancers in the world.[26] Infection with *H. pylori* is very common, as about 50% of adults in North America are infected and virtually 100% of adults are infected in many developing nations. Although *H. pylori* infection is curable with antibiotic therapy, it is quite likely that a cured individual would quickly become reinfected, since the proportion of infected adults is so high. Therefore, it may be reasonable to propose vaccination as a preventive measure for *H. pylori* infection and gastric cancer. This is potentially very difficult because the immune system, which is responsible for long-term immunity to a virus or bacterium, is most effective at dealing with those disease-causing agents to which it has direct access. The *H. pylori* bacterium normally resides on the stomach lining, which is topologically external to the body. Therefore immune system access to the bacterium may be limited. However, antibodies are normally secreted into the digestive tract, and antibodies directed against *H. pylori* were found in about 96% of infected individuals.[27] Therefore, it is possible that the immune system could be stimulated by a vaccine to mount an attack against *H. pylori*.

Research into a vaccine against *H. pylori* will likely not be driven by an effort to eradicate stomach cancer, since infection with *H. pylori* is believed to be responsible for most ulcers. About 90% of the time ulcers are treated with the antiacids Tagamet or Zantac, yet these drugs are not very effective; the relapse rate for ulcers with conventional treatment is about 50% over six months, and as high as 95% over two years.[28] Yet, in 1992, these drugs accounted for $4.4 billion in total sales. Antibiotic treatment is generally more successful at curing ulcers, with a long-term recurrence rate less than 20%. Yet if vaccination against *H. pylori* is able to further reduce the recurrence rate of ulcers, this may mean that vaccination will become standard therapy. This, in turn, could have the benefit of reducing the incidence or mortality of stomach cancer.

Currently a number of vaccines are under development that are proposed as therapy for cancer.[29] Most of these vaccines are intended to stimulate the immune system to attack an established tumor, using crude extracts of tumor cells that are then injected back into the patient. However, a few of the vaccines under development are more sophisticated, and rely upon injection of antigens, or molecules, that are characteristic of a specific tumor type. For example, a gene was recently identified which codes for antigens present on the surface of melanoma cells, and these antigens are apparently not found elsewhere in the body. If it is possible to make an effective vaccine against an established melanoma, then it may be simply a matter of time before there is a process of generalization, so that therapeutic vaccines will eventually assume a preventive role.

RADIATION PREVENTION OF CANCER

Prophylactic radiation therapy has been used to prevent the development of cancer of the eye in certain children with familial retinoblastoma.[30] This again seems like a radical preventive measure, but the risk of retinal cancer in children with a mutated retinoblastoma gene approaches 95%. Therefore, any child of a parent with retinoblastoma is at very high risk of developing this cancer. If treated early the survival for this cancer is generally fairly good, but therapy can involve surgical removal of the affected eye. If a prophylactic measure could be developed that spared vision while being reasonably successful at preventing the development of cancer, this would become a very attractive alternative for children afflicted with retinoblastoma.

Radiation therapy has been used in the treatment of early stage retinoblastoma for more than a decade, with generally good results.[31] An effort is made to avoid irradiating the uninvolved eye, because patients with retinoblastoma appear to be at an elevated risk of radiation-induced cancer. However, even when the uninvolved eye is not irradiated, the incidence of second primary tumors in this eye is quite high. Therefore, if radiation can be shown to lessen the incidence of second primary tumors, without causing undue side effects, then the possibility of a radiation-induced tumor becomes less compelling. A small prospective study examined the effect of radiation therapy on the incidence of second primary tumors in infants with retinoblastoma. A total of 44 healthy appearing eyes were irradiated with external beam radiotherapy. The incidence of retinoblastoma in these eyes was compared to the incidence of retinoblastoma in a control group of 14 eyes that were not irradiated. It was found that 86% of the control eyes later developed retinoblastoma, which compares reasonably well with the 95% incidence of retinoblastoma in historical controls. Yet only 14% of the eyes that were irradiated later developed retinoblastoma, and the radiation technique was sufficiently advanced that very few side effects were reported. Prophylactic radiation therapy may thus be appropriate in certain infants at high risk of developing retinoblastoma, although it is unknown whether prophylactic radiation therapy will find a role in prevention of any other cancers.[32]

BIOLOGICAL PREVENTION OF CANCER

The principle of biological prevention of cancer is fairly simple: since certain cellular and genetic factors predispose to cancer, deliberate manipulation of these factors may suppress cancer. Thus, biological prevention can be defined as any cancer preventive strategy that acts primarily through the natural defense mechanisms of cells, or by the administration of substances that naturally occur in cells. There have already been several notable successes with cancer therapies based on biology: interferon-α is now the treatment of choice for hairy cell leukemia, hematopoietic growth factor is commonly used to augment red blood cell production in cancer patients undergoing chemotherapy, and interferon-α and interleukin-2 can be directly toxic to tumor cells.[33] But biological approaches to cancer prevention are quite novel, and few attempts have been made to investigate this type of cancer prevention. Biological prevention of cancer could be based upon modulation of the immune system, as we discussed in the section on cancer vaccination, or it could be based upon modulation of genes within cells, in a process called gene therapy. Modulation of the immune system is now better established than gene therapy in cancer treatment, but both approaches are evolving so rapidly that it is impossible to predict which will achieve more success in cancer prevention.

In gene therapy, mutated genes within cancer-prone cells could be specifically replaced by normal genes of the same type, or the expression of cancer-causing genes within cells could be specifically blocked. This might be accomplished using a newly developed technology called antisense RNA, which permits scientists to delete the function of a single gene within the living cell. The power of this technique was demonstrated recently in experiments using cultured human breast tumor cells. Researchers used a type of breast tumor cell that is dependent upon added estrogen to stimulate cell growth.[34] When estrogen is added to these cells, a gene known as c-*myc* is turned on. Yet when c-*myc* expression was specifically blocked in the tumor cells with antisense RNA, this also blocked cell growth in response to estrogen. Antisense RNA for c-*myc* even inhibited the growth of another type of breast tumor cell that is not normally dependent upon estrogen for growth. This suggests that c-*myc* expression may be required for growth of all breast tumor cells. Therefore, blocking expression of this gene might result in long-term suppression of tumor cell growth. These findings are potentially very important because c-*myc* amplification is present in about 27% of all human breast tumors, and c-*myc* amplification is generally correlated with poor long-term prognosis.[35]

Gene therapy could also be used to introduce new genes into healthy, noncancerous cells to augment the ability of those cells to resist cancerous transformation. Recently, scientists were able to introduce a gene for superoxide dismutase (SOD) into the cells of some fruit flies.[36] SOD is an enzyme that is able to detoxify a highly toxic chemical called superoxide, which is derived from oxygen. Superoxide can damage DNA, so if it is not detoxified, cells run the risk of becoming cancerous. When the expression of SOD within fruit fly cells was augmented, it was found that the flies lived about 33% longer than normal, and the degree of life extension was closely correlated with the level of expression of SOD. Flies with a 50% higher level of SOD expression also showed a lower level of oxidative damage of proteins and a delayed loss of physical performance. This probably occurred because augmentation of SOD within cells would make cells better able to resist damage to DNA. Thus, it is reasonable to propose that augmented SOD expression might also make cells more resistant to cancerous transformation.

Perhaps the most intriguing application of biological prevention of cancer would be to introduce a normal "tumor suppressor gene" into cells that have only abnormal or mutated versions of these genes. Since a gene called p53 is mutated in more than half of all human cancers, a technique to introduce a normal functional p53 gene into mutated cells would be particularly exciting. The best way to introduce a functional p53 gene into specific cells in the body is not known, but it could be as simple as incorporating the gene into a disabled virus, then allowing the virus to infect cells and import the new gene. For example, mutations of the p53 tumor suppressor gene are frequently found in a type of human leukemia called T-cell acute lymphoblastic leukemia (T-ALL), especially when patients are in relapse.[37] To determine whether human tumor cell growth could be suppressed by the p53 gene, a T-ALL cell line that lacked the normal p53 gene was infected with an engineered virus that carried a functional p53 gene. Expression of a normal p53 gene in the tumor cells reduced tumor cell growth rate, suppressed the ability of cells to form colonies in culture, and blocked the ability of these cells to form tumors in mice. This suggests that suppression of acute leukemia cells via transfection with a wild-type p53 gene may be a viable therapeutic strategy for T-cell ALL.[38] Furthermore, if cells with an abnormal p53 gene could be identified before they became cancerous or at least before they formed a tumor, it should become possible to insert a functional p53 gene into these abnormal cells. In a sense this is just presymptomatic treatment of cancer, but this could also be a very effective way of reducing the incidence and mortality of cancer. A further exciting possibility is that drugs can be found that mimic or stimulate the function of the tumor suppressor genes.

SOCIAL AND PSYCHOLOGICAL PREVENTION OF CANCER

It is well-known that the socio-economic status (SES) of women can have a potent effect on the risk of poor-prognosis breast cancer. A study in Connecticut showed that women of low SES were more likely to be diagnosed with late stage cancer and were more than twice as likely to die from a curable breast cancer, as women of high SES.[39] These results have been confirmed by a study of 28,486 breast cancer cases in Los Angeles County.[40] Women of low SES were 35% more likely to have late stage breast cancer than women of high SES, despite the fact that low SES women are actually less likely to get breast cancer overall. The high incidence of late stage cancer in women of low SES may be explained by the fact that low SES women were 56% more likely to tolerate symptoms for longer than a month. This suggests that low SES women have less access to health care and may have less awareness of the importance of early detection of breast cancer. It is a failure of the social system when poverty itself is a risk factor for fatal cancer. If there is to be a serious effort to reduce the toll of cancer, then breast cancer early detection programs should give special attention to women of low SES.

A great deal of controversy surrounds the idea that psychological factors play a role in cancer causation. Yet it is well-known that high-risk behaviors such as smoking are a major cause of cancer. Since high-risk behaviors are psychologically motivated, at least in part, it seems self-evident that psychological factors can play a key role in cancer causation. This suggests that psychological factors can potentially be manipulated to reduce the incidence or mortality of cancer.[41]

Social isolation is known to be a risk factor for many diseases, including cancer, and several recent studies have shown that social integration promotes health.[42] Several prospective studies, which have controlled for health and the presence of high-risk behaviors at study enrollment, have shown that there is an increased risk of death for persons with a low quantity or quality of social relationships. Experimental work with social animals such as monkeys and dogs has shown that there are psychological and even physiological consequences to living in isolation, and that chronic stress often leads to poor health in isolated animals. These findings have led to the emergence of "social support theory," which argues that humans are intrinsically social and that the social network is protective of individual mental and physical health. This theory is potentially of broad significance because of sweeping changes in the American lifestyle over the last several generations. By comparison with adults in the 1950s, adults in the 1970s were less likely to be married, more likely to be living alone, less likely to belong to volunteer organizations, and less likely to visit informally with others.[43] These trends were further exacerbated through the 1980s, so that there has been an increasing degree of social isolation for most Americans.

Psychological stresses can affect the immune system to the point that stress can even increase one's susceptibility to the common cold.[44] This was shown by studying a group of 394 healthy volunteer subjects who were deliberately exposed to respiratory virus after filling out a questionnaire that explored sources of stress. Volunteers were then quarantined, to determine what proportion of those exposed would actually develop a cold. Both the rate of infection and the severity of symptoms were found to be closely associated with the degree of psychological stress. Infection rates ranged from 74% to 90%, depending upon stress level, and stress led to a nearly six-fold increase in the risk of infection. Even when the effects of smoking, alcohol consumption, exercise, diet, quality of sleep, white blood cell count, allergic status, and viral exposure prior to the experimental exposure were eliminated, it was found that people suffering increasing levels of stress were increasingly likely to develop colds. The mechanism by which stress depresses the immune system remains unknown. Yet, if chronic stress is able to increase the risk of an acute illness like a cold, it seems likely that chronic stress could also increase the risk of a chronic illness like cancer.

The effect of marital status on cancer survival was examined using a database that included information on 27,779 cancer patients.[45] It was found that unmarried persons were 23% more likely to die of cancer than married persons. The poorer survival of singles was due to three separate reasons. Unmarried persons were about 19% more likely to be diagnosed with late stage cancer. After adjustment for stage, it was found that unmarried persons were also 43% more likely to receive no treatment for their cancer. Finally, after correction for both stage and treatment, it was found that unmarried persons were still more likely to die of their cancer. Considering only those cancers that were local at diagnosis, and excluding all patients who received less-than-adequate treatment, single persons were still 20% more likely to die of their cancer than married persons. Results show clearly that married persons have a decreased death rate from a range of different cancers, suggesting that an adequate social support network can contribute to good health.[46] Yet, clearly, marriage is not the only way to obtain social support, and finding other ways to enhance social support might lessen cancer mortality.

Scientists recently studied the effect of a social support group on survival of women diagnosed with metastatic breast cancer.[47] Eighty-six women with metastatic breast cancer were randomly assigned to one of two different treatment groups. The control group of 36 women received standard breast cancer therapy at a leading medical center, while the experimental group of 50 women received the same therapy plus a year of weekly group therapy sessions. Each session lasted only an hour and a half, and was designed to help women confront their fears of death and dying, to provide practical guidance through common coping problems, and to provide a supportive environment for the venting of strong emotion. Women in the support group were found to be less anxious and depressed, less likely to suffer from fatigue and loss of vigor, and better able to cope with cancer pain. Four years after the program began, all of the women in the control group had died, but one-third of the women in the support group were still alive. The mean survival time for control women was 18.9 months, while the mean survival time of women in the support group was 36.6 months. In fact, three of the women in the support group were still alive 10 years after the beginning of the intervention. The reasons for this increased survival are unknown, but several mechanisms have been proposed: perhaps group-support patients who feel less isolated and depressed are better able to obtain a good diet, regular sleep, and exercise; or perhaps group support patients are better able to obtain quality medical care; or perhaps unsupported patients suffer more harmful effects of stress on the endocrine or immune systems. An argument can be made for each of these possibilities but, in truth, no one knows why the group support women did so much better than the women who received treatment only. In any case, these results suggest that the mind and body have been too long dichotomized,[48] and that Western medicine must deal with the patient as a whole, rather than as a collection of body parts with symptoms.

The potent effect that stress can have on cancer survival was confirmed by a study of women with operable breast cancer who were at risk of relapse.[49] Life history data were collected from a group of 50 case women who developed recurrences after surgery for breast cancer, and these women were matched with 50 control women with breast cancer who did not develop recurrence after surgery. Case and control women were matched with respect to all of the clinical variables known to be predictive of breast cancer recurrence, including age, menopausal state, SES, histological type of breast cancer, tumor size and location, extent of surgery, evidence of local and metastatic spread, and type of adjuvant therapy. It was found that the relative risk of relapse was nearly six-fold higher among women who suffered a severely threatening life event following treatment for their cancer. Severely threatening life events included death of a husband or child, divorce, or a complete breakdown of family relations that persisted for more than six months. The relative risk of relapse was also nearly five-fold higher among women who suffered life difficulties following their treatment. Life difficulties included all life conditions that were major problems and that persisted for more than six months, such as having an alcoholic, quarrelsome, or spendthrift spouse. Life events and difficulties that were not rated as severe were not related to breast cancer relapse. This was a small study, and it was not prospectively done, so the results may be biased. Nevertheless, these results do suggest that severe stress can play a role in recurrence of breast cancer.[50]

Since social support clearly plays a role in reducing cancer mortality, this implies that enhanced social support networks should be provided for those at high risk of cancer due to psychological factors. Persons of low SES, or those suffering chronic isolation, or those undergoing extreme stresses may all be at a substantially higher risk of cancer. Stresses such as bereavement, divorce, loss of employment, forced relocation, or recent diagnosis of a life-threatening disease in a loved one do not disturb psychological equilibrium only, they seem capable of disturbing physical equilibrium as well.

SUMMARY

Prospects are very good for hormonal prevention of cancer to become a routine and highly effective way to reduce the incidence and mortality from endometrial, ovarian, and breast cancer. In fact, careful formulation of a hormonal supplement could potentially reduce the incidence of all three cancers simultaneously. Side effects are likely to be rather minimal, which would make this kind of cancer preventive effort appropriate for most women. It has been estimated that if women used a GnRH blocker for 10 years, such use could reduce lifetime risk of breast cancer by 47%, risk of ovarian cancer by 65%, and risk of endometrial cancer by 33%.[51] For 15 years of use, the risk of breast cancer would decline by 70%, risk of ovarian cancer would decline by 79%, and risk of endometrial cancer would decline by 45%. Clinical trials of hormonal supplements will be completed soon, and if the final results are as convincing as the initial results were intriguing, then hormonal supplements will probably be on the market within a decade.

Vaccine prevention of cancer is another preventive measure that may become generally applicable. This is especially true in the case of vaccines against the hepatitis B virus (HBV), a major cause of liver cancer, human papilloma virus (HPV), a major cause of cervical cancer, and perhaps even *Heliocobacter pylori*, a major cause of stomach cancer and ulcers. Since a vaccine against HBV is already available, the major obstacle at this point is cost. Given that the cost of caring for a patient dying of liver cancer is quite high by comparison to the cost of immunizing large numbers of people, it may become feasible and even economically compelling to begin immunization programs in the near future.

Social and psychological prevention of cancer is an option that has never been seriously considered by society because, until very recently, no data suggested this approach would have efficacy. However, in light of several new research findings, it may be time for us to consider such options as enhanced social support networks for those at risk of isolation or depression.

The remaining cancer preventive measures discussed in this chapter will likely never become routinely applied, but rather will be reserved for persons known to be at high risk for a particular cancer. In much the same way that blood pressure medication is reserved only for those people with sharply elevated blood pressure, cancer prevention methods such as surgery and radiation will likewise be reserved for those people with a sharply elevated cancer risk. An exception to this may be tubal sterilization, which has promise as a mass preventive strategy for ovarian cancer.

However, these various, rather extreme, cancer preventive strategies will probably never be as generally effective as mass behavioral changes. It would be very foolish to spend billions of dollars to institute mass cancer screening programs or mass vaccination programs without first doing everything in our power to eradicate tobacco smoking. Tobacco use is, without a doubt, the single most important cause of human cancer. Since tobacco is an addictive substance with many harmful side effects and no known benefits, recent efforts by the Federal Drug Administration to regulate this drug make a great deal of sense.

NOTES TO CHAPTER 16

1. J.R. Harris, M.E. Lippman, U. Veronesi, W. Willett, "Breast cancer" (Part 3), *N. Engl. J. Med.* 327 (1992): 473–480.
2. B.E. Henderson, R.K. Ross, M.C. Pike, "Hormonal chemoprevention of cancer in women," *Science* 259 (1993): 633–638.
3. *Ibid.*
4. *Ibid.*
5. D.V. Spicer, M.C. Pike, A. Pike, R. Rude, D. Shoupe, J. Rishardson, "Pilot trial of a gonadotropin hormone agonist with replacement hormones as a prototype contraceptive to prevent breast cancer," *Contraception* 47 (1993): 427–444.
6. *Ibid.*
7. B. E. Henderson, "Hormonal chemoprevention of cancer in women," 633–638.
8. *Ibid.*
9. *Ibid.*
10. S.G. Nayfield, J.E. Karp, L.G. Ford, F.A. Dorr, B.S. Kramer, "Potential role of tamoxifen in prevention of breast cancer," *J. Natl. Cancer Instit.* 83 (1991): 1450–1459.
11. *Ibid.*
12. M. Henderson, "Current approaches to breast cancer prevention," *Science* 259 (1993) 630–631.
13. B.E. Henderson, "Hormonal chemoprevention of cancer in women," 633–638.
14. L. Seachrist, "Restating the risks of tamoxifen," *Science* 263 (1994): 910–911.

15. M-C. King, S. Rowell, S.M. Love, "Inherited breast ovarian cancer: What are the risks? What are the choices?," *J. Amer. Med. Assoc.* 269 (1993): 1975–1980.
16. Harris, "Breast cancer," 473–480.
17. King, "Inherited breast ovarian cancer," 1975–1980.
18. B.E. Henderson, "Hormonal chemoprevention of cancer in women," 633–638.
19. S.E. Hankinson, D.J. Hunter, G.A. Colditz, W.C. Willett, M.J. Stampfer, et al., "Tubal ligation, hysterectomy, and risk of ovarian cancer: A prospective study," *J. Amer. Med. Assoc.*, 270 (1993): 2813–2818.
20. D-S. Chen, "From hepatitis to hepatoma: lessons from Type B viral hepatitis," *Science* 262 (1993): 369–370.
21. *Ibid.*
22. *Ibid.*
23. M. Fortuin, J. Chotard, A.D. Jack, N.P. Maine, M. Mendy, et al., "Efficacy of hepatitis B vaccine in the Gambian expanded programme on immunisation," *Lancet* 341 (1993): 1129–1131.
24. M.H. Schiffman, H.M. Bauer, R.N. Hoover, A.G. Glass, D.M. Cadell, et al., "Epidemiologic evidence showing that human papillomavirus infection causes most cervical intraepithelial neoplasia," *J. Natl. Cancer Instit.* 85 (1993): 958–964.
25. M.H. Schiffman, "Recent progress in defining the epidemiology of human papillomavirus infection and cervical neoplasia," *J. Natl. Cancer Instit.* 84 (1992): 394–398.
26. J. Parsonnet, G.D. Friedman, D.P. Vandersteen, Y. Chang, J.H. Vogelman, et al., "*Helicobacter pylori* infection and the risk of gastric carcinoma," *N. Engl. J. Med.* 325 (1991): 1127- 1131.
27. J. Guarner, A. Mohar, J. Parsonnet, D. Halperin, "The association of *Helicobacter pylori* with gastric cancer and preneoplastic gastric lesions in Chiapas, Mexico," *Cancer* 71 (1993): 297–301.
28. J. Alper, "Ulcers as an infectious disease," *Science* 260 (1993): 159–160.
29. J. Cohen, "Cancer vaccines get a shot in the arm," *Science* 262 (1993): 841–843.
30. P.N. Plowman, J.E. Kingston, J.L. Hungerford, "Prophylactic retinal radiotherapy has an exceptional place in the management of familial retinoblastoma," *Br. J. Cancer* 68 (1993): 743–745.
31. *Ibid.*
32. *Ibid.*
33. S.A. Aaronson, "Growth factors and cancer," *Science* 254 (1991): 1146–1153.

34. P.H. Watson, R.T. Pon, R.P.C. Shiu, "Inhibition of c-*myc* expression by phosphorothioate antisense oligonucleotide identifies a critical role for c-*myc* in the growth of human breast cancer," *Cancer Res.* 51 (1991): 3996–4000.
36. W.C. Orr, R.S. Soha, "Extension of life-span by overexpression of superoxide dismutase and catalase in *Drosophila melanogaster*," *Science* 263 (1994): 1128–1130.
37. J. Cheng, J-K. Yee, J. Yeargin, T. Friedmann, M. Haas, "Suppression of acute lymphoblastic leukemia by the human wild-type p53 gene," *Cancer Res.* 52 (1992): 222–226.
38. *Ibid.*
39. T.A. Farley, J.T. Flannery, "Late-stage diagnosis of breast cancer in women of lower socioeconomic status: public health implications," *Am. J. Public Health* 79 (1989): 1508–1512.
40. J.L. Richardson, B. Langholz, L. Bernstein, C. Burciaga, K. Danlyey, R.K. Ross, "Stage and delay in breast cancer diagnosis by race, socioeconomic status, age and year," *Br. J. Cancer* 65 (1992): 922–926.
41. D. Spiegel, "Psychosocial intervention in cancer," *J. Natl. Cancer Instit.* 85 (1993): 1198–1205.
42. J.S. House, K.R. Landis, D. Umberson, "Social relationships and health," *Science* 241 (1988): 540–545.
43. *Ibid.*
44. S. Cohen, D.A. Tyrrell, P.A. Smith, "Psychological stress and susceptibility to the common cold," *N. Engl. J. Med.* 325 (1991): 606–612.
45. J.S. Goodwin, W.C. Hunt, C.R. Key, J.M. Samet, "The effect of marital status on stage, treatment, and survival of cancer patients," *J. Amer. Med. Assoc.* 158 (1987): 3125–3130.
46. *Ibid.*
47. Spiegel, "Psychosocial intervention in cancer," 1198–1205.
48. *Ibid.*
49. A.J. Ramirez, T.K.J. Craig, J.P. Watson, I.S. Fentiman, W.R.S. North, R.D. Rubens, "Stress and relapse of breast cancer," *Brit. Med. J.* 298 (1989): 291–293.
50. *Ibid.*
51. B.E. Henderson, "Hormonal chemoprevention of cancer in women," 633–638.
52. *Ibid.*

Appendix

COMPENDIUM OF CANCER RISK FACTORS

MASTER TABLE				
RISK FACTOR	**RELATED CANCER**	**RELATIVE RISK**	**RELATIVE FREQUENCY**	**WEIGHTED RISK**
Rb gene mutation	Retinoblastoma	28,500	1	28,500
Ataxia-telangiectasia (AT)	Leukemia	769	2	1,538
Xeroderma pigmentosum	Skin	1,000	1	1,000
High radon (mines) × tobacco	Lung	194	5	970
Tobacco × alcohol	Larynx	330	2	660
Breast cancer suscept. gene	Ovary	300	2	600
Ataxia-telangiectasia (AT)	All cancers	100	5	500
Hepatitis B virus (HBV)	Liver	223	2	446
Tobacco (≥2 pks/day, 10 yrs)	Lung	81	5	406
Thoratrast infusion	Liver	126	2	252
Tobacco × asbestos	Lung	50	5	250

MASTER TABLE				
RISK FACTOR	RELATED CANCER	RELATIVE RISK	RELATIVE FREQUENCY	WEIGHTED RISK
Lung cancer suscept. × smoking	Lung	42	5	210
High radon (home) × tobacco	Lung	32.5	5	163
Rb gene mutation	Brain	73.7	2	147
Tobacco smoke (>30 cigs/day)	Larynx	59.7	2	119
Rb gene mutation	Bladder	28.8	4	115
Tobacco × alcohol (40 cigs+5 drinks/dy)	Oral	38	3	114
Heavy drinking × smoking	Oropharyngeal	37.7	3	113
Tobacco smoke (men, any use)	Lung	22.4	5	112
Chronic immunosuppression	Lymphoma	35	3	105
HPV-16 or 18	Cervical	51.0	2	102
Familial adenomatous polyposis	Colon	20	5	100
DES (*in utero* exposure)	Vaginal	~100	1	~100
Rb gene mutation	Lung	16.4	5	82
Rb gene mutation	Skin (melanoma)	73.3	1	73
Human papilloma virus (HPV)	Cervical	33.6	2	67
HPV-31, 33, 35, or 39	Cervical	33.0	2	66
HPV-45, 51, or 52	Cervical	33.0	2	66

MASTER TABLE				
RISK FACTOR	RELATED CANCER	RELATIVE RISK	RELATIVE FREQUENCY	WEIGHTED RISK
High radon (mines)	Lung	12.7	5	64
Average radon (home) × tobacco	Lung	11.6	5	58
Rb gene mutation	All cancers	9.9	5	50
BRCA1 susceptibility gene	Breast	8.6	5	43
Salted fish consumption	Nasopharynx	38	1	38
Father and uncle with disease	Prostate	8.8	4	35
Saturated fat	Lung	6.1	5	31
Low intake of folate	Cervical	10	3	30
AT gene carrier × radiation	Breast	5.8	5	29
Late pregnancy × family cancer	Breast	5.8	5	29
Li-Fraumeni syndrome	Soft tissue	27.8	1	28
Tobacco smoke (10 yr smoker)	Oral	8.9	3	27
Heavy drinking (any alcohol)	Oropharyngeal	8.8	3	26
AT gene carrier	Breast	5.1	5	26
Li-Fraumeni syndrome	Breast	4.5	5	23
Li-Fraumeni syndrome	Brain	11.5	2	23
Tobacco smoke	Larynx	10.3	2	21
Thoratrast infusion	Leukemia	10	2	20
AT gene carrier	All cancers	3.6	5	18
DDT in pesticides	Breast	3.5	5	18
Arylamines	Bladder	4.6	4	18
Frequent meat consumption	Colon	3.6	5	18

MASTER TABLE				
RISK FACTOR	RELATED CANCER	RELATIVE RISK	RELATIVE FREQUENCY	WEIGHTED RISK
Hp infection (black Americans)	Stomach	9.0	2	18
Long-term drinking (vodka)	Larynx	9.0	2	18
Phenoxyacetic acid in pesticides	Lymphoma	5.5	3	17
Mastitis therapy	Breast	3.4	5	17
HPV-6, 11, or 42	Cervical	8.7	2	17
Heavy drinking (hard liquor)	Oropharyngeal	5.5	3	17
Stressful life events (> 2)	All cancers	3.3	5	17
Low intake of vitamin E	Colon	3.1	5	16
Low intake of vitamin C	Cervical	5	3	15
High-level Hp infection	Stomach	7.6	2	15
Nulliparous × family cancer	Breast	3.0	5	15
Heavy drinking (beer)	Oropharyngeal	4.7	3	14
Thoratrast infusion	Gall bladder	14	1	14
OC use at 40–44 years age	Breast	2.7	5	14
ERT × benign breast disease	Breast	2.8	5	14
Tobacco smoke (for 25 yrs)	Urinary tract	4.5	3	14
Chlorophenols in pesticides	Lymphoma	4.8	3	14
Diuretic use (regular use)	Kidney	4.5	3	14
Neurofibromatosis (NF-1)	Brain and CNS	7	2	14
Mother & sister with disease	Breast	2.5	5	13

MASTER TABLE				
RISK FACTOR	RELATED CANCER	RELATIVE RISK	RELATIVE FREQUENCY	WEIGHTED RISK
Use of black hair dye	Lymphoma	4.4	3	13
High ratio of red:white meat	Colon	2.5	5	13
Low intake raw fruits and vegetables	Lung	2.5	5	13
Low intake of vitamin E	Breast	2.5	5	13
Obesity	Colon	2.4	5	12
Hp infection (Japanese American)	Stomach	6.0	2	12
Low carbohydrate intake	Colorectal	2.5	5	12
Tobacco smoke (current smoker)	Bladder	2.9	4	12
Second-hand smoke (>22 years)	Lung	2.4	5	12
Sister with disease	Breast	2.3	5	12
Li-Fraumeni syndrome	Leukemia	6	2	12
HRAS1 cancer gene	Colon	2.2	5	11
Mother with disease by age 40	Breast	2.1	5	11
Li-Fraumeni syndrome	All cancers	2.1	5	11
Obesity x family cancer	Breast	2.2	5	11
Tobacco smoke (smokers only)	Cervix	3.4	3	10
Dietary fat	Colon	1.9	5	10
Red meat consumption	Prostate	2.6	4	10
Low fiber intake	Colorectal	1.9	5	10

MASTER TABLE				
RISK FACTOR	RELATED CANCER	RELATIVE RISK	RELATIVE FREQUENCY	WEIGHTED RISK
Total caloric intake	Prostate	2.5	4	10
Low fruit and vegetable intake	All cancers	2	5	10
Low intake of selenium	Lung	2	5	10
Low intake of peas and beans	Lung	1.9	5	10
Low fiber intake	Colorectal	1.9	5	10
Whole-body irradiation (1 Gray)	Leukemia	4.9	2	10
Whole-body irradiation (1 Gray)	Breast	2.0	5	10
Age at first birth > 30 years	Breast	1.9	5	10
Nulliparous (no children)	Breast	1.9	5	10
Late pregnancy (≥ 30 years)	Breast	2.0	5	10
Low activity (<1000 kcal-/week)	Colorectal	2.0	5	10
Female obesity	Kidney	3.3	3	10

Only risk weightings greater than or equal to 10 are included in this compendium, so that only 103 risk factor-cancer pairs are shown (of the 224 risk factor-cancer pairs in this book).

INDEX

This index is arranged alphabetically letter-by-letter.
Tables are indicated by *t* following the page number.

A

acquired immune deficiency syndrome *see* AIDS
adenoma 66, 93–94, 119–120, 123, 136, 237–238, 243
adenoma, familial *see* familial adenomatous polyposis (FAP)
aflatoxin 107
AFP *see* alpha fetoprotein (AFP)
Agent Orange 69–71
AIDS (acquired immune deficiency syndrome) 211, 215, 219, 273, 290–291
air pollution 11t, 247–249
Alar 8
alcohol
    and caloric intake 89
    combined with tobacco 9, 16, 24, 65, 77–78, 254–255t, 264t, 265t, 344
    consumption linked to stress 270
    excessive consumption as risk factor 34, 36, 254–255t, 265t, 266, 268t, 269t
    linked to various cancers 234–239
    as root cause of death 273
alpha fetoprotein (AFP) 318, 325t
alpha-tocopherol *see* vitamin E
analgesics 72, 81t, 241–243, 254t, 255t, 341t, 348–349
animal research 18, 19–23, 25, 34, 63, 93–94, 346, 350
anti-inflammatory agents 241–243, 348–349
antioxidants 133–134, 337–338
arylamines 71–72, 80t, 268t
asbestos 11t, 70t, 78, 202–203, 206, 265t, 287–289, 337
ascorbate *see* vitamin C
ascorbic acid *see* vitamin C
aspirin *see* analgesics
AT *see* ataxia-telangiectasia
ataxia-telangiectasia (AT) 51–52, 56t, 57t, 177, 264t
atomic bomb 152–155

B

bacteria *see* microbes
benzene 70t
beta-carotene
    dietary 11t, 67, 125, 126t, 128–133, 137, 143, 145t, 146
    supplementary 333–337, 340, 344, 348–350
bioassay 19–23, 34
bladder cancer
    chemical hazards 2t
        arylamines 71, 80t, 268t
        fluoride 72–73
    diet and prevention of
        beta-carotene 126t, 130
        selenium 126t, 133, 145t
    genetic factors
        ataxia-telangiectasia (AT) 51
        HRAS1 57t
        rare alleles 48
        Rb mutation 56t, 264t
        retinoblastoma carrier 41
    racial differences in incidence of 53
    radiation and 153, 178t
    survival rate 27
    tobacco and 62, 67, 81t
body mass index (BMI) *see* obesity
bone cancer 2t, 155, 166, 179t, 206
brain cancer
    dental X-rays and 164–165
    dietary factors
        beta-carotene possibly protective against 128–129
        maternal diet and incidence in offspring 135, 139, 145t
    electromagnetic fields and 175–176, 179t
    genetic factors 2t
        Li-Fraumeni syndrome 41, 57t
        Rb mutation 56t, 264t
    injuries and 2t, 205t
BRCA1 gene 43, 56t, 264t, 321–322, 360–361

L

laboratory research 18, 19–23, 25, 34, 93–94
lactation *see* breast feeding
laryngeal cancer
  alcohol and 77, 80t, 236, 254t, 264t, 265t, 268t, 344
  chemical hazards 2t
  diet and prevention of 118, 126t
  survival rate 27
  tobacco and 62, 65, 77, 80t, 236, 254t, 264t, 265t, 268t, 344
leukemia
  electromagnetic fields and 175
  genetic factors
    ataxia-telangiectasia (AT) 56t, 264t
    HRAS1 57t
    Li-Fraumeni syndrome 57t
    p53 mutations 367
  radiation and 2t, 69, 153, 156, 163–166, 168, 170–172, 178–179t, 268t
  tobacco and 62, 68, 69, 81t
  viral link to (HTLV-1) 212–213
Li-Fraumeni syndrome 41–42, 56t, 57t
lip cancer *see* oral cancer
liver cancer
  alcohol and 255t
  chemical hazards 2t, 69
  diet and prevention of 127t
  diet implicated in 107, 112t
  oral contraceptives and 199
  radiation and 163–164, 178t
  screening for 318
  tobacco and 178t, 255t
  vaccination against *see* hepatitis B virus (HBV)
  viral link to *see* hepatitis B virus (HBV)
lung cancer
  air pollution and 11t, 247–248, 255t
  asbestos and 11t, 80t, 202–203, 265t
  chemical hazards 2t
  diet and prevention of 126–128t
    beta-carotene 11t, 126t, 129–132, 145t, 336–338, 340
    citrus juices 144t
    fiber 123, 127t
    fruits and vegetables 112t, 118, 269t
    peas and beans 144t, 269t
    selenium 11t, 126t, 144t, 269t
    vitamin E 11t, 126t, 142, 144t, 340
  dietary fat implicated in 11t, 100–101, 112t, 268t, 269t
  fluoride and 73

genetic factors
  family susceptibility 38–39, 50–51, 78–79, 265t
  Rb mutation 41, 56t, 265t
  high-dose retinoid treatment for 346
  racial differences in incidence of 53
  radiation and 2t, 11t, 158, 160–163, 170, 178–179t, 265t, 268t
  screening for 315–316, 319–320
  survival rate 27
  tobacco and 4, 11t, 56t, 62–65, 73, 78–79, 80–81t, 178t, 202–203, 265t, 268t, 269t, 279–280
lymphoma
  chemical hazards
    black hair dye 72, 80t, 269t
    organic solvents 81t
    pesticides and herbicides 74–75, 80–81t, 268t
  chronic immunosuppression linked to 215, 219, 224t, 264t, 265t, 268t
  electromagnetic fields and 175
  radiation and 2t, 164, 170–172
  rheumatoid arthritis linked to 242
  viral factors 2t
    Epstein-Barr virus 214–216, 224t
    HIV-1 219
    HTLV-1 212–213

M

magnetic fields *see* electromagnetic fields (EMFs)
magnetic resonance imaging (MRI) 52, 181, 315
malnutrition 107, 143
mammography 32, 51–52, 169, 177, 181, 274, 296, 299–309, 325t
mastectomy 11, 321, 360–361
meat consumption 36, 90–95, 97–98, 112, 112t, 121, 268t, 269t, 274
media *see* news media
Medicaid 4, 321
Medicare 4, 321
melanoma 2t, 41, 130, 277, 364
memory bias 16, 175, 198
menopause 191–193, 195–196, 197, 204t, 205t, 231
menstruation 190–191, 195–198, 205t, 206–207, 233–234, 244, 357–358
mesothelioma 202–203, 287–288
meta-analysis 118, 122, 137–138, 141, 193, 237, 238, 245–246, 304, 359
methionine 136, 145t, 238
microbes 54–55, 219–222, 224t, 225, 271, 272t